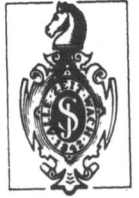

G.W.H. Stamp • N.A. Wright

Advanced Histopathology

Foreword by Colin L. Berry

Springer-Verlag
London Berlin Heidelberg New York
Paris Tokyo Hong Kong

G.W.H.Stamp, MBChB, MRCPath
Clinical Research Fellow, Imperial Cancer Research Fund, Royal College of
Surgeons, 35–43 Lincoln's Inn Fields, London WC2A 3PN, UK and Honorary
Consultant in Histopathology, Hammersmith Hospital, Du Cane Road,
London W12 0HS, UK

N.A.Wright, MA, DSc, MD, PhD, FRCPath
Professor and Director, Department of Histopathology, Royal Postgraduate Medical
School, Hammersmith Hospital, Du Cane Road, London W12 0HS, UK and Associate
Director and Head of Histopathology Unit, Imperial Cancer Research Fund, Royal
College of Surgeons, 35–43 Lincoln's Inn Fields, London WC2A 3PN, UK

With contributions from:

Dr T. Clarke, MA, MBBChir, MRCPath, Senior Registrar in Histopathology,
Royal Devon and Exeter Hospital, Exeter, Devon EX2 5AD, UK

Dr F. Barker, MA, MBBS, MRCPath, Senior Registrar in Histopathology and
Dr M.B. Prentice, BMedSci, MBBS, FRCPathAust, Registrar in Histopathology
Hammersmith Hospital, Du Cane Road, London W12 0HS, UK

ISBN-13:978-3-540-19589-4   e-ISBN-13:978-1-4471-1753-7
DOI: 10.1007/978-1-4471-1753-7

British Library Cataloguing in Publication Data
Stamp, G.W.H. (Gordon W.H.), *1955–*
   Advanced histopathology.
   1. Medicine. Histopathology
   I. Title   II. Wright, N.A. (Nicholas Alcwyn), *1943–* 611'.018
   ISBN-13:978-3-540-19589-4

Library of Congress Cataloging-in-Publication Data
Stamp, G. W. H. (Gordon W. H.). 1955–
   Advanced histopathology/ G.W.H. Stamp and N.A. Wright.
   p.   cm.
   ISBN-13:978-3-540-19589-4 (U.S. alk. paper)
1. Histology, Pathological–Examinations, questions, etc.   2. Histology,
Pathological–Outlines, syllabi, etc.   I. Wright, N. A. (Nick A.), 1943–   II. Title.
RB43.S73 1989
611'.018—dc20   89-26119
                                                                          CIP

Typeset by Fox Design, Surbiton

2128/3916-543210 Printed on acid-free paper

Foreword

It is easy to be confident that an appropriate body of advice is available to candidates about the content of an examination once you have passed it. Prospectively, the Primary and Final Examinations of the Royal College of Pathologists will appear to most to involve the assimilation of what seems at the time an inexhaustible volume of data, and the recent change in the College examination system has not diminished this concern for the majority of candidates. The guidelines for training for the new Part I examination state that this is the "major hurdle of the MRCPath" and it is clear that it will determine whether candidates are suitable for training which will permit them to practise independently as consultants after Part II.

These general aims and objectives do not answer questions such as "How much do I need to know about glomerulonephritis?" or "Where do I stop with the lymphomas?" This text attempts to resolve the difficulty of knowing what standard to aim at, using College questions as its starting point. It concentrates on the essential basis of any single answer; many candidates for the new three-year examination will know more about individual topics than is stated here. However, it is the breadth of information required which is a feature of College examinations and this text should help with this problem.

There are a number of important additional points. You will not pass if you do not do an adequate post-mortem or present it clearly, if you do not know something about special techniques, if you have ignored cytology, or if you suppose surgical pathology can be learned by picture matching. Many slides are put into practical examinations to see how you think about problems – it is not necessary to know all the answers but you do have to behave sensibly when confronted with something difficult.

The Government White Paper on the National Health Service should have convinced you that it is important to know about management issues and to be able to evaluate your own work pattern critically (and financially). If you pass the examination(s) you can be confident that this phase of your training has been satisfactorily completed and that you have demonstrated a high standard of proficiency – an important achievement.

London   Colin L.Berry, PhD, FRCPath
October 1989   Professor of Morbid Anatomy
                        The London Hospital Medical College

Preface

We assume you have bought, or are thinking of buying, this book because you are faced, *horribile dictu*, with the Histopathology examinations of the Royal College of Pathologists, or some related ordeal.

If you have not taken the examination before, then, apart from advice from your seniors (who may not have taken the examination personally, being Grandfathers, or even worse, achieved their MRCPath status through *research*) and mythology prevalent among your peers, you will not know what to expect. If you have taken the examination, then you have obviously been failed, albeit by biased and intransigent examiners. Take comfort: help is on the way.

Following an initial discussion between Nick Wright and Colin Berry, it was decided to attempt a *vade-mecum* for prospective examination candidates. Gordon Stamp prepared the initial and final drafts, enlisting the substantial help of Fred Barker, Tom Clarke and Mark Prentice; Colin Berry's continuing guidance has been invaluable and without Susan Chandler, who deciphered our holographic offering, this book would not have been possible.

Keep this book beside you during your revision effort, take careful heed of the advice given, and behave in the examination in the manner suggested, and if you don't pass this time, then there is obviously something wrong with the examination system, and you should join the serried ranks of those who clamour for examination reform (again).

Unless you positively enjoy examinations, then you will certainly not be looking forward to the event. We hope that this book will to some extent allay your fears, give you encouragement, and help minimise your negative feelings.

We would like to take this opportunity of wishing you luck (an important ingredient in these examinations) and stay off the ß-blockers.

London,   Gordon Stamp
September 1989   Nick Wright

Contents

Introduction

The final part of the examination for membership of the Royal College of Pathologists was introduced in 1962 in order to provide a professional qualification which would establish whether a candidate was capable of undertaking the duties and responsibilities of a consultant. As such, the examination was intended to be set at a relatively greater degree of difficulty than other professional examinations for membership of the other medical colleges, which are taken relatively early in training, assessing suitability for training. The Primary examination was designed to fulfill this role, success in which enabled candidates to pursue more advanced training in registrar and senior registrar posts.

Naturally, over the years the examination has been refined and expanded with the advances in histopathology and morbid anatomy, in common with most medical and scientific disciplines, and it is true to say that a higher standard is expected than say ten or fifteen years ago, especially with the emergence of a more science-based approach to pathology which has greatly increased our understanding of the pathogenesis of disease.

Unfortunately, little advice is available to prospective candidates and the onus on preparation for the examination has remained largely up to the individual concerned. This is to a large extent a consequence of the broad scope of skills and knowledge expected of a modern pathologist, so that revision courses along the lines of those offered for MRCP or FRCS examinations are impractical because of the difficulties in organising the complex material required. It could, however, be argued that the examination is intended to assess the results of five or more years of training to a satisfactory level of competence in all respects, which could not possibly be achieved during a 'crammer' course. Instead, individual courses in aspects of histopathology, morbid anatomy or specialised disciplines such as paediatric pathology are available, but they are not a compulsory requirement of training, and attendance is selective, based on the trainee's perception of need, measured against financial considerations and utilising a finite amount of study leave.

As many candidates are not made aware of the format of the Final examination during their junior appointments (especially if based overseas) it is not surprising that many do not have an organised general training covering all important aspects, which allows the practice and perfection of certain of the skills required. This cannot be left until the last minute as part of the revision programme. For instance, those who have tried to remove a spinal cord for the first time or made a serious attempt to understand the classification of lymphomas in the few weeks heading up to the examination will know the folly of leaving preparation too late.

Therefore it seemed obvious that an explanatory overview of both the examination and preparation requirements, aimed at potential candidates, would be of value, to enable the optimal planning of a training programme. As such we do not intend to provide anything approaching a comprehensive account of disease states, but instead suggest some approaches to the problems encountered during the examination, with guidance to more detailed sources of information where appropriate. Considerable emphasis is placed on the ability to provide clinically useful information in a succinct, relevant fashion, the hallmark of a competent histopathologist in routine hospital service and teaching commitments, as well as in the examination.

A relatively informal style is used, since this is not designed to be a conventional textbook of pathology. This may provoke some criticism from the more intellectual reader, especially as it could be argued that the obvious is being stated in some sections. However, while these views may appear superfluous when the examination is some way off, it often happens that the finer points of self-discipline and perception are the first faculties to be lost in a stress situation. The more capable readers may want to exercise their critical ability by taking issue with some of the ideas and views expressed, which is often of greater benefit.

This book is divided into sections to cover all aspects of the examination, including both the written papers and various parts of the practical sessions. Within this framework there is an attempt to cover most of the problems commonly encountered by trainee pathologists and examination candidates, and those areas which are identified by examiners as serious deficiencies. It is hoped that the advice given will enable a candidate to direct revision in a coordinated, logical fashion, avoiding unnecessary repetition or over-emphasis, and moreover enable the principles outlined to be applied to sound histopathological practice.

Preparation for the Examination

The Final examination is essentially an exercise to try to establish whether a candidate has achieved a satisfactory level of competence during his training, which will enable him to function as a consultant. As such, there is need to display a broad base of knowledge, and the ability to apply it in a practical manner. Nevertheless it is important to realise that the examination is very much a 'game situation' with limited relevance to the way histopathology is actually done. Like all games, it has its rules, subtleties, refinements, and indeed fools; it is necessary to win, as, besides ignominy, the price of losing is expensive, if nothing else. This book might be regarded as a guide to 'winning' within the rules, but only just within the rules. The main problem, for many candidates, is that few indeed know the rules.

A further concern is that most histopathology training in this country is carried out by accident, so to speak. Trainees wait in departments, and are taught on, and learn about, those cases which happen to come their way. Consequently, whatever the deficiencies of such a process, the choice of training positions becomes critical.

In order to achieve the required standard, it it essential to try to choose registrar and senior registrar posts which will cover most aspects of pathology, or will give access to some specialised areas (e.g. paediatric pathology, neuropathology, renal pathology) which may otherwise not be covered. There is a tendency for some trainees to stay at one particular institution and apply for more senior positions within it, with the more able pathologists encouraged to go for research positions. While this may be suitable for some trainees, some might be pressed to do research for not entirely altruistic reasons by their superiors and others may find that they will have serious deficiencies in their experience by the time the Final examination comes. In general it can be recommended that candidates have worked in at least two university departments or Regional Health Authorities by the time the examination comes around, which should enable a broader degree of experience to be obtained, because it is the usual practice to link district general hospital posts with a university department, certainly at senior registrar level, and with many registrar posts.

If this is not possible, it may be possible to attend specialist units by personal arrangement with the pathologists concerned, to gain some practical experience. This is often the case with university lecturers, who may remain in post for up to six years, with restricted provisions for rotation to other units or departments. If further experience is required, it is most important to plan this early on, and not leave it until six months or so before the examination when the dreadful day is looming. The need to revise several areas means that full attention to the subject would be impossible, and such trainees often end up being a nuisance rather than an asset to a particular unit, especially if some of their colleagues have the same idea.

The choice of training posts is a highly individual business, but make sure that the more junior positions will give a good grounding in general pathology, perhaps with some specialist applications as a bonus. It is a mistake to specialise in a particular discipline (e.g. neuropathology or paediatric pathology) until some time after successfully taking the Primary examination, and even when this decision is made it is important to ensure that adequate access to the general aspects of routine work is included. In general, most departmental heads recognise this and make allowances, but it is largely up to the individual concerned to assess their own progress and particular requirements, and not become too obsessed with the specialty pathology at the expense of the general ability which is so important in the examination.

Another important component of training is to attend various courses both within and outside the region. Most university hospitals within a particular Regional Health Authority conduct training courses for both the Primary and Final examinations, and it is essential to attend these if at all possible. It will also enable the establishment of valuable contacts with colleagues, against whom trainees are able to gauge their own progress. Other general and specialist courses are available on a national basis and again, there is probably an optimal time to attend these. It is often advisable to consider going well in advance of taking the examination so any areas of ignorance can be corrected and practised. Most trainees learn about the value of these courses by personal recommendations of contemporaries or more senior colleagues, but it is important to look for the advertisements in the British Medical Journal, major pathology journals, the Royal College of Pathologists' Bulletin or symposia organised by Pathological Societies to see if there are any which fulfil particular requirements, or which may be newly organised. In addition, remember that most of the more useful courses are frequently oversubscribed, and therefore early application is essential. Many candidates ignore this every year and are disappointed. A detailed list of courses, with a brief summary of their content and organisation is provided in Appendix 2.

It is naturally very difficult to provide anything more than general recommendations in respect of training posts, and a trainee's own assessments and those of predecessors should act as a guide to senior colleagues and department heads who are responsible for ensuring that a reasonable level of comprehensive experience can be acquired. It is recommended that each trainee critically reviews their position every six months, taking steps to improve on 'grey' areas on a gradual basis, without having to cram everything in just before the examination. This requires more self-discipline than might be imagined at first!

Pathology Textbooks and Journals

During the period of training, candidates will have access to a wide range of books and journals, and it is sometimes very difficult to assess which are more or less essential as a basis for revision, and which are more detailed and require selective reading, or perhaps are less relevant to the examination. It is difficult to make specific recommendations on every Pathology textbook or journal available, as each individual's requirements and preferences will be different (e.g. a university lecturer versus a registrar in a district general hospital), but the lists of textbooks cited in Appendix 1 (and of Journals in Appendix 3), may provide a basis upon which each candidate could start to evaluate his or her own needs. Most trainees would be familiar with all of these by the time of the examination, but many are specialised and are better read at leisure than for revision purposes for reasons already stated. The following section inevitably contains a degree of bias according to personal experience with these texts, and must therefore be evaluated with a degree of circumspection by the reader.

Some of the larger textbooks which cover aspects of general and systematic pathology are invaluable, providing a very good basis for further reading, and having an adequate amount of information for undergraduate or some postgraduate pathology teaching, and even contain enough material for answering many essay questions. Used as a standard referral, it is possible to add in information from other more specialised sources to provide sufficiently comprehensive accounts of most entities. One way to assimilate this information is to work on cases encountered during routine surgical pathology or necropsies, always reading up on these subjects at the time, which retains the interest due to the clinical relevance.

Among these texts, *Muir's Textbook of Pathology* (ed. J.R. Anderson, 1985) is rather basic, although admirably comprehensive and very readable. Quickly scanning through the pages can enable a swift identification of those areas with which a candidate may not be fully conversant, and can revise accordingly. It might be reasonable to say that a Final examination candidate should have a standard of knowledge of any subject to the level of this text as a minimum requirement.

Pathologic Basis of Disease (eds. Robbins, Cotran & Kumar, 1989) has established itself as a superbly concise account of general and systematic pathology, which contains sufficiently detailed material for most undergraduate and basic postgraduate teaching requirements, and to answer many questions in the written section of the Final examination; this is reflected in the number of times this work is cited in the references in this book. It is important not to become over-reliant on such texts however, because although comprehensive, they are not geared towards the working surgical pathologist, and thus require supplementation.

Systemic Pathology (ed. W. St. C. Symmers, 3rd edition Vols. 1–6 1978) is still a useful source of reference, but is now rather dated. However, it fulfilled the requirement of a textbook which was equally applicable to necropsy pathology or surgical histopathology. The fourth edition is now being published as several volumes, emerging at the rate of about two per year, and considerably more detailed as a consequence. Only three volumes are available to date, but these will eventually form a substantial basis for all Departmental libraries, and may be essential reading for the dedicated pathologist.

There are innumerable works on surgical histopathology, but *Ackerman's Surgical Pathology* (ed. J. Rosai, 1989) is a superb example and widely regarded as a standard 'bench' book in most Pathology departments, if not for personal ownership. Some of the examination questions could be comprehensively answered by information derived from this text, especially from some of the less frequently consulted chapters (such as the mediastinum). However, it should be noted that many areas (such as renal, pulmonary and CNS biopsy pathology) are not covered to any degree, and it would be necessary to recognise this is the case before deciding on the choice of other books for training and revision.

The Armed Forces Institute of Pathology 'fascicles' are too detailed for revision purposes (except for selective review of certain volumes where information is comprehensive, e.g. tropical and extraordinary pathology, tumours of the salivary glands etc.) or conversely where specialised pathological texts are often more detailed than necessary for the required standard (e.g. tumours of the central nervous system). These fascicles are invaluable for reference purposes in a Departmental library, especially when working on current problems rather than examination revision, and are sufficiently inexpensive when ordered direct from the Institute's publishers for most pathologists to seriously consider adding them to their personal collections.

With regard to necropsy pathology, there are a few textbooks which deal with the technical details of the procedure but one concise, well-illustrated book which also covers aspects of post mortem room facilities, safety, forensic and specialised techniques is *Post Mortem Procedures* (Gresham & Turner, 1979). It is surprising that there are so few works on this subject. Books covering macroscopic pathology are of some use in this respect, but are often limited for the more advanced pathologist as they, of necessity, can only illustrate the typical example, whereas most problems arise from the complex cases with atypical features.

More specialised textbooks are a greater problem for the trainee, for it is difficult to know to what level of detail and complexity to delve into any particular system or subspecialty, and there is a bewildering variety of texts now available on any particular subject, from equally eminent authors. It is of little value to document all of the available choices, but the references cited at the end of some of the sections have been consulted during the preparation of this book. The titles in Appendix 1 are recommended as a minimum available for consultation in a Departmental or personal collection, although it is acknowledged that others equally deserving of consideration have not been cited. The choice of specialist books should ideally be made after consultation with a respected senior colleague with experience in that field, or amongst contemporaries. It is often best to consult the book in a hospital library before purchasing it, however. It is recommended that at least one text on each major system should be available for consultation during training and revision.

Having obtained such a text, try to use it as a practical book relating to routine practice as far as possible. Relatively few of these books are conducive to light reading, and reading through 100–200 pages in a session will result in very little retention of information unless the reader is fortunate enough to have a 'photographic' memory. Even if this could be the case, it is a different matter to know how to apply this knowledge.

An essential set of books for all examination candidates are the *Recent Advances in Histopathology* (Appendix 1), and it is most important to obtain the most recent edition as soon as it is published. Not only do they contain a wealth of up-to-date information on a variety of topical subjects, generally in a very readable form, but more importantly the written examination questions are frequently related to the contents of the recent editions. The more recent volumes are a valuable source of information on various trends and entities in surgical pathology, and such examples often appear in the practical examination. Volumes 10 onwards should be acquired (and sections of Volume 9 consulted if possible), and it should be noted that they are as useful for day-to-day work as for examination revision.

One of the other main ways which will help to accumulate information and understand it, is to have a teaching commitment. A great deal of factual information can be learned by preparing undergraduate lectures or post mortem presentations, and it is recommended that all candidates grasp these opportunities. It is far easier for lecturers, who have to teach on a regular basis, but even registrars and senior registrars should have ample chances to teach in most rotating posts, certainly in university departments. Even in a district general hospital, there are often medical students, junior colleagues or surgeons who would appreciate pathology tuition. Although there is a tendency to try to avoid such teaching, regarding it as an imposition or even a chore, it should be remembered that the benefits will become obvious later when communicating with clinical colleagues, and in the examination situation where a fluent and relevant discourse on various subjects is required.

In addition to textbooks, it is advisable that you keep up with current advances described in the major pathology journals. There are many journals to choose from, and some are certainly very specialised and more suited to the specialist. As a start, it is recommended that the general reviews in *Histopathology, Journal of Pathology, Human Pathology* and the *American Journal of Surgical Pathology* are consulted on a regular basis. Reading the major original articles takes up relatively little time provided some time is left aside for this every month. This has to be a regular commitment, otherwise a large backlog will accumulate and defeat the object of the exercise. Providing it is possible to adhere to this plan, a surprisingly large spread of knowledge can be accumulated after only a few months.

Editorials often provide a very useful overview of the more important articles, and are well worth reading because they are more concise and place the articles in a broader context.

The articles in *Histopathology* and the *American Journal of Surgical Pathology* have a very heavy emphasis on diagnostic surgical pathology, and are a rich source of information on newly described entities and application of modern techniques to diagnosis. The *Journal of Clinical Pathology* contains a broad spread of articles concerning the other major pathological disciplines as well as histopathology, so that selection is necessary. This is a useful reference for technical methods which are of practical use in surgical pathology. The *Journal of Pathology* concentrates more on experimental pathology and the theoretical basis of disease, but contains very useful review articles and editorials, as well as papers on more general aspects of pathology. *Human Pathology* carries papers of general histopathological interest which are relevant to all levels of experience, and some of the largest series of particular entities may be found in this journal, with abundant illustration. *Archives of Pathology* and *Laboratory Medicine* contain articles and reviews in a similar vein, but are usually somewhat more concentrated.

In general, it is difficult to select and assimilate the information from more detailed journals such as *Laboratory Investigation*, specialist cancer journals, *American Journal of Pathology* or *Virchows Archivs* to name but a few, because these assume a high standard of knowledge on the part of the reader, and often fail to provide the background perspective which is necessary for the less experienced pathologist. Attempting to read the relatively technical articles in these Journals may well be counter-productive, squandering energies which could be directed into absorbing more basic and general aspects which are often included in the recommended journals.

It may prove impossible to read all of the original articles in the Journals selected, but a useful compromise may be to read the abstract thoroughly, combined with an examination of the illustrations, which are the focal point of many pathological articles. (The review articles are designed to be read in full however.) A swift 'scan' of the discussions may reveal some background information which is also of value. It is probably true that the message of any such article could be summarised in one or two sentences in the vast majority of cases.

Another very useful device for general reference, and for revision purposes when a specific article or subject is required, is to photocopy the subject indexes in the major journals, (which are found in the December issues) and keep these in a separate file. Copies of the previous five years should be sufficient. It is important not to be too ambitious, restricting the choice to the major journals previously recommended, otherwise the amount of information becomes too unwieldy and defeats the purpose.

Rather than mechanically wading through a number of articles in any one session, a useful 'aide mémoire' is to make short notes or paragraph summaries of the more important current advances in pathology. The more relevant articles may also be identified after informal discussion with colleagues, or in the context of a journal review 'club' organised on a Departmental or Regional basis.

Membership of the Association of Clinical Pathologists and of the Pathological Society of Great Britain and Ireland entail automatic subscription to the *Journal of Clinical Pathology* and the *Journal of Pathology* respectively. *Histopathology* is sent to members of the International Academy of Pathologists. Application details can be obtained from the sources in Appendix 3. As well as other benefits, membership of these organisation entails access to other very useful publications, especially the ACP who have completed a series of broad-sheets on a various topical subjects, the Model Training Programme (currently under review) and the Education supplement. These can be supplied on request. All of these organisations arrange symposia and international meetings which are frequently highly relevant to trainees, details of which are sent automatically to members.

Associate membership of the Royal College of Pathologists brings with it the *College Bulletin*, which often contains very useful review articles and views on current problems. The College also issues handbooks on various subjects which may not be adequately covered elsewhere, such as health service laboratory management and safety. Such issues may assume a much higher profile in future examinations, and should not be overlooked in preparation or training.

Health and safety considerations in pathology have come to receive much greater emphasis in recent years, culminating in the publication of the *Howie Report* (HMSO 1982). This is mandatory reading for all trainee pathologists, and is surprisingly concise. Examination questions have been set directly relating to this Report, and it contains advice on conduct during post mortem examinations and in the laboratory, which candidates will be expected to know in detail and carry into practice, for the protection of others as much as themselves. It is most important to be aware of any future recommendation on laboratory safety and management which may be published or implemented.

It is very difficult to keep up with many of the advances or sources of information when working alone, and candidates are urged to join a group of contemporaries working for the examination in order to share information on symposia, meetings and courses, and to set up 'slide clubs' and 'journal clubs'. Regular meetings (usually once a month) to present and review cases and articles are invaluable. Although it requires some effort to organise such meetings, especially for trainees working at district hospitals within a Region, the benefits to be gained far outweigh any minor inconveniences.

The preceding ideas are not intended to be comprehensive guidelines for the ideal training post or examination preparation, but it is often difficult to identify those areas which may be under-represented or over-emphasised within any particular appointment. The ACP Model Training Programme contains more detailed and considered opinion on these aspects. The interchange of ideas among colleagues at a similar level of training is however of far more value in terms of self-advancement than the information which can be gleaned from any book. It is also suggested that every chance to teach others in pathology is taken, both in formal lectures and in informal tutorials or necropsy demonstration, for this is where the most valuable preparation is done. Finally, avoid reading books or journals as a chore – this is a certain way to become disillusioned and disheartened with the task in hand!

Application for the Final Examination

For trainees who have entered histopathology before December 1988, the Final examination is held in Spring and Autumn each year, and the dates are advertised in advance in the Bulletin of the *Royal College of Pathologists* which is distributed to Associate Members. There are strict closing dates for formal applications which are usually mid-February for the Spring of that year, and mid-May for the Autumn (the longer interval required because of the intervening academic vacation period).

Trainee pathologists are eligible to sit the written part of the Final examination after obtaining the Primary MRCPath and completing at least three years full-time in recognised posts, (and candidates must always ensure that these posts are suitable by checking with the College before appointments if the situation is unclear). Different arrangements apply to those working in part-time posts, and candidates working overseas should write to the College for advice.

Application forms may be obtained from the Examinations Secretary at the College. The present fee payable for both parts of the examination is £150. A member of the College must act as a sponsor (preferably the head of department) and be able to certify that the applicant is capable of cutting and staining a frozen section, and has completed three months formal experience in cytopathology. Candidates who wish to withdraw their application after the closing date may forfeit a proportion of the fee.

As from January 1989, new regulations are applied. There will be no Primary examinations; the main examination will be taken after three years full-time experience in histopathology, and will be of the same format as the current Final examination, and at the same standard. However, candidates will only be expected to perform at a level commensurate with their experience, whatever that might mean. There follow two further years of higher professional training, and to acquire the magic letters of MRCPath, a further 'exit' component is required: this can be (i) the presentation of a successful MD/PhD in an appropriate subject, (ii) the passing of a practical examination slanted towards one of the specialties, such as dermatopathology or gynaecological pathology, or (iii) a practical examination in what might be called general histopathology.

We suspect that *all* candidates, with an eye on consultant selection committees, will choose the last option. Some few able individuals will take (i) and (iii), or (ii) and (iii), and the odd academic or monomaniac will elect to do (i) or (ii) only. The merits of this new system are unknown and debatable; this examination-ridden training period is certainly not what the proponents of freeform envisaged. One thing is certain, histopathology trainees will have to get used to taking examinations, like it or lump it. Whether you regard examinations as a necessary or unnecessary evil there is no doubt that the MRCPath examination will loom large on the horizons of trainees for generations to come. In essence therefore, this book is suitable for both groups of trainees.

The Written Examination

General Preparation

The preceding chapter dealt with much of the general preparation for achieving a satisfactory standard in histopathology. The written examination is intended to ascertain whether a candidate has achieved a certain degree of broad theoretical knowledge, and in recent years there has been an increasing tendency to set questions which are related to mechanisms of disease and their clinical relevance, or to the practical application of scientific observations. The papers now tend to strike a balance between diagnostic and 'academic' pathology (see e.g. April 1988, Oct 1985). The first paper is devoted to principles of pathology to ensure that the candidate has a clear understanding of the pathogenesis of disease. Questions may be included on principles of techniques used in histopathology but details of technical methods are not expected. The second paper is devoted to clinical aspects of histopathology. Questions should cover a wide range of the conditions seen in consultant histopathological practice including autopsies and cyto-pathology. A question on the organisation or management of a histopathology laboratory is appropriate for this part of the examination. We recommend that all candidates review some of the papers early on in training, in order to cover many of the areas in question, and obtain some idea of the standards required. As the examination approaches, it is important to establish that this knowledge can be converted into a reasonable written answer, which like all skills is a result of both planning and practice.

The earlier this is started, the more proficient a candidate will become, but few have the inclination to begin much before a year in advance of the examination, and the majority will start in earnest around five to six months beforehand. It is naturally very difficult to assess how much time is required to prepare, as some candidates will have achieved much more than others during the course of their training, and learning abilities vary enormously. However, at this stage an individual should at least have a rough idea of their learning capacity and how much time will need to be devoted.

Comparisons with colleagues' progress can often prove to be disheartening, because they often appear to be achieving that much more. However, it is surprising how distorted their recollection of the amount of revision work completed can be! Each candidate must decide how much work they can *reasonably* be expected to achieve within the timetable they have set themselves and work steadily, while remembering that few achieve all that was originally intended.

Assuming the decision has been made to apply for the written examination, the general aspects should be considered first. Even for revision, good writing instruments and paper are essential, and the work should be conducted in a relatively peaceful environment. An assessment of the general writing style should be made at this stage, since this is the time to try to correct bad or illegible handwriting, and improve the layout of the work. Always check that spelling is correct, and that correct grammar is being used. These factors are important, because a badly handwritten, poorly laid out answer will always be looked on less favourably than a well presented one, even if the content is identical, and some examiners will even ignore illegible sections of an answer. Colleagues or secretaries should be asked to comment on whether improvements can be made on this score. If so, it follows that such alterations will require to be consistently put into effect.

A distinctive and neat layout could be introduced when taking lecture notes, or writing up post mortem or surgical pathology reports. Other details such as underlining, side headings, neatly crossing out mistakes, etc. can be practised. If a writing style looks 'professional' it will inevitably create a better impression.

Essay Format

Most of this book is concerned with the approach to the written answers, both to illustrate technique and to provide revision exercises. Past papers can be obtained from the Examinations secretariat at the Royal College of Pathologists, for which a small charge is made. Whether or not the ability of medical graduates to express themselves clearly in written prose has been eroded by years of inspired guess-work imposed by the computer-besotted, literacy-debasing protagonists of the MCQ, the experience of most examiners in the written part of the Final Examination is that candidates do not know how to approach the planning and execution of an essay. Please, therefore, do not skip this section; it is as important as any. Assuming that a candidate has established a reasonable essay writing style, the recommended approach is to construct essay 'plans', using side headings and key words to represent contents of a sentence or paragraph. The alternative is to write out essays in full, but this is generally a tedious and time-consuming business. An essay plan can be constructed within a shorter period of time using appropriate articles or texts, and will enable an assessment of balance and emphasis in an essay.

It is vital that the ability to translate a plan into an essay style is acquired, and should be a matter of regular practice, starting with a plan, then writing the essay, within a reasonable time limit. At first this may taken in excess of an hour, but you should aim to complete both within 45 minutes, the time allowed in the examination itself. (The plan may be written on the answer papers, as long as it is indicated quite clearly that it is only an outline, which is left as such or neatly crossed through.)

The outline has another benefit, in that few examiners will resist reading it. They will see the general organisation and grasp the answer swiftly, and note that the candidate has (hopefully) included all the major points. In the event that an answer cannot be completed, the examiner might take into account the general direction of the answer, and what was intended as the remainder.

One major advantage is that all the planning is concentrated into one 5–7 minute session at the beginning, rather than as a more diffuse, sustained effort which often leads to inconsistency and inaccuracy. It is less tiring to construct paragraphs of a suitable length to fit the overall framework, without having to continually recall complex detail while writing. This avoids problems with 'freestyle' essays which very often result in distorted answers, with over-detailed description at the beginning, and gradual deterioration towards the latter half as time begins to run out.

In addition, facts are often recalled out of 'sequence' or in an illogical fashion. These can be more easily slotted into an essay plan, but it is very difficult to adopt prose-style answers to take account of these variations. It is important to attempt to estimate how much time might be required for each section and adhere to it. The plan should also be laid out neatly, with enough gaps to add in information which comes to mind during the course of writing the answer.

Some candidates do not have the confidence to spend five minutes or so preparing an outline, believing it to be time better spent on the actual answer.

Ultimately, this is a matter for personal preference but, certainly for revision purposes, plans save much effort in writing and allow concentration on the important principles and key words necessary, and so we have used this construction in our approach in this book.

Papers back to 1969 have been examined and the questions have been arbitrarily grouped into broad categories such as cardiovascular system and lung, central nervous system, alimentary system, etc. We have obviously emphasised the more recent questions, and where the subject has appeared more than once, an outline which could provide the basis for an essay is usually suggested. In general, plans have been considered for about a quarter of the total number of questions. For the remainder there are paragraph summaries suggesting possible approaches to the answer, including observations on the wording of the question which may affect the emphasis on particular aspects of a subject. The suggested outlines are not attempting to provide compehensive answers, and issue might be taken with some points, but in general it is believed these should lead to an adequate pass mark if properly expanded.

Essay Plans

The examples generally occupy 1 to 1.5 pages, and are usually based on one or two reference articles. Wherever possible attempts have been made to identify any questions apparently related to recently published material just prior to the examination of that year (e.g. Chapters in *Recent Advances in Pathology*, Journal review articles or subjects of 'topical' interest at that time). These outlines are probably longer than the reader as an individual would construct in practice (and some would certainly take more than 5 minutes to write out), but there has been a deliberate attempt to avoid using too many abbreviations in order to make them more readable. In practice each person would devise their own abbreviation style, although it should not be too incomprehensible, remembering that it is for the examiner's benefit as much as their own.

A notation style of format has been used for the sections following the introduction, subdividing the answer into sections which are generally labelled 1), 2) 3) etc. with subsections a) b) c), and even smaller subheadings i) ii) iii). In this way the information has been laid out to put the appropriate degree of weighting on the answers, concentrating on the more important entities at the beginning, and gradually introducing less common or perhaps less relevant ones.

If the side headings are underlined, it usually indicates a paragraph or more of writing is required. Adjacent to this, some key words have been inserted, which need to be expanded to anything from a sentence to a whole paragraph. The bare minimum of factual information has been introduced, but if it is not clear exactly how to expand a particular section it is an indication to read up about the subject from the reference or other sources. Enough space has been left in order to introduce other ideas as the reader feels appropriate or when more recent information comes to hand.

Naturally, the pathological aspects figure predominantly in most of the answers, but in many of the questions, subheadings such as Gross Pathology, Microscopic Features, Immunohistochemical Findings, etc. have been left without further key words. This is because, in some situations, the reader would be expected to know how to provide the necessary expansion for these sections or the necessary information would usually be found in the reference.

The overall result is intended to be a skeleton plan, addressing most of the ground intended by the question. A distinctive layout to the plan makes it easier to recall the content of certain parts of this structure while continuing to write the essay, avoiding the need to continually keep referring back to it. Theoretically you only require to look up small subsections whose presence you recall by the 'pattern' created by the plan, but have forgotten the content. This may become clearer once it has been practised a few times.

The introductory paragraphs should include an indication of the clinical background to some diseases, including the age range, rare incidence, frequency of disease in the population, distinction from other diseases, clinical relevance of the pathological diagnosis and importance for patient management, etc. In more theoretical questions the exact meaning of terms used should be explained and the relevant aetiological factors and pathogenetic mechanisms should be outlined as appropriate.

In general, the introductory paragraph should include

a) an appraisal of the scope of the question
b) definition of the terms used in the question
c) an explanation of the background to the problem
d) an indication of the general direction(s) of the answer if only a selection of the possible aspects are to be discussed.

The only 'hard' facts which need to be included at this stage are statistical (e.g. epidemiological and clinical data). The introduction has not been expanded in many of the plans because in an examination situation the subjects in section a) and c) require a descriptive approach, and d) is merely a brief overview of the following plan. The introduction is an essential part of a structured answer and, being the first section the examiners will read, a demonstration of a grasp of the essential aspects of the question will undoubtedly influence their attitude to the remainder.

You will find that there is generally too much information to be included in the answer to have time for a concluding paragraph, but on occasion this may be appropriate. It is probably of much less importance than the introductory paragraph, merely because the examiner will have already formed an opinion about the essay by this stage.

The majority of the questions have not been formulated as essay plans, but there is an explanatory paragraph illustrating various points which may relate to the wording of the question, or assessments of the general direction of the answer and possible areas of misunderstanding, and suggestions as to the content of the essay. They are not intended to be comprehensive, and it is suggested that the questions are used for practice essay plans and essay writing, as well as reading up on the suggested references and any other source the reader is aware of, which has not been cited.

It would be reasonable to ask why one should cover in detail previous essay questions, rather than cover areas on which questions have not been asked. The answer is of course that there are only a limited number of subjects in pathology about which sufficient detailed knowledge could be expected for a candidate to write for 40 minutes or so. It is also worthwhile noting that 20 questions per annum need to be set, which means that subjects can be covered more than once, and often are. However, although it is unusual for identical questions to be set, subtle alterations in the wording of the questions may mean radical alterations in the answer. Nevertheless, diligent study of previous papers, coupled with an elementary knowledge of probability, enabled one of the contributors to have prepared more or less specimen answers to no less than six out of the eight required questions in the two papers. There is no reason why you should not do at least as well.

In addition to repeated questions, most aspects of pathology would be covered by using these plans and paragraphs as revision exercises for the written examination. The knowledge gained will not only help in routine work, but there are other sections of the examination where it may prove useful, including the *viva voce* examination. Logical, structured answers to questions guided by a recalled plan are more impressive than ill thought-out answers. These sorts of frameworks are a basis for all parts of the examination, and can be adapted to each circumstance.

However, it is inadvisable to try to memorise the plans and adhere rigidly to them for the reasons outlined in the preceding paragraphs, in that an alteration in a wording of a question may alter the content of the answer. The examination should be approached with the intention to construct an entirely new plan for each question, perhaps using sections or subsections previously revised, but with the introduction of new ideas relevant to the question. This is easier than it sounds, but practice is essential!

The emphasis has been placed on the more recent questions, and it should be appreciated that some older questions are outdated, and do not lend themselves to an adequate answer in the light of current knowledge (e.g. on lymphomas). It would be a useful exercise to try to 'update' such questions, or construct a question which may be set on this or a closely related subject, but this has not been attempted in this book.

Regarding the practical aspects of writing the actual answer, while it is suggested that the divisions outlined in the plan are followed in general, this may be difficult to introduce in some circumstances. Strictly speaking, an essay should not include side and subheadings, etc. but it is justifiable in this situation to make some division and organisation in most cases in order to break up what would otherwise be long tracts of writing. If nothing else, it stops the tendency for overlong and repetitious discussion, which provides few marks for a lot of effort. Experience indicates that examiners vary considerably in their appreciation of headings and subheadings. Remember, because of the vicissitudes of time and commitments, examiners are usually marking against the clock, and there is nothing more daunting in this situation than to be confronted by page after page of handwriting, unredeemed by space, heading or indeed paragraph.

Diagrams and illustrations may be very useful as part of an answer and should be included if at all possible. It is a good idea to make a file of drawings and diagrams on a variety of subjects. If these are relevant to the question, ensure that they can be reproduced quickly, accurately and above all neatly. Scruffy, 'thumbnail' sketches on the other hand definitely detract from an answer. So, if a diagram is to be attempted, it should occupy at least half a page and be drawn boldly. A descriptive title is necessary but more important subjects in each system need to be practised in advance of the examination.

It would be a mistake to try to construct a novel diagram or illustration during the course of the answer in the actual examination, as it would be unlikely to be a success at the first attempt, and the time involved in considering it would far outweigh any benefit.

There is also a temptation to include them where they are not strictly relevant in certain circumstances, but this should be resisted. Diagrams are most useful where they avoid the necessity for long tracts of explanatory text, and must relate to the most central aspects of the question.

A few suggested examples for diagrams include the following:

1) *Gastrointestinal tract*
   a) Architecture of various polyps
   b) Duke's classification of carcinoma of the rectum
   c) Portal circulation and effects of portal hypertension
   d) Early gastric cancer – microscopic patterns

2) *Cardiovascular system*
   a) Types of dissecting aneurysms
   b) Myocardial infarction – anatomical and topographic distribution
   c) Patterns of emphysema
   d) Atherosclerosis – general microscopic architecture

3) *Genitourinary system*
   a) Dysplasia and intraepithelial neoplasia – grading patterns
   b) Sites of urinary obstruction

4) *Lymphoreticular system*
   a) Architecture of lymph node and spleen (and involvements by disease)
   b) Morphology of lymphoid cells – normal and neoplastic
   c) Morphology of granulomas

5) *Central nervous system*
   a) Location of intracranial haemorrhage – gross anatomical patterns
   b) Structure of the eye and location of pathology
   c) Cerebral arterial circulation

6) *Musculoskeletal system*
   a) Sites and effects of osteosarcoma
   b) Normal bone and metabolic bone disease – microscopic architecture

7) *Skin*
   a) Classification of melanoma – types and invasive patterns
   b) Cutaneous lymphoid proliferation
   c) Bullous disease of the skin – location of bullae

Other ideas may come to mind during revision. It would be a useful exercise to compile a list of about ten diagrams for each category. One way of doing this is to consider providing one potential diagram for each essay plan attempted during revision.

Up to three references are provided with each outline plan or explanatory paragraph in the following sections, and where possible they are related to the question around the time it was set, if the appropriate article is identified. Generally speaking, they are taken from the most popular and easily available texts for both general and diagnostic work, together with the review articles and journals outlined previously and under Appendix 1. Single articles in journals or other texts are referenced in full. Every candidate should be able to add to the list as articles are encountered during training or revision.

All of the written examination questions back to 1969 have been included in the following sections, dividing them in a systematic basis into the following groups. It is acknowledged that there will be overlap between some of the groups.

1) General Pathology
2) Neoplasia
3) Lymphoreticular System
4) Alimentary Tract
5) Cardiovascular and Respiratory Systems
6) Endocrine System
7) Renal Pathology
8) Central Nervous System
9) Osteoarticular Pathology
10) Reproductive System
11) Dermatopathology
12) Miscellaneous
13) Short notes questions

About one in four of the answers are in the form of outline plans, and the remainder are as explanatory paragraphs. The questions are set out in reverse order chronologically, but some questions are grouped with others on a similar theme from previous years. Where a topic has recurred there is usually an essay plan on the question having the broadest scope, and the differences in emphasis and approach in the other variants are compared by short explanatory paragraphs.

One disadvantage to grouping the questions in this way is that it does not give much insight into the 'balance' of individual examinations, hence the recommendation that the actual papers are reviewed to retain some idea of this.

By the time the examination is near, a candidate should feel able to mentally construct a reasonable outline to most of the questions when perusing the papers. Having said this, it is important not to feel demoralised if the perfect approach to the answer is not immediately apparent, as is common with most people; ideas come to mind during actual formulation of the plan and to a lesser extent during the essay writing itself. What is important is the ability to get started and have some idea of the direction. Those whose approach is to look at a question and announce they can answer it with little difficulty almost always turn out to have a very superficial grasp of the subject. It is important not to take any notice of such colleagues, as they may unnecessarily reduce one's level of confidence. One final word of advice: answer the question! There are few things more irritating for examiners than candidates who regard even the most clearly formulated question as an excuse to unselectively regurgitate the sum total of their knowledge of that subject.

MRCPATH ESSAY QUESTIONS

1969–1989

1. General Pathology

Give an account of amyloidosis

Introduction

General features of amyloidosis

Gross appearances

  a) localised, systemic
  b) iodine staining

Microscopic appearances

  a) conventional – cellular distribution
  b) special stains – Congo Red, dichroism, thioflavine T, metachromatic dyes
  c) ultrastructure
  d) X-ray diffraction – beta pleated sheet

Associated protein

  a) amyloid-P

Classification of amyloid

  a) AL (immunological associated)
  b) AA (reactive systemic)
  c) AA (hereditary – FMF)
     AF (neuropathic)
  d) AE (localised-endocrine)
     AS (localised-cardiac)
     AS (localised-cerebral)

Distribution

AL –   heart, nerves, tongue, skin, kidney

AA –   liver, spleen, kidney

Distinction

KMnO$_4$ preincubation abolishes Congo Red binding to AA

Associations

AL

  a) myeloma/occult immune dyscrasia
  b) serum – M band
  c) urine – Bence-Jones protein/light chains

AA

    a) chronic disorders (e.g. osteomyelitis, RA)

    b) neoplasms (e.g. renal adenocarcinoma)

Heredofamilial

    a) rare

    b) fever and recurrent serositis

Localised

    a) nodular (lung, larynx, skin, etc.)

    b) endocrine tumours (?conversion of hormone secretion)

    c) cardiac (senile)

    d) cerebral (Alzheimer's plaques)

Pathogenesis

AL

    a) light chains

    b) unknown 'amyloidogenic' factors

    c) immunohistochemical evidence

AA

    a) serum AA (acute phase reactant)

    b) ?defective breakdown

    c) reduced degrading activity in FMF & RA

Complications

1) Cardiac

2) Renal

3) GIT

(October 1981, Paper 1, Question 4)

References

1) Cohen, A.S., Connors, L.H. The pathogenesis and biochemistry of amyloidosis. J. Pathol. (1987) 151: 1–10.

2) Hind, C.R.K., Pepys, M.B. Amyloidosis. Hospital Update (1984) 10(7–9): 593–597; 637–648; 737–747.

Discuss the aetiology of amyloid

The wording of this question makes it difficult to know exactly what is required as the distinction between aetiology and pathogenesis is necessarily rather blurred in this subject. The sections on aetiology (pathogenesis) given in the previous answer, including classification and a description of the nature of amyloid could be expanded, avoiding pathological appearances and consequences since this is clearly not required. This illustrates a need for an essay plan, since it would be very easy to drift off the central theme.   *(October 1984, Paper 1, Question 1)*

What is known of the fine structure and chemical composition of amyloid? Comment on the distribution of this substance in primary, secondary and senile amyloidosis
(November 1976, Paper 1, Question 4)

Discuss the nature and pathogenesis of the various types of amyloidosis

These questions could be answered in a very similar way to the essay outline.
(April 1975, Paper 2, Question 1)

What are mast cells? Describe how you would demonstrate them in histological sections. In what disease processes are they involved?
(November 1974, Paper 1, Question 1)

Discuss the role of the mast cell in health and disease

Questions which are clearly designed to assess the breadth of knowledge of a candidate, and their ability to integrate material gleaned from a variety of sources into a potentially interesting account. It is probably of value to compile an essay plan on this subject for general revision purposes if nothing else, and the series of articles given in references 2 and 3 are eminently readable. The essay should cover normal morphology, function and demonstration of mast cells, and the pathology would either cover the role in various sites in the body (as in the given references) or under involvement in various pathogenetic mechanisms and pathology, e.g. Type I hypersensitivity reactions, angiogenesis, neoplasia, etc.
(October 1981, Paper 1, Question 2)

References

1) Taussig, M.J. Hypersensitivity. In: Processes in Pathology and Microbiology. 2nd edition. p153–157. Blackwell Scientific Publications, Oxford (1984).
2) Mitchell, E.B. The mast cell: structure and function. Hospital Update (1984) 9: 1367–1378.
3) Holgate, S.T., Kay, A.B. Mast cells and the lung. Hospital Update (1984) 10: 151–162.

Give an account of the role of the macrophage in tuberculosis and neoplasia

In spite of having been the subject of investigation for many years, the functions of the macrophages and their regulation are only partly understood. This incompleteness of knowledge is reflected in the difficulty of composing an answer to this question. The first part is the easier as it requires a description of the well-known morphology of tuberculous inflammation, and the first reference provides some information about the mononuclear phagocyte system, about ultrastructure and speculation upon the function of the macrophage in granulomatous inflammation. The pathologist searching the general texts for an account of macrophages in neoplasia will be disappointed. The immune response is a very complicated subject, in which the macrophage plays a role in antigen presentation to T cells, antibody production by B cells, and phagocytosis.

(November 1977, Paper 2, Question 2)

References

1) Robbins, S.L., Cotran, R.S., Kumar, V. The mononuclear phagocyte system, and immune response and immunosurveillance. In: Pathologic Basis of Disease, 4th edition. p61–63; 374–376; 296–298. W.B. Saunders, Philadelphia (1989).
2) Taussig, M.J. The immune response and neoplasia. In: Processes in Pathology and Microbiology, 2nd edition. p114–117; 745–749. Blackwell Scientific Publications, Oxford (1984).

Discuss the role of products synthesised by the macrophage in disease

Introduction

Nomenclature
Distribution and role in mononuclear phagocyte system
General functions   1) Phagocytosis and bacterial killing
                    2) Immune response
                    3) Wound healing and chronic inflammation
                    4) Neoplasia

Products synthesised in each group

1) *Phagocytosis and bacterial killing*

a) C3b and Fc receptors – engulfment after opsonisation
b) lysozyme – glucosidase affecting cells walls
c) other lysozymal hydrolases
d) O_2 dependent mechanism for killing? H_2O_2 or OH^-

2) *Immune response*

a) MHC + processed Ag presentation to T lymphocytes
   Role of HLA DR
   Relation to antibody production
b) IL-1 – T_4 lymphocyte stimulation

3) *Wound healing and chronic inflammation*

a) neutrophil chemotactic factor
b) arachidonic acid metabolites – vasodilatation
                                  – vascular permeability
c) haemostasis – coagulation activated by tissue thromboplastin
d) enzyme release – fibrinolysis (plasminogen activator)
                   – collagenase
                   – elastase
e) IL-1
   i)   release of PgE in hypothalamus? resets thermoregulatory centre (i.e. fever)
   ii) ↑ muscle catabolism
   iii) ↑ haemopoiesis
   iv) collagenase production by fibroblasts
   v)   fibrogenesis
f) TNF
   i)   endotoxic shock
   ii) angiogenesis

4) *Neoplasia*

a) non-specific cytotoxicity
   ? lysosyme enzymes following activation
   ? complement or proteases
b) TNF – cytotoxic to cells *in vitro*
   γ interferon sensitises cells to killing

(October 1988, Paper 1, Question 2)

References

1) Auger, M.J. Mononuclear phagocytes. Br. Med. J. (1989) 298: 546–548
2) Robbins, S.L., Cotran, R.S., Kumar V. Inflammation and repair. In: Pathologic Basis of Disease, 4th edition. p39–86. W.B. Saunders, Philadelphia (1989).
3) Taussig, M.J. Inflammation and the immune response. In: Processes in Pathology and Microbiology, 2nd edition. p23; 114–117; 147–148; 745–749. Blackwell Scientific Publications, Oxford (1984).

Discuss the role of the eosinophil in disease

Introduction

Origin and lineage
Morphology
Histochemical staining
General disease associations – 'allergic' disease,
parasitic disease, neoplasia, unknown

Normal function

Surface IgG and Fc receptors

Granule content
a) basic proteins (EBP)
b) PAF
c) leukotrienes
d) phospholipase D
e) arylsulphatase B
f) histaminase
g) eosinophil cationic protein (ECP)

Pathological states

'Allergic'

a) asthma and mucosal inflammation
    i)   mast cell – IgE binding
    ii) eosinophil chemo-attraction (ECF-A)
    iii) granules
        – leukotrienes
        – bronchoconstriction
        – vascular permeability
    iv) anti-inflammatory
b) eosinophilic gastroenteritis
c) drug reaction – idiosyncrasy
d) hypereosinophilic syndrome
e) endocardial fibrosis
    i)   peripheral eosinophils – degranulated
                             – dysmorphic
    ii) action of EBP
    iii) thrombosis   – PAF

Parasitic disease

   a) IgG binds to parasite
   b) eosinophil binding (Fc receptors)
   c) EBP and ECP released
   d) IgE production (mast cell binding)
   e) ECP-A released
   f) also IgE-mediated parasite binding
   g) Fc receptors on eosinophils

Neoplasia

1) Primary
   a) eosinophilic leukaemia
2) Reactive
   a) Hodgkin's disease
      i) IgE fixation
      ii) chemoattractants
      iii) ? interleukin 5
   b) squamous ca lung
      i) uterine cervix
      ii) ? mechanism
      iii) chemoattractants (good prognostic indicator)
   c) metastatic carcinoma
      i) blood eosinophilia
   d) epithelioid haemangio-endothelioma
   e) unknown
      i) e.g. histiocytosis X
      ii) T cell lymphoma
      iii) ? IL5

Idiopathic skin diseases

1) Eosinophilic cellulitis
   a) flame figures
2) Eosinophilic spongiosis
   a) pemphigus prodrome
3) Eosinophilic fasciitis

(October 1984, Paper 2, Question 1)

References

1) Spry, C.J.F. New properties and roles for eosinophils in disease. J. Royal Soc. Med. (1985) 78: 844–848.
2) Lowe, D., Jopizzo J., Hutt, M.S.R. Tumour-associated eosinophilia: a review. J. Clin. Pathol. (1981) 34: 1343–1348.
3) Taussig, M.J. Inflammation and immune response. In: Processes in Pathology and Microbiology, 2nd edition. p 145–146; 153–156. Blackwell Scientific Publications, Oxford (1984).

Write an essay on the clinical manifestations and histopathological changes in graft versus host disease

At present this subject has received surprisingly scant attention in the major textbooks, and comprehensive reviews are hard to find. The organs predominantly affected are skin, gut and liver, and latterly respiratory tract changes are described, and both acute and chronic types of the disease could be described for each of these sites. This is one subject where, at present, a candidate who is up to date with the literature or has attended symposia on the subject would have a distinct advantage.   *(April 1987, Paper 2, Question 2*

Reference

1) Snover, D.C. Acute and chronic graft versus host disease. Human Pathol. (1984) 15: 202–205.

Discuss the morphological features and pathogenesis of sickle cell disease

This question does not require discussion of the aetiology of this disease, which is known (but which could be mentioned in the introduction). The pathogenesis of the disease should ideally be considered first, as the morphological changes are a consequence. The biochemical abnormalities and the effects of oxygen tension, presence of other haemoglobins, MCHC or pH all require consideration, and how the rheological effects in the cells are produced. The morphological features include the effects of anaemia on various organisms, and consequences of erythrohyperplasia of bone marrow and other sites. The consequences of chronic sickling are due to capillary stasis, thrombosis and infarction affecting bone, liver, lung, brain, spleen and kidney, with the more florid effects in acute cases. Other considerations include the general association of chronic diseases such as growth retardation and susceptibility to infection.   *(April 1973, Paper 2, Question 3)*

Reference

1) Robbins, S.L., Cotran, R.S., Kumar, V. Sickle cell disease and the kidney. In: Pathologic Basis of Disease, 4th edition. p666–670; 1070. W.B. Saunders, Philadelphia (1989).

Discuss the role of lysosomes in pathological processes

Lysosomes contain a variety of toxic degradative enzymes which normally are contained safely within the lysosomal membrane and are released into a phagolysosome under physiological conditions. Asbestos, silica and copper ions cause disruption of macrophage lysosomal membranes with subsequent cell damage and fibrosis following repair. Histiocyte lysosomes can also act as 'dustbins' when macromolecules (sphingolipids, for example) accumulate due to lack of specific lysosomal enzymes, so a description of the major types of 'storage disorders' could comprise a major part of the answer. Other aspects could include a consideration of deficient lysosomal function as found in chronic granulomatous disease of childhood where there is a lack of myeloperoxidase killing in neutrophils.

(April 1970, Paper 1, Question 4)

Reference

1) Allison, A.C. Lysosomes in pathology. In: Recent Advances in Histopathology 10. N. Woolf, P.P. Anthony (eds.). Churchill Livingstone, Edinburgh (1978).

Discuss the effects of ionising radiation on human tissue
(October 1986, Paper 1, Question 2)

Discuss the effect of ionising radiation on cells and tissues

Introduction

Definition of ionising radiation
Radiation measurement – grays/rads
Types of ionising radiation
Energy transfer
Linear

Extent of radiation injury

a) type
b) dose
c) sensitivity
d) genetic susceptibility

Effects of injury

1) Acute

a) single large dose
    i)   10 000 rad – death < 2 hours
    ii) 2–5000 rad – death 2–5 days (GIT damage)
    iii) 300–1000 rad – death 10–14 days (haemopoietic failure)
b) multiple smaller doses
    i)   50–300 rad – haemopoietic suppression
    GI crypt cell damage

2) *Chronic*

- a) lung
  - i) 3–6 months post dose, vascular changes and fibrosis
- b) kidney
  - i) tubular damage
- c) colon
  - i) ? vascular damage with muscular fibrosis and strictures
- d) lymphoedema
  - i) lymphatic fibrosis
- e) skin
  - i) atrophy, elastosis, appendage loss and telangiectasia, 'radiation' fibroblasts
- f) bone
  - i) necrosis
- g) eye
  - i) cataract formation
- h) gonads
  - i) atrophy of germ cells

Carcinogenesis

1) Leukaemia
   a) post therapeutic and atomic bomb survivors

2) Thyroid carcinoma
   a) head and neck irradiation

3) Osteosarcoma
   a) 'dial' painters – radiation

4) Bronchial carcinoma
   a) uranium miners

(November 1969, Paper 1, Question 1)

Reference

1) Robbins, S.L., Cotran, R.S., Kumar, V. Neoplasia and environmental pathology. In: Pathologic Basis of Disease, 4th edition. p273–275; 504–511. W.B. Saunders, Philadelphia (1989).

Describe the pathological effects of radiation

While ionising radiation should again comprise the major part of this essay, consideration should also be given to other forms of radiation, especially ultraviolet radiation and to a lesser extent infrared radiation.

(April 1984, Paper 1, Question 4)

Describe the late complications of radiotherapy in different organs

This question requires greater attention to the chronic effects of radiation detailed previously, with greater description of the microscopic features and vascular changes, together with tumours produced, although the mechanisms producing tumours are not required.

(April 1971, Paper 2, Question 5)

Discuss the spectrum of pathology and pathogenesis of diseases associated with alpha-1-antitrypsin deficiency

Introduction

Nature of alpha-1-antitrypsin
Genetic features   – autosomal co-dominant inheritance
                   – multiple alleles at each locus
                   – significance of M & Z alleles
                   – Z gene frequency (4%) and homozygote PiZZ
                     frequency (0.03–0.006)

Disease associations and pathology

1) Acute cholestatic hepatitis in infancy
2) Cirrhosis in adolescence
3) Hepatocellular carcinoma
4) Pulmonary emphysema

Pathogenesis

1) Emphysema

  a) effect of smoking
     i)   heterozygotes
     ii) homozygotes
     iii) antielastase activity
     iv) neutrophil activity (e.g. smoking) in basal lobes
     v)   distribution of alveolar walls – panacinar emphysema

2) Liver disease

  a) heterozygote
     i)   liver cell globules – non secreted aIAT
     ii) ? association with chronic liver disease homozygote
  b) i)   normal
     ii) infantile intrahepatic cholestasis – unknown pathogenesis
     iii) cirrhosis – ? deficient antiprotease activity
     iv) hepatocellular carcinoma ? related to cirrhosis

(October 1982, Paper 1, Question 5)

References

1) Garver, R.I. et al. Alpha-1-antitrypsin deficiency and emphysema caused by homozygous inheritance of non-expressing alpha-1-antitrypsin genes. New Engl. J. Med. (1986) 314: 762–766.
2) Scheuer, P.J. Causation of liver disease: recent developments. In: Recent Advances in Histopathology 10. N. Woolf, P.P. Anthony (eds.). p179–192. Churchill Livingstone, Edinburgh (1978).

Discuss the pathology and pathogenesis of iron overload states

Introduction

1) Definitions

   a) haemochromatosis
   b) haemosiderosis

2) Normal Fe metabolism

   a) absorption
   b) transport
      i)   enterocyte
      ii) plasma
      iii) hepatocyte
   c) storage
      i) ferritin
      ii) haemosiderin

3) Histochemical identification

Primary Fe overload

   a) excessive
   b) HLA A3, B14 linkage
   c) gene frequency (5%) and prevalence (0.3%)
   d) chromosome 6p

1) TBI

   a) up to 80 g (n 5 g)

2) Sites

   a) parenchymal organs
   b) skin
   c) joints

3) *Clinical features*

   a) cirrhosis
   b) diabetes
   c) skin pigmentation
   d) cardiomyopathy

4) *Pathology*

   a) liver
      i) cirrhosis
      ii) hepatocellular carcinoma
   b) pancreas
      i) exocrine
      ii) endocrine
   c) myocardium
   d) pituitary
      i) trophic atrophy, e.g. testis
   e) skin
      i) melanin pigmentation
      ii) Fe deposits
   f) joints
      i) pyrophosphate arthropathy

Pathogenesis

1) *Experimental evidence*

   a) superoxides and free radicals – peroxidation of lysosomal lipid membranes
   b) ferric ions – hepatic and pancreatic fibrogenesis

Secondary Fe overload

   a) no genetic association
   b) clinical features similar or less marked
   c) TB1 normal

Pathogenesis

1) *Excessive Fe intake*

   a) transfusion in chronic dyserythropoiesis
   b) alcoholism
   c) diet (e.g. Bantu beer)

(October 1980, Paper 2, Question 4)

Reference

1) Powell, L.W., Bassett, M.L., Halliday, J.W. Haemochromatosis: 1980 update. Gastroenterology (1980) 78: 374–381.

Write an essay on hydatid disease

(October 1978, Paper 1, Question 4)

Describe in detail the structure of a hydatid cyst and give an account of the life cycle of the parasite responsible for it

Introduction

Echinococcus granulosus and E. multilocularis
Epidemiology

Life cycle

1) Primary host

a) canines

2) Intermediate host

a) herbivores

3) Accidental host

a) man
   i) ingestion of ova
   ii) duodenal hatching
   iii) larvae invade bowel wall
   iv) cyst formation after 5–10 years

4) Sites of parasitic cysts

a) liver
b) lungs, bone, brain and others

5) Cyst structure

a) macroscopic
   i) E. granulosus
   ii) E. multilocularis
b) microscopic
   i) host inflammatory reaction
   ii) fibrous capsule
   iii) outer non-nucleated layer
   iv) inner germinative layer
   v) human +/- brood capsules
   vi) calcification and atrophy

Complications

1) Rupture and anaphylaxis
2) Pressure effects
3) Secondary bacterial infection
4) Membranous glomerulonephritis
5) Cholecystitis
6) Pathological fracture
7) Embolism
8) E. multilocularis – invasion and metastasis

(November 1974, Paper 1, Question 3)

Reference

1) Robbins, S.L., Cotran, R.S., Kumar, V. Fungal, protozoal and helminthic diseases and sarcoidosis. In: Pathologic Basis of Disease, 4th edition. p421; 422. W.B. Saunders, Philadelphia (1989).

Describe the life cycle of the parasite responsible for hydatid disease, and the histological features of the cysts. How does this disease differ from cysticercosis?

As well as outlining hydatid disease as for the previous essay, the differences in the life cycle of the pork tapeworm together with its pathological appearances, including distribution and complications of the cysts, should be outlined. This will probably comprise a quarter to a third of the total essay time, and the hydatid section should be abbreviated accordingly.

(October 1979, Paper 2, Question 2)

Describe the pathological changes that may be produced by infection with Toxoplasma gondii

(November 1971, Paper 2, Question 3)

Give an account of the pathology of toxoplasmosis. Which subjects are particularly susceptible to this infection? How is it transmitted?

Introduction

T. gondii – parasitic protozoon
Epidemiology
Prevalence (antibody studies)
Morphological features   a) tachyzoite
                          b) bradyzoites/cysts

Life cycle

Primary host :   cats
Intermediate host : rodents and birds (ingestion of faecal oocysts)
Accidental host :   human (ingestion of faecal oocysts)

Clinical features

1) *Adult*

    a) mononucleosis syndrome (cf EBV, CMV)
       i)   cervical lymphadenopathy
       ii) lymphocytosis
       iii) fever

2) *Congenital*

    a) transplacental infection
       i)   death
       ii) microcephaly
       iii) choroidoretinitis
       iv) hydrocephalus

3) *Infantile*

    a) pneumonia
    b) myocarditis

4) *Reactivation*

    a) encephalitis (immunosuppression)
    b) choroidoretinitis

Pathological features

1) *Lymphadenopathy*

    a) follicular hyperplasia with sinus histiocytosis
    b) epithelioid granulomas

2) *CNS*

    a) microglial nodules with tachyzoites
    b) necrosis, thrombosis
    c) hydrocephalus
    d) cysts

3) *Myocardium*

    a) inflammatory reaction to parasites

4) *Retina*

    a) granulomatous inflammation

(April 1982, Paper 1, Question 1)

References

1) Robbins, S.L., Cotran, R.S., Kumar, V. Fungal, protozoal and helminthic diseases and sarcoidosis. In: Pathologic Basis of Disease, 4th edition. p410; 411. W.B. Saunders, Philadelphia (1989).
2) Anon. Toxoplasmosis. Br Med J (1981) 282: 249–250.

Outline the clinico-pathological features of leprosy in terms of immune response to Mycobacterium leprae

Introduction

Epidemiology
Transmission
General clinical features

Cutaneous leprosy

1) Tuberculoid TT

Clinical features

Pathology
a) Granulomata
b) Perineural disease
c) Wade-Fite-Bacilli +/- or -
d) Lepromin test and immunohistochemistry
e) T4 cells predominate

2) Lepromatous leprosy (LL)

Clinical features

a) poor immunological response

Pathology

a) Grenz zone
b) Lepra cells, no granulomas
c) Wade-Fite-Bacilli +ve
d) Lepromin test -ve
e) Immunohistochemistry – T8 cells (few)

Systemic spread

Variants

1) Borderline BB
   Others BL, BT
2) Indeterminate (early)
   Perineural lymphocytes +ve
3) Erythema nodosum leprosum
   Immune complex disease following treatment of LL
   Leucocytoclastic vasculitis
   Glomerulonephritis
4) Histoid leprosy
   Post treatment
   Dermatofibroma-like lesion – Wade Fite +ve

(April 1985, Paper 1, Question 3)

References

1) Hutt, M.S.R., Spencer, H. Tropical diseases in Britain. In: Recent Advances in Histopathology 10. N. Woolf, P.P. Anthony (eds.). p303–324. Churchill Livingstone, Edinburgh (1978).
2) Lucas, S.B. Histopathology of leprosy and tuberculosis – an overview. Br. Med. Bull. (1988) 44: 584–599.

Discuss the immunopathological basis of the lesions found in leprosy

To answer this question the lesions which may be seen in leprosy need to be identified. This may be confusing as leprosy is classified by both clinical appearances and by the histopathological changes present in a biopsy. It is best in this answer to use a pathological classification, thus the lesions occurring in leprosy may be classified as follows – Indeterminate leprosy, Tuberculoid leprosy, Borderline leprosy, Lepromatous leprosy and Reactional leprosy.

The specific cellular composition of the infiltrates, as demonstrated by immuno-histological analysis, can be described for each, and as well as cell mediated responses, the humoral factors and hypersensitivity reactions in reactional leprosy should also be considered.   *(April 1988, Paper 1, Question 2)*

Discuss the pathology of human T cell lymphotrophic virus III (HTLV III/LAV) infection

Introduction

Nature of virus
Routes of infection
Cellular receptor (CD4)
Life cycle – T4 lymphocyte – permissive and lytic
          Monocyte/macrophage – permissive

Pathological effects

1) *Reticuloendothelial system*

   a) immunosuppression and decreased T4 lymphocytes
   b) polyclonal B cell stimulation (? envelope derived gp120 glycoprotein)
   c) autoimmune haemolytic anaemia
   d) NHL high grade extranodal
   e) lymph node
      i)   hyperplastic
      ii) diffuse hyperplasia
      iii) lymphocyte depletion

2) *CNS*

   a) toxoplasmosis
   b) cryptococcal meningitis
   c) subacute encephalitis
   d) ? multiple sclerosis
   e) PMLE (JC virus)
   f) CMV encephalitis and retinitis
   g) CNS lymphoma

3) *Respiratory system*

   a) pneumocystis pneumonia
   b) mycobacterium tuberculosis (and atypical mycobacteria)
   c) pneumococcal pneumonia
   d) alveolar proteinosis
   e) lymphoid interstitial pneumonia

4) *Alimentary tract*

   Mouth and oesophagus

   a) candidiasis
   b) herpes simplex
   c) CMV

   Intestine

   a) cryptosporidiosis
   b) isopora belli
   c) herpes simplex
   d) CMV
   e) Atypical mycobacteria

Anal

 a) herpes simplex
 b) genital warts

Neoplasms

 a) Kaposi's sarcoma
 b) NHL

5) *Skin*

 a) seborrhoeic dermatitis
 b) molluscum contagiosum
 c) Kaposi's sarcoma

(April 1986, Paper 2, Question 3)

References

1) Ho, D.D. et al. Pathogenesis of infection with human immunodeficiency virus. New Engl. J. Med. (1987) 317: 278–286.
2) Millard, P.R., Chapel, H.M. Immunodeficiency states including AIDS. In: Recent Advances in Histopathology 13. P.P. Anthony, R.N.M. MacSween (eds.) p129–158. Churchill Livingstone, Edinburgh (1987).

Discuss the pathological lesions which may develop in the gastrointestinal tract in a patient with AIDS

Introduction

Definition of AIDS
Clinical features of gut disease
Frequence and epidemiology

Infections

1) *Protozoal*

 a) cryptosporidiosis
  i)   sites – (SI +/- LJ)
  ii) microscopic
 b) entamoeba histolytica
  i)   site (LI +/- liver)
  ii) microscopic
 c) strongyloidiasis
  i)   sites (SI)
  ii) microscopic

2) *Fungal*

    a) candida
       i)   sites (mouth, oesophagus)
       ii) macroscopic
       iii) microscopic
    b) aspergillus
       i)   disseminated disease

3) *Bacterial*

    a) mycobacterium avium
       i)   site (SI, stomach)
       ii) intracellular – microscopic
    b) spirochaetosis
       i)   site (LI)
    c) others

4) *Viral*

    a) CMV
       i)   site (whole GIT)
       ii) microscopic
    b) HSVI
       i)   sites (mouth, oesophagus, rectum)
    c) HPV
       i)   sites (mouth, anus)
    d) HBV
       i)   sites (liver)

Tumours

1) *Kaposi's sarcoma*

    a) sites
    b) macroscopic
    c) microscopic
    d) behaviour

2) *Lymphoma*

    a) NHL primary and secondary involvement

(April 1988, Paper 2, Question 5)

References

1) Millard, P.R., Chapel, H.M. Immunodeficiency states including AIDS. In: Recent Advances in Histopathology 13. P.P. Anthony, R.N.M. MacSween (eds.) p129–158. Churchill Livingstone, Edinburgh (1987).
2) Rotterdam, H., Sommers, S.C. Alimentary tract biopsy lesions in the acquired immune deficiency syndrome. Pathology (1985) 17: 181–192.

Describe the macroscopic and microscopic appearances of the lesions of primary gout and discuss their pathogenesis

Notice the wording in this question, whereby only primary gout should be considered in terms of pathogenesis. An outline knowledge of purine metabolism would clearly be essential to answer this question adequately, but there are a large number of pathological changes which can occur in this condition, which should provide more than enough for an essay length answer given due consideration.

(April 1978, Paper 1, Question 3)

Reference

1) Robbins, S.L., Cotran, R.S., Kumar, V. Gout and gouty arthritis. In: Pathologic Basis of Disease, 4th edition. p1355–1360. W.B. Saunders, Philadelphia (1989).

Write an essay on arteritis

(April 1983, Paper 1, Question 5)

Write an essay on arteritis

Perhaps a question set to catch out those who believe they are never repeated! It is, fortunately, a relatively straightforward answer that is required, but it is important to try to show some flair by subdividing the primary arteritides into granulomatous and non-granulomatous and large, medium or small vessels, and then highlight the major diagnostic and pathogenetic differences between each condition, rather than list each condition and describe them in a 'repetitive' fashion. Vasculitic processes secondary to infection or other cause should also be included.

(October 1984, Paper 1, Question 5)

References

1) Mitchinson, M.J. The vasculitis syndromes. In: Recent Advances in Histopathology 12. P.P. Anthony, R.N.M. MacSween (eds.) p223–240. Churchill Livingstone, Edinburgh (1984).
2) McCluskey, R.T. et al. Vasculitis in primary vasculitides, granulomatoses and connective tissue diseases. Human Pathol. (1983) 14: 305–315.

Tabulate the causes of abnormal pigmentation. Outline the procedure you would adopt to identify an abnormal pigment seen in a histological section of liver (details of method are not required but the principles of the techniques should be indicated)

This question should appeal to any diagnostic histopathologist, and although the table requires some thought, given that all pigments throughout the body should be considered, the remainder of the question is really a 'bench mark' for the examination – if candidates cannot answer this adequately without revision, they would probably not have the standard of experience required.

(November 1976, Paper 1, Question 1)

Reference

1) Bancroft, J.D., Cook, H.C. Manual of Histological Techniques. Churchill Livingstone, Edinburgh (1984).

Discuss the role of the HLA system in the pathogenesis of disease

This is a complex issue and one which is quite difficult to answer given the wide range of diseases with which the HLA associations are thought to play a part. It is probably best to discuss the theoretical functions of the HLA molecules, and discuss how these may be deranged or contributory in general terms, rather than taking specific diseases and attempting to explain the individual possible mechanisms.

(April 1984, Paper 1, Question 2)

Reference

1) Dick, H.M., Powis, S.H. HLA and disease: possible mechanisms. In: Recent Advances in Histopathology 13. P.P. Anthony, R.N.M. MacSween (eds.) Churchill Livingstone, Edinburgh (1987).

Give an account of genetically determined immunodeficiencies

This is a particularly difficult question to answer for those who do not have a particular interest in this field, as the area is complex. It would be better to group the diseases according to the specific immune defect rather than the mode of inheritance. A preliminary diagram illustrating the particular level of the defect would be of value to avoid unnecessary repetition. The pathological changes of the primary condition should be defined in each case, along with the sequelae of the immunodeficiency.

(November 1977, Paper 2, Question 1)

References

1) Paradinas, F. Primary and secondary immune disorders. In: Lymph Node Biopsy Interpretation, A.G. Stansfeld (ed.). p159–163. Churchill Livingstone, Edinburgh (1985).
2) Berry, C.L. Spleen, lymph nodes and immunoreactive tissues. In: Paediatric Pathology, p565–606. Springer-Verlag, Berlin (1989).

Discuss the visible abnormalities of human karyotype and their relation to disease

The introduction to this essay should include methods of karyotyping and an explanation of the terms used in cytogenetic disorders such as trisomy, mono-somy, mosaicism, translocation, inversion, deletion, etc. This question excludes genetic disorders e.g. sickle cell disease or multifactorial inherited disorders such as congenital heart disease. One or more examples from each group should be included with discussion of their major associated conditions (e.g. trisomies with associated congenital heart disease, leukaemia and Alzheimer's disease), together with descriptions of the sex chromosome disorders and their possible consequences (e.g. malignancy developing in cryptorchid testes) to ensure a comprehensive assessment.   *(April 1981, Paper 1, Question 2)*

Reference

1) Robbins, S.L., Cotran, R.S., Kumar, V. Genetic disorders. In: Pathologic Basis of Disease, 4th edition. p121–136. W.B. Saunders, Philadelphia (1989).

Discuss the causation of congenital malformation
(April 1970, Paper 1, Question 3)

Discuss the aetiology of congenital malformation

This question requires a systematic approach to the answer, dividing the known aetiological factors into groups such as chromosomal, infections, toxins and drugs and their effects at various stages in embryogenesis and foetal development. Speculation on the so-called multifactorial causes would be appropriate.
(April 1971, Paper 1, Question 4)

References

1) Robbins, S.L., Cotran, R.S., Kumar, V. Diseases of infancy and childhood – congenital malformations. In: Pathologic Basis of Disease, 4th edition. p519–523. W.B. Saunders, Philadelphia (1989).
2) Berry, C.L. Congenital Malformations. In: Paediatric Pathology, p41–61. Springer-Verlag, Berlin (1989).

Discuss the pathology of chronic alcoholism

Introduction

Definition
Incidence
Acute alcoholism   – clinical features
Chronic alcoholism – clinical features
                   – associated deficiencies

1) *Liver*

   a) Steatosis
      i)   pathogenesis
      ii) morphology
   b) Alcoholic hepatitis
      i)   morphology
   c) Alcoholic cirrhosis
      i)   morphology

2) *Pancreas*

   a) Chronic pancreatitis
      i)   incidence
      ii) morphology

3) *Gastrointestinal tract*

   a) Mouth
      i)   carcinoma
   b) Oesophagus
      i)   Mallory-Weiss syndrome
      ii) carcinoma
   c) Stomach
      i)   gastritis
      ii) peptic ulceration

4) *Heart*

   a) Cardiomyopathy
      i)   macroscopic
      ii)   microscopic
      iii) ultrastructure

5) *Nervous system*

   a) Neuritis and SACD
      i)   pathogenesis
      ii) microscopic
   b) Cerebellar atrophy
   c) Wernicke's encephalopathy
      i)   microscopic features
   d) Trauma
      i)   e.g. subdural haematoma
   e) Korsakoff's psychosis
      i)   chronic lesions
      ii) neuronal degeneration (chromatolysis and lipofuscin accumulation)

(April 1978, Paper 1, Question 2)

Reference

1) Robbins, S.L., Cotran, R.S., Kumar, V. Environmental pathology – ethyl alcohol. In: Pathologic Basis of Disease, 4th edition. p490–492. W.B. Saunders, Philadelphia (1989).

Discuss the pathological effects of prolonged alcohol in organs other than the liver

This question only allows a brief résumé of all the possible effects, since these are so widespread, but the more significant in clinical terms should be emphasised. In the alimentary system, acute and chronic pancreatitis, gastric and oesophageal inflammation and Mallory–Weiss syndrome are important, but although liver pathology is specifically excluded, the effects of portal hypertension such as varices, ascites and splenomegaly should be included. Central nervous system effects are important and varied, including indirectly associated conditions such as subdural haematomas. Other organs affected include the heart (cardiomyopathy), endocrine system, haemopoietic system, respiratory system (tuberculosis and aspiratic pneumonia) among others. Thus this essay requires considerable organisation with the use of a plan, and some element of selection.

(April 1988, Paper 2, Question 3)

Reference

1) Edmondson, H.A. Pathology of alcoholism. Am. J. Clin. Pathol. (1980) 74: 725–742.

Describe the lesions of sarcoidosis and discuss the aetiology of this condition

The lesion of sarcoidosis should be described firstly in general terms of the granulomas, with their characteristic features (e.g. asteroid and Schaumann bodies, fibrosis) and their evolution, and then consider the effects on various organs in order of clinical importance and frequency (e.g. lungs, lymph node, eyes etc.). It is always difficult to answer questions such as this where the aetiology is unknown, but there is opportunity to discuss the immunological abnormalities and proposed aetiologies with the arguments against them.

(November 1970, Paper 1, Question 4)

References

1) Robbins, S.L., Cotran, R.S. & Kumar, V. Fungal, protozoal and helminthic diseases and sarcoidosis. In: Pathologic Basis of Disease, 4th edition. p427–429. W.B. Saunders, Philadelphia (1989).
2) Anon The immune response in sarcoidosis. Lancet (1987) ii: 195–196.

Describe the reaction of tissues to minerals containing silica

This question requires some knowledge of mineralogy as well as pathology, and as well as acute, subacute and chronic silicosis, there are materials such as glass and, more importantly, asbestos to consider. The pathological reactions associated with the latter would constitute an essay on their own.

(November 1971, Paper 2, Question 4)

References

1) Gibbs, A.R. Industrial lung disease. In: Recent Advances in Histopathology 13. P.P. Anthony, R.N.M. MacSween (eds.) p109–129. Churchill Livingstone, Edinburgh (1987).
2) Dunnill, M.S. Industrial lung disease. In: Pulmonary Pathology. p399–438. Churchill Livingstone, Edinburgh (1982).

Give an account of the pathological changes which may be found in systemic sclerosis (generalised scleroderma)

This would constitute a straightforward essay which is easily divided up into the general aspects of the disease, and how it affects different organ systems. Ensure that in an answer such as this you would start with the most frequent organs involved (e.g. skin, gut) and those which have the most serious clinical consequences (kidney), before considering those with relatively minor or infrequent involvement. Consideration of the pathogenesis and aetiology of the disease is not needed in questions worded like this, but some insight into these aspects would almost certainly be required in future questions on this subject.

(April 1972, Paper 1, Question 5)

References

1) Jayson, M.I.V. Systemic sclerosis: a collagen or microvascular disease? Br. Med. J. (1984) 288: 1855–1857.
2) Robbins, S.L., Cotran, R.S. & Kumar, V. Diseases of immunity. In: Pathologic Basis of Disease, 4th edition. p204–209. W.B. Saunders, Philadelphia (1989).

Describe and discuss the histological changes produced by pathogenic fungi

Introduction

Fungal types
Pathogenicity (immunodeficiency)
Range of tumour responses

Deep mycoses

1) *Candidiasis*

    a) fungal morphology and staining

    b) tissue response
        i)   mucocutaneous   – acute & chronic inflammation
                                          – abscesses
                                          – granuloma
        ii) systemic   – microabscesses
                                          – endocarditis

2) *Mucormycosis*

    a) fungal morphology and staining

    b) tissue response
        i)   rhinocerebral   – osteomyelitis
                                          – vascular invasion
        ii) pulmonary
        iii) gastrointestinal

3) *Aspergillosis*

    a) fungal morphology and staining

    b) tissue response
        i)   allergic   – asthma
                                          – alveolitis
                                          – bronchopulmonary
                                          – aspergillus
        ii) colonising   – aspergilloma
        iii) invasive

4) *Cryptococcosis*

    a) fungal morphology and staining

    b) tissue response
        i)   meningeal   – granulomatous
                                          – immunosuppression
        ii) pulmonary   – early
                                          – late

5) *Coccidioidomycosis*

    a) fungal morphology and staining

    b) tissue response
        i)   primary pulmonary – suppurative
                                          – granulomatous
        ii) progressive   – suppurative/granulomatous

6) *Histoplasmosis*

    a) fungal morphology and staining

    b) tissue response
        i)   latent
        ii) primary
        iii) disseminated

7) *Chromomycosis*

    a) fungal morphology and staining
    b) tissue response
       i) dermal inflammation
       ii) epidermal hyperplasia

Superficial mycoses

1) *Candida*

    a) tissue responses
       i) suppurative (thrush)
       ii) chronic

2) *Tinea*

    a) tissue responses
       i) chronic inflammatory response

(This question could equally well be answered by taking the various tissue responses e.g. suppurative, granulomatous, etc. and enumerating the causative organisms.)   *(October 1985, Paper 1, Question 4)*

References

1) Robbins, S.L., Cotran, R.S., & Kumar, V. Fungal, protozoal and helminthic diseases and sarcoidosis. In: Pathologic Basis of Disease. 4th edition. p385–396. W.B. Saunders, Philadelphia (1989).
2) Anthony, P.P. A guide to the histological identification of fungi in tissues. J. Clin. Pathol. (1973) 26: 828–831.

Describe the pathology of neurofibromatosis

In such a question, the best approach would be to split up the various aspects into side headings with brief descriptions, very closely following the essay plan style. There should really be a concentration on the most frequent findings such as the neurofibromas, café au lait spots and Lisch nodules, followed by a description of the abnormalities in the skeleton and other organs, and finally the most clinically significant complications such as malignant transformation of neurofibromas and other neoplasms.   *(April 1976, Paper 2, Question 1)*

References

1) Robbins, S.L., Cotran, R.S. & Kumar, V. Genetic disorders. In: Pathologic Basis of Disease, 4th edition. p139; 140. W.B. Saunders, Philadelphia (1989).

2. Neoplasia

Outline the criteria necessary to establish a viral aetiology for tumours and discuss these in respect of human carcinogenesis

Introduction

Evidence for viral aetiology

    a) animal studies – contagious examples rare
    b) human   – HPV only proven example

Criteria for establishing viral aetiology

Koch's postulates a) always associated with disease
                  b) isolated and grown in pure culture
                  c) late pure culture produces diseases in susceptible animal
                  d) organism isolated from latter

Problems in application to human tumour viruses

Human tumour viruses

1) HPV

    a) skin tumours
        i)   experimental studies
        ii) isolation of virus
        iii) localisation of viral DNA
        iv) in situ hybridisation
    b) cervical carcinoma
        i)   epidemiology
        ii) cytological features
        iii) immunochemical and DNA analytical studies

2) Herpes viruses

    a) EB virus
        i)   Burkitt's lymphoma
                  – epidemiology
                  – cell culture isolation of viruses
                  – hybridisation studies
                  – in vitro lymphoid cell transformation
        ii) nasopharyngeal carcinoma
                  – epidemiology
                  – isolation of virus
                  – hybridisation studies
        iii) immunosuppression and lymphoma
                  – evidence
    b) Herpes simplex type 2
        i)   cervical carcinoma
                  – epidemiology
                  – hybridisation studies
                  – virus isolation studies

3) *Hepatitis B virus (HBV)*

    i)   hepatocellular carcinoma
- epidemiology
- serological studies
- temporal relationship of HBV infection and cirrhosis to development of tumour
- animal model (Woodchurch hepatitis virus)
- DNA integration

4) *HIV I and III*

    a) HIVI
       i)   Caribbean lymphoma
    b) HIVIII
       i)   Kaposi's sarcoma in AIDS – Ab to HIV
       ii) African KS – 17% Ab to HIV
       iii) do not fulfill Koch's postulates

(October 1981, Paper 1, Question 5)

References

1   Taussig, M.J. Viruses and neoplasia. In: Processes in Pathology and Microbiology, 2nd edition. p776–802. Blackwell Scientific Publications, Oxford (1984).
2   Brescia, R.J. et al. The role of human papilloma viruses in the pathogenesis and histologic classification of precancerous lesions of the cervix. Human Pathol. (1986) 17: 552–558.

Discuss the contribution of epidemiological studies to our understanding of the causes of malignant tumours

Much of the early insight on cancer causation came from epidemiological studies and further advances have come from investigation of ideas generated therefrom. To encompass all epidemiological factors is a difficult task, but could be approached by illustrating the current theories of cancer development, as in the previous two examples, but emphasising the components of the theory which have a base in epidemiological study. Bronchogenic carcinoma is the classic example, reflecting the work of Professor Sir Richard Doll, but alimentary cancers and the influence of diet could provide abundant material for consideration in addition. *(November 1969, Paper 1, Question 4)*

Comment on the World Health Organisation's statement that about 80% of human cancer is environmentally induced

This type of question is difficult to answer in an examination because it requires considerable organisation. In reality such a question can only be attempted satisfactorily if the candidate has made an effort to be conversant with current theories of cancer pathogenesis, and their supportive data. One possible approach would be to briefly outline the multistep theory of neoplasia with emphasis on the ultimate alteration of the DNA code or alteration of gene expression which produces an established permanent malignant phenotype. The role in these processes of chemical carcinogens, radiation and viruses, all of which are environmental agents, should be highlighted. To complete the answer one or two individual tumours could be selected to illustrate the points made. Squamous cell carcinoma of the uterine cervix or bronchus are good well-studied examples of malignant neoplasms with unquestionable environmental associations.

(October 1979, Paper 1, Question 2)

References

1   Paul, J. Oncogenesis. In: Recent Advances in Histopathology 13. P.P. Anthony, R.N.M. MacSween (eds.), p13–31. Churchill Livingstone, Edinburgh (1987).
2   Medline, A., Farber, E. The multistep theory of neoplasia. In: Recent Advances in Histopathology 11. P.P. Anthony, R.N.M. MacSween (eds.) Chapter 6, p19–34. Churchill Livingstone, Edinburgh (1981).
3   Robbins, S.L., Cotran, R.S., Kumar, V. Neoplasia. In: Pathologic Basis of Disease, 4th edition. p262–282. W.B. Saunders, Philadelphia (1989).

Discuss the part played by non-biological environmental factors in the aetiology of human cancer

This question is similar to October 1979, Paper 1, Question 2 and can be approached in a similar way. The discussion needs to commence with description of current cancer formation theory highlighting the role of non-biological agents. Chemical carcinogenesis and radiation of various sorts will form the main discussion points. Illustration of the above can be provided by discussing bronchogenic carcinoma or skin cancers, and the neoplastic lesions associated with asbestos as alternative examples.   *(April 1977, Paper 1, Question 2)*

Reference

1   Gibbs, A.R. Industrial lung disease. In: Recent Advances in Histopathology 13. P.P. Anthony, R.N.M. MacSween (eds.) p109–117. Churchill Livingstone, Edinburgh (1987).

State one general theory of carcinogenesis. Discuss the main lines of evidence for and against the theory you choose

The problem here lies with choosing a particular theory, but at the current time most people would concentrate on the oncogene theory, which is now better understood. Moreover there is now sufficient data available to call into question its universal application as the cause of cancer. The essay could be commenced by defining the term carcinogenesis (malignant transformation), with brief outlines of other theories such as chemical carcinogenesis, radiation, etc. The conclusion should reiterate the current idea that abnormal gene expression and its consequences are considered the main pathway to malignant change.

(April 1972, Paper 2, Question 3)

References

1   Robbins, S.L., Cotran, R.S., Kumar, V. Neoplasia. In: Pathologic Basis of Disease, 4th edition. Chapter 6, p260–296. W.B. Saunders, Philadelphia (1989).
2   Taussig, M.J. Neoplasia. In: Processes in Pathology and Microbiology, 2nd edition. p689–810. Blackwell Scientific Publications, Oxford (1984).

Discuss the oncogene hypothesis

Introduction

Definition
Viral oncogene
Cellular oncogene
Proto-oncogene
Anti-oncogenes

Relationship of v-onc to c-onc with examples (e.g. RSV)

1) *Transformation*

    a) recognition and induction
    b) oncogenic retroviruses, 'rapid' vs. 'slow'
    c) helper viruses

2) *Identification of proto-oncogenes*

    a) v–onc probes
    b) transfection experiments

3) *Oncogene activation*

    a) transduction e.g.
       i) FeLV
    b) chromosomal rearrangement e.g.
       i) Burkitt's lymphoma
       ii) ph.Chr 9–22 (ber-abl)
    c) point mutation e.g.
       i) Ha-ras
       ii) c-myc translocated from 8–2, 8–14
       iii) 8–22
    d) gene amplification e.g.
       i) c-myc, N-myc

4) *Viral oncogenes*

    a) DNA viruses e.g. SV40 T antigen

5) *Oncogene products*

    a) regulatory functions
       i)   growth factors e.g. sis gene (PGDF)
       ii) receptors e.g. erb-B (EGF)
       iii) G protein (intracellular messenger) e.g. h-ras
       iv) Nuclear acting proteins e.g. c-myc

6) *Anti-oncogenes*

    a) chromosome 13 deletion in constitutional retinoblastoma

7) *Role of oncogene activation*

    a) ? stage in multistep process
    b) initiation and promotion
    c) role of immune suppression

(April 1981, Paper 1, Question 1)

References

1   James, N., Sikora, K. Oncogenes and cancer. Hospital Update (1988) 14: 1261–1270.
2   Paul, J. Oncogenesis. In: Recent Advances in Histopathology 13. P.P. Anthony, R.N.M. MacSween (eds.) p13–31. Churchill Livingstone, Edinburgh (1987).
3   Goudie, R.B. Editorial: What are anti-oncogenes? J. Pathol. (1988) 154: 297–298.

Discuss the role of oncogenes in carcinogenesis
(October 1986, Paper 1, Question 1)

Discuss the role of growth factors in neoplasia

Introduction

Definition (miscellaneous group of molecules acting in a paracrine fashion)
Relationship to oncogene products
General characteristics (low mw <80 kD; local action; specific cell surface receptors; affect cell differentiation ± growth)

Types of growth factors (GFs)

1) *Epidermal GF*

2) *Colony stimulating factors (CSF)*

3) *Platelet derived GF*

4) *Fibroblast GF*

5) *Interleukins*

6) *Transforming GF*

Functions of GFs

'Signal' molecules influencing differentiation and growth
GF binding to membrane receptor activates intracellular pathway
Normal function control ? receptor saturation ± feedback
Excessive production or deficiency influences cellular behaviour

GF in malignancy

1) *Mechanisms*

    a) 'autocrine' hyperstimulation (e.g. bombesin in small cell lung ca)

    b) receptor alterations e.g.
        i)   EGF ↑ in squamous Ca skin + gliomas ? gene amplification
        ii) ↑ IL2 receptor in T cell leukaemia ? transcriptional deregulation
        iii) mutation causing activation e.g. c-erb B1 oncogene product
             resembling truncated EGF receptor in breast and gastric ca

    c) intracellular pathways – oncogene relations e.g.
        i)   ras group – signal transducers (activated by mutation)
        ii) fos, myc groups – nuclear transcriptional regulators

    d) inhibitory function
        i)   loss of gene function
        ii) loss of responsiveness to GF e.g. TGFβ

(normally inhibits cell growth) receptor deficient in retinoblastoma cell lines

    e) induction of other GFs e.g. TNF, ILs

    f) unknown e.g. CSFs

(October 1986, Paper 1, Question 1)

References

1   Green, A.R. Peptide regulatory factors: multifunctional mediators of cellular growth and differentiation. Lancet (1989) i: 705–707.

2   Waterfield, M.D. Altered growth regulation in cancer. Br. Med. Bull. (1989) 45: 570–581.

3   Anon. Growth factors in malignancy. Lancet (1986) ii: 317–318.

What factors determine the metastatic potential of tumours?

Introduction

Definition of metastasis
Relationships of morphology to biological behaviour
Historical aspects of 'benign' vs. 'malignant'
Classifications in tumour pathology

Mechanisms of metastasis

1) *Cellular detachment from primary*

2) *Penetration of basement membrane* (? Type IV collagenase)

3) *Stromal invasion* (proteolytic enzymes)

4) *Vascular penetration* (enzymic/mechanical)

5) *Transport to metastatic site*
   a) aggregation
   b) coagulation

6) *Endothelial attachment, vascular penetration* (?Plasminogen activator)

7) *Growth and desmoplasia*

'Metastatic inefficiency'

Heterogeneous metastatic capability in primary tumours

(Experimental observations)

Factors influencing metastatic capacity

1) *Host immune response*
   a) specific-MHC expression and tumour Ags
   b) non-specific – NK cells, granulocytes

2) *Oncogene expression*   e.g. fos gene increases MHC expression
                            ras transfection experimentally increases
                            metastatic ability

3) *?Site specific cellular receptors*
   a) autopsy studies (Paget (1889) seed/soil hypothesis!)
   b) animal models

4) *Cell structural alterations*
   a) membrane
      e.g. carbohydrates, enzymes, antigens putative associations (e.g. helix
      pomatia lectin binding in breast ca)
   b) cytoskeleton – ? 'deformability' ↑ invasive/metastatic ability

Histological parameters enabling assessment of metastatic potential

1) *Size (e.g. renal adenocarcinoma, various sarcomas)*

2) *Differentiation*

    a) grading systems (e.g. breast, skin, prostate ca)

    b) other cytological features (e.g. pleomorphism, cellular maturations, ? 'nucleolar organiser regions'

3) *Mitotic index* (e.g. uterine smooth muscle tumours)

4) *Extent of tumour* (e.g. malignant melanoma, colorectal ca)

5) *Vascular invasion* (e.g. follicular thyroid tumours, breast ca)

6) *?Host immune response* (e.g. colorectal ca, nasopharyngeal ca)

(October 1988, Paper 1, Question 5)

References

1   Feldman, M., Eisenbach, L. What makes a tumor cell metastatic? Sci. Am. (1988) 259: 40–47.
2   Hill, R.P. Metastasis. In: The Basic Science of Oncology, Chapter 10, p160–175. Pergamon Press, Oxford (1987).
3   Robbins, S.L., Cotran, R.S., Kumar, V. Neoplasia. In: Pathologic Basis of Disease, 4th edition. Chapter 6, p255–260. W.B. Saunders Co, Philadelphia (1989).

Discuss the value of electron microscopy in the differential diagnosis of tumours

The introduction to this answer should include some appraisal of the use of EM in conjunction with conventional microscopy and immunocytochemistry, and advantages it may offer. Many of the applications hinge on the identification of subcellular particles which cannot be identified by other means (e.g. neurosecretory granule presence and morphology, Z-band material, melanosomes, etc.) and in the delineation of certain tumours which have similar appearances on conventional microscopy (e.g. synovial sarcoma vs. leiomyosarcoma, or small cell tumour of childhood). Some of the discussion could centre on the cost effectiveness of EM diagnosis, and the organisation of such a service for diagnostic purposes. It would also be reasonable to discuss certain research applications.   *(April 1982, Paper 2, Question 3)*

Reference

1   McLay, A.L.C., Toner, P.G. Diagnostic electron microscopy. In: Recent Advances in Histopathology 11. P.P. Anthony, R.N.M. MacSween (eds.) p241–261. Churchill Livingstone, Edinburgh (1981).

What do you understand by the term 'fibromatosis'? Give a brief account of the entities you would include under this heading

The introduction to this answer should clearly define the fibromatoses, as fibrous tissue proliferations intermediate in behaviour between benign fibrous tumours and fibrosarcoma. Entities such as fasciitis or localised nodular fibrous proliferation are clearly excluded. The classification includes the superficial (e.g. palmar fibromatosis) and deep (e.g. extra-abdominal desmoid tumour) types, but in addition the fibromatoses characteristic of infancy and childhood should be described (including infantile digital fibromatosis, infantile myelofibromatosis, fibromatosis colli and juvenile hyaline fibromatosis). In view of the common appearances in the superficial and deep forms, one example of each should be described microscopically, and then the characteristic location and clinical behaviour outlined for the remainder in each group. The infantile and childhood forms have fairly characteristic appearances which might merit individual description. Fibromatoses are a common source of difficulty in pathological diagnosis, and it is perhaps surprising that this subject has not been chosen more often in the examination.   *(October 1978, Paper 1, Question 2)*

Reference

1   Enzinger, F.W., Weiss, S.W. Fibromatous and fibrous proliferation of infancy and childhood. In: Soft Tissue Tumors, 2nd edition. p136–200. C.V. Mosby Co, St Louis (1988).

Discuss the differential diagnosis in a child with a small cell tumour involving the maxilla

This question relates to the likelihood of finding a small cell tumour of childhood in this particular site. Lymphoma might be the most likely diagnosis, especially over the age of ten years, and the site provides an opportunity to describe Burkitt's lymphoma and its associations. Embryonal rhabdomyosarcoma may well occur at this site, whereas Ewing's sarcoma and metastatic neuroblastoma are less likely. The differential diagnostic considerations should include ultrastructural features and, as a more recent advance, immunohistochemistry.
                                                   (April 1974, Paper 1, Question 4)

Reference

1   Variend, S. Small cell tumours in childhood: a review. J. Pathol (1985) 145: 1–25.

Using illustrative examples, discuss the current clinicopathological importance of the terms 'histogenesis' and 'differentiation' as applied to tumour pathology

The terms should be defined in the introductory paragraphs, histogenesis being the presumed cell or tissue of origin of a tumour, and differentiation being the extent to which the tumour resembles a mature cell or tissue. A current rather emotive argument concerns whether the expression of what were previously considered as tissue-specific antigens reflects cell lineage or mere expression of a particular locus by the neoplastic process, e.g. cytokeratin expression in smooth muscle tumours. This is a question which requires quite a sophisticated approach in consideration of these concepts. Examples are fairly easy to think of (e.g. carcinoid tumours and oat cell carcinoma, ductal and lobular carcinoma of the breast, leiomyosarcoma and rhabdomyosarcoma, etc.). The first two references given are excellent overviews of this subject.   *(April 1987, Paper 1, Question 1)*

References

1   Gould, V.E. Histogenesis and differentiation: a re-evaluation of these concepts as criteria for the classification of tumours. Human Pathol. (1986) 17: 212–215.
2   Mendelsohn, G. et al. Divergent differentiation in neoplasms: pathologic, biologic and clinical considerations. Path. Ann. (1986) Part 1: 91–119.
3   Gatter, K.C. et al. Human lung tumours: a correlation of antigenic profile with histological type. Histopathology (1985) 9: 805–823.

Discuss the problems, in principle and in practice, associated with separating benign from malignant lesions. Use examples of endocrine tumours to illustrate the points which you make.

This should be a relatively straightforward essay question to answer, without specific revision, for most histopathologists and may be regarded as another example of a 'bench-mark' question, since if the examinee cannot provide a comprehensive answer on the basis of personal experience, then they are probably not up to the required standard.   *(April 1986, Paper 1, Question 1)*

Discuss critically the concepts of hyperplasia and neoplasia in relation to endocrine cells

This is a difficult essay to write in terms of achieving a good balance, and avoiding a long-winded and not very relevant discourse. It is probably better to introduce with the standard definitions of hyperplasia and neoplasia, and then discuss various examples in the endocrine system such as thyroid, parathyroid and adrenal glands, with an example from the diffuse (neuro) endocrine system. The functional, behavioural and therapeutic implications of the distinction between hyperplasia and neoplasia should be thoroughly considered in each case.
                                         (April 1983, Paper 1, Question 2)

Discuss the concepts of conditioned (hormone-dependent) and autonomous neoplasia

In answering this question, the introduction should clearly outline the differences between hyperplasia and neoplasia, and discussion centred on the tumours, benign and malignant, which show a response to hormones either experimentally, during normal physiology or as a result of therapeutic administration, including uterine leiomyoma, breast fibroadenoma and carcinoma, prostatic carcinoma, endometrial and ovarian carcinomas.   *(November 1974, Paper 2, Question 3)*

Discuss aberrant ('ectopic') hormone production by tumours

It is clearly important to define what the term 'ectopic' means in this context, and indeed clearly state what is understood by the term hormone, otherwise there is a danger of drifting off the topic (e.g. 5H-T synthesis, by carcinoid tumours, which is not a hormone). The best idea is to list all the hormones which are associated with inappropriate synthesis, and the tumours which may produce them. A useful table is found in the reference on page 295. In addition, a brief discussion of the pathological consequences of these disorders (e.g. ectopic ACTH production) and the histochemical and immunochemical methods used in their detection would be useful.   *(November 1972, Paper 1, Question 2)*

Reference

1   Robbins, S.L., Cotran, R.S., Kumar, V. Neoplasia and Clinical Aspects of Neoplasia. In: Pathologic Basis of Disease, 4th edition. Chapters 6 and 7, p243–245; 294–296. W.B. Saunders, Philadelphia (1989).

What evidence is there in man that immunological factors are involved in malignant disease?

This is undoubtedly a very difficult question to answer in the light of current knowledge, as the issues involved are highly complex. The wording of the question is rather vague (it depends on opinion as to what constitutes an 'immunological factor' or 'involvement' for instance), and it is unlikely that such a question would emerge again.   *(November 1970, Paper 1, Question 1)*

Discuss the role of the immune process in the development and spread of neoplasms

This question has rather more information than November 1970, Paper 1, Question 1, indicating two separate areas, carcinogenesis and progression of neoplasia. With respect to the former, while there is little evidence of a direct role in carcino-genesis, defects in immunity may allow neoplasms to proliferate, e.g. immunosuppressive states such as AIDS, renal transplantation, etc. The spread of tumours may be affected by the host response to the tumour, as demonstrated in breast and rectal carcinomas or melanomas for instance. The role of tumour antigens and markers should be discussed.   *(April 1975, Paper 1, Question 3)*

Discuss the MEN syndromes

The introduction should include an explanation of the term and the general features present, including an explanation of the differences and difficulties of distinguishing between hyperplasia and neoplasia. The features of the three major MEN syndromes, MENI and MENIIa and IIb should be discussed, with the pathological features of their components, and some speculation as to the associations, and ways of investigating these syndromes (e.g. gene mapping).

(April 1988, Paper 1, Question 1)

Reference

1   Robbins, S.C., Cotran, R.S., Kumar. V. Multiple endocrine neoplasia syndromes. In: Pathologic Basis of Disease, 4th edition. p1007; 1008. W.B. Saunders, Philadelphia (1989).

Discuss teratomas

This question could still arise, but possibly in a slightly different format, since there has been a marked increase in the volume of research on this subject in recent years. As it stands, it would probably be best to approach this in a general fashion, defining the term and giving data on gonadal and extragonadal teratomas, with some paragraphs giving the major clinical and pathological features, and perhaps a comparison of ovarian and testicular teratomas. However, the rest of the essay should be devoted to a discussion of the theories of the origin of teratomas, and their relationship to carcinogenesis and embryogenesis.

(April 1970, Paper 1, Question 5)

Reference

1   Fox, H. Biology of teratomas. In: Recent Advances in Histopathology 13. P.P. Anthony, R.N.M. MacSween (eds.). Chapter 3, p 33–43. Churchill Livingstone, Edinburgh (1987).

What are the principal similarities and differences between teratomas and blastomas? Illustrate your answer by examples from each group

The introduction to this answer should include descriptive definitions of the terms teratoma and blastoma, which may be found in reference 1. The major differences could be summarised in tabulated form, occupying half to a full A4 page, and then discussions centred upon the features of the tumours found in the most common sites e.g. gonads (teratoma), adrenal gland, kidney, lung, liver (blastomas). The histogenetic theories for each of these entities could be introduced but should not occupy a major segment of the answer, as the second half of the question implies considerable emphasis should be given to the morphological features.

(November 1975, Paper 1, Question 5)

References

1   Fox, H. Biology of teratomas. In: Recent Advances in Histopathology 13. P.P.
    Anthony, R.N.M. MacSween (eds.). Chapter 3, p33–43. Churchill Livingstone,
    Edinburgh (1987).
2   Berry, P.J. Paediatric solid tumours. In: Recent Advances in Histopathology
    13. P.P. Anthony, R.N.M. MacSween (eds.). Chapter 12, p203–232. Churchill
    Livingstone, Edinburgh (1987)

Discuss the differential diagnosis of an anterior mediastinal mass in a man aged 17

The differential diagnosis should be strictly related to the age in terms of
likelihood, and weighted according to frequency and clinical importance. Since
this is not a common clinical problem, these decisions require some careful
thought. However, a candidate familiar with the cited reference should be able to
formulate a comprehensive answer. It also lends itself to a rather easier type of
essay plan construction, with a separate subheading for each entity, and this is
one of the better questions on which to practise this technique.

(October 1981, Paper 2, Question 1)

Reference

1   Rosai, J. Mediastinum. In: Ackerman's Surgical Pathology, 7th edition.
    p345–390. C.V. Mosby Co, St Louis (1989).

Discuss the problems in the diagnosis of neoplasms of soft tissue

This question should be approached from several aspects. Firstly the problem area
should be defined, excluding the lesions with easily recognisable differentiated
features e.g. rhabdomyomas, well-differentiated fatty tumours, etc. Then the
general aspects of dividing benign from malignant neoplasms in soft tissue are
addressed. It would then perhaps be an idea to divide the problems of the
distinctive childhood tumours and their diagnosis, and then consider the
commoner problems in the adult. A discussion of the more common diagnostic
problems in adults should include an appraisal of subtle diagnostic features on
conventional staining, together with use and limitations of immunohistochemistry
and electron microscopy. Examples of tumours should be given but the overall
discussion kept in a general basis.   *(April 1983, Paper 2, Question 2)*

How do you classify malignant tumours of soft tissue? Discuss the role of specific techniques in classifying an anaplastic spindle cell tumour

Malignant tumours of soft tissue are best classified according to features in the
tumour which resemble differentiation characteristics in adult tissues or their
embryonic precursors. This enables a reproducible classification, with diagnostic
criteria that can be understood and used by the practising histopathologist. In

some cases the differentiation described is only assumed to represent a certain adult tissue for purposes of classification e.g. malignant fibrous histiocytoma. In some tumours there is no feature which resembles mature or embryonic non-neoplastic tissues, these lesions can be classified as STT of uncertain histogenesis. In using a classification such as this one does not necessarily imply that the cell of origin of the neoplastic growth was a committed cell to the lineage, expressed in the differentiation of the tumour. The most accepted classification is found in the first reference, but this would only be reproduced somewhat broadly, but the question does not require a regurgitation of the classification, more a discussion as above, citing specific examples from the groups selected by Enzinger and Weiss.

The specific techniques include conventional histochemistry (which is often overlooked), immunohistochemistry and electron microscopy. Note that the 'anaplastic spindle cell tumour' could be a carcinoma or melanoma (or even rare spindle cell lymphomas) as much as a sarcoma. In addition, it would not be appropriate to discuss non-spindle cell sarcomas – a point which might be overlooked in an examination.   *(April 1988, Paper 2, Question 4)*

References

1   Enzinger, F.M., Weiss, S. General considerations and immunohistochemistry of soft tissue lesions. In: Soft Tissue Tumors, 2nd edition. p1–18; 83–101. C.V. Mosby Co, St. Louis (1988).
2   Gatter, K.C., Falini, B., Mason, D.Y. The use of monoclonal antibodies in histopathological diagnosis. In: Recent Advances in Histopathology 12. P.P. Anthony, R.N.M. MacSween (eds.) p35–67. Churchill Livingstone, Edinburgh (1984).

What processes underlie hypercalcaemia which may occur in association with malignant neoplasms?

Introduction

Definition of hypercalcaemia
Paraneoplastic syndrome–incidence (15/100 000/year)
Detection/clinical presentation

Mechanisms

1) *Metastatic disease*

   a) tumour types – lung, breast, renal, endometrial ca
   b) patterns
       i)   osteolytic
            – peritumoural lysis of bone–hypercalcaemia
            – but some lytic bone mets (e.g. oat cell ca) normocalcaemic
   c) mechanisms
       i)   PGE synthesis (e.g. breast ca, melanoma)
       ii) TGF alpha and beta (e.g. breast ca)
       iii) as for non-metastatic disease

    d) osteosclerotic
       i) osteoblast stimulation
      ii) mechanism unknown

2) *Non-metastatic disease*

    a) 25 – 50% of solid tumours no obvious bony metastases
    b) mechanisms
       i) PTH-like activity ('ectopic' PTH)
          – e.g. squamous/large cell ca lung
                renal cell ca
                small cell ca ovary
          – action of PTH – bone
                       – kidney
                       – gut
      ii) hypersecretion of PTH
          – parathyroid carcinoma

3) *Primary bone involvement*

    Myeloma
    a) mechanisms
       i) osteoclast activating factors (lymphokines e.g. IL-1)
      ii) reduced renal excretion in 'myeloma kidney'
     iii) ? increased 1,25 (OH)2 D3 production

    Non-Hodgkin's lymphoma/leukaemia
    a) mechanisms
       i) ?1,25 (OH)2, D3 production
      ii) osteoclast activating factors

(April 1985, Paper 1, Question 4)

Reference

1   Strewler, G.J., Nissenson, R.A. Non-parathyroid hypercalcaemia. Adv. Intern.
Med. (1987) 32: 235–258.

Describe the pathological conditions that give rise to hypercalcaemia; discuss the effects on other tissues of the body

This essay encompasses the ground covered in the previous answer, together with other non-parathyroid causes of hypercalcaemia (e.g. sarcoidosis, milk-alkali syndrome etc.), which are also covered in the previous reference. A major section also needs to be included on hyperparathyroidism, where the abnormalities of the endocrine glands rather than the bony changes require description according to the wording of the question. In all essays like this, it is usually of value to include a précis of the control of normal calcium and phosphate absorption and excretion in the introduction, or even as a line diagram. This will aid the explanation of the tissue effects (renal complications, metastatic calcification, etc.).

April 1975, Paper 2, Question 5)

How would you examine a mastectomy specimen for a suspected carcinoma? What macroscopic and microscopic criteria do you use to assess the prognosis of breast cancer?

A question which would be relatively easy for those trainees who had undertaken a meticulous approach to these specimens in routine practice. Different types of mastectomy should be described (e.g. simple, radical, etc.) along with procedures to ensure prompt fixation. The macroscopic features are fairly straightforward (e.g. size, site, resection margins, etc.) but details of lymph node dissection should be detailed since this is the most important prognostic indicator. Much of the information on microscopic features is contained within the previous answers. Grading of breast carcinoma is contentious but provides an opportunity for discussion. *(October 1984, Paper 1, Question 2)*

References

1 Rosai, J. Guidelines for handling of most common and important surgical specimens. In: Ackerman's Surgical Pathology, 7th edition. 1868–1872. C.V. Mosby Co, St Louis (1989).
2 Haybittle, J.L. et al. A prognostic index in primary breast cancer. Br. J. Cancer (1982) 45: 361–366.

What pathological features assist in determining the prognosis in mammary carcinoma?

(April 1980, Paper 1, Question 1)

Discuss the histopathological (including histochemical and immunohistochemical) features that may be related to prognosis in carcinoma of the breast

(April 1981, Paper 1, Question 4)

Give an account of the various types of breast cancer. What role has the pathologist to play in the management of this malignancy?

(October 1982, Paper 1, Question 2)

What features enable a pathologist to venture an opinion on prognosis in a case of carcinoma of the female breast?

These questions require some expansion of the second part of the previous answer, relating to the classification and its relationship to behaviour (especially the better prognostic types such as papillary, mucoid, some medullary, tubular and adenoid cystic carcinomas), location in the breast and staging, and certain histological features which may have a bearing on behaviour (e.g. vascular invasion). It is also important to include an assessment of nodal involvement, and discuss the relevance (or otherwise) of grading systems. More recent advances such as oestrogen and progesterone receptor status and indeed /EGF receptor and c-erb B protein expression could also be included within the discussion.

(October 1979, Paper 2, Question 4)

Reference

1   Robbins, S.L., Cotran, R.S., Kumar, V. Carcinoma of breast. In: Pathologic Basis of Disease, 4th edition. p1192–1201. W.B. Saunders, Philadelphia (1989).

Discuss the correlation between pathological features and prognosis in mammary carcinoma

Introduction

Incidence of breast carcinoma
Overall mortality rate
Changes in therapy
Influence of breast screening

Role of the Pathologist

Management of specimens

   a) naked eye examination
   b) specimen radiography
   c) resection margins for lumpectomy
   d) mastectomy specimens

Classification of breast carcinoma

1) *Invasive carcinoma with average or poor prognosis*

   a) ductal
   b) lobular
   c) carcinoma NOS

2) *Invasive carcinomas with above average prognosis*

   a) tubular
   b) medullary with lymphoid infiltration
   c) papillary
   d) 'minimal' cancer
   e) mucinous/colloid

3) *In situ carcinoma*

   a) ductal
   b) lobular
   Implications for management and risk of invasive cancer

Spread of disease (and staging)

1) Local factors

    a) tumour size

    b) vascular invasion

    c) local invasion and resection margins

2) Metastatic disease

    a) local lymph nodes and sites

    b) recurrence and extramammary deposits

(April 1971, Paper 2, Question 1)

References

1   Azzopardi, J.G. Problems in Breast Pathology. Chapters 11-13, p240–333. W.B. Saunders, Philadelphia (1979).

2   Robbins, S.L., Cotran, R.S., Kumar, V. The breast. In: Pathologic Basis of Disease, 4th edition. Chapter 25, p1192–1201. W.B. Saunders, Philadelphia (1989).

Describe the appearances of lobular carcinoma of the breast and give a critical account of its natural history

Introduction

Description of normal breast lobule
Putative 'origin' of lobular and ductal carcinoma

Lobular carcinoma in situ

1) Microscopic features

    a) uniform cells

    b) nucleoli

    c) lobular distention

    d) 'intracytoplasmic' lumina

    e) Pagetoid spread

2) Clinical features

3) Behaviour

    a) risk of malignancy

    b) bilaterality

    c) comparison with intraductal carcinoma

Atypical lobular hyperplasia A

Distinction from LCIS

Invasive lobular carcinoma

1) Macroscopic features

2) Microscopic features

   a) LCIS
   b) invasive patterns – solid, alveolar, mixed features
      i)   targetoid spread
      ii) indian filing
      ii) desmoplasia
      iv) intracytoplasmic lumina
      v)   signet ring cell type
   c) immunohistochemistry
   d) oestrogen receptors

3) Clinical features

4) Behaviour

5) Identification of metastases

6) Comparison with ductal carcinoma

(October 1983, Paper 2, Question 4)

References

1   Azzopardi, J.G. Underdiagnosis of malignancy, and special problems in breast pathology. In: Problems in Breast Pathology. p216–233; 278–285. WB Saunders, Philadelphia (1979).
2   Howell, A., Harris, M. Infiltrating lobular carcinoma of the breast. Br. Med. J. (1985) 291: 1371–1372.

Discuss critically the evidence which led to the decision to introduce a national screening programme for breast cancer. What impact do you think the implementation of such a programme will have upon the histopathology laboratory?

Introduction

Highest level of breast cancer mortality in UK
'Static' mortality in breast cancer patients in last 50 years
Assessment of screening benefits (Forrest Report)
National programme – one view mammography every three years in 50–64 age group

1) *'Early' detection of breast cancer*

2) *Assessment and management of premalignant breast disease*

Evidence

1) *↓ mortality in 50–65 yr age group (US/Swedish trials) of 30–50%*

2) *↓ morbidity (more modest surgery)*

Criticisms

1) *'Lead-time'; bias*

2) *False positive results (mammographic)*

3) *False negative results*

4) *Evidence of long term benefit not established*

5) *?Theoretical radiation risk*

Implications for histopathology laboratories

1) *Workload*
   a) FNA cytology
   b) surgical biopsy

2) *Management implications*
   a) funding of laboratory
   b) quality control procedures
   c) computer processing and registration for regional and national evaluation

3) *Specimen radiography*
   a) liaison with surgeon/radiologist
   b) ? laboratory x-ray facilities
   c) interpretation of results
   d) localisation of lesion (?pre-operative) and sampling procedures
   e) excision margins and multifocal disease
   f) fixation and dissection
   g) staging and classification

4) *Interpretation of histopathological abnormality*
   a) training programmes and courses
   b) evaluation of atypical hyperplasias
   c) management of epithelial proliferative diseases
   d) assessment of small cancers

(October 1988, Paper 2, Question 2)

References

1   Gad, A. Screening for breast cancer: examination and reporting of histopathological preparations. Lancet (1988) ii: 953.
2   Anderson, T.J. The pathologist and breast cancer screening. J. Pathol. (1987) 153: 309–310.
3   Reidy, J., Hoskins, O. Controversy over mammography screening. Br. Med. J. (1988) 297: 932–933.

Give an account of carcinoid tumours

Since the appearance of this question significant advances have been made in this field. Carcinoid tumours are now generally regarded as a component of the spectrum of neoplasia arising from the diffuse endocrine and neuroendocrine system. The biological activity of tumours of this group and their histochemical, immunohistochemical and ultrastructural features are now extensively described. An examination question posed today would almost certainly be more specific, for example – 'Discuss the pathology of diffuse endocrine tumours of midgut origin'. The question requires an introduction with brief description of the current concept of the diffuse endocrine and neuroendocrine system together with a macroscopic and microscopic description of the tumours to include histochemistry and immunohistochemistry. A discussion of hormone production and secretion, and a description of the behaviour of the lesions in question must be included.   (*April 1972, Paper 2, Paper 4*)

References

1   Polak, J.M., Bloom, S.R. Pathology of peptide producing neuroendocrine tumours. Br. J. Hosp. Med. (1985) 33: 78–88.
2   Dawson, I.M.P. Diffuse endocrine and neuroendocrine cell tumours. In: Recent Advances in Histopathology 12. P.P. Anthony, R.N.M. MacSween (eds.) p111–128. Churchill Livingstone, Edinburgh (1984).

Write an essay on endothelial cell neoplasia

Introduction

Neoplasms vs. malformations/reactive lesions e.g. Masson's tumour, haemangiomas
Pleomorphic nature of endothelial cell reflected in neoplasia
Exclude leiomyoma and haemangiopericytoma
Endothelial cell markers in diagnosis e.g. laminin
Factor VIIIr Ag, UEA1

Benign tumours

1) Epithelioid haemangioma

- a) clinical features
- b) histological appearance
- c) distinction from Kimura's disease
- d) confusions in nomenclature

2) CNS haemangioblastoma

- a) age, location
- b) microscopic appearance
- c) associations (phaeochromocytoma, renal cell carcinoma)

Low grade malignancy

1) Epithelioid haemangioendothelioma

- a) terminology, (inc IVBAT, 'sclerosing cholangiocarcinoma')
- b) clinical features
- c) microscopic features
- d) differential diagnosis
- e) behaviour

2) Malignant endovascular papillary angioendothelioma

- a) Dabska tumour
- b) clinical and microscopic features

Malignant tumours

1) Angiosarcoma

- a) clinical features
- b) aetiology (arsenic, vinyl chloride, thorotrast)
- c) macroscopic
- d) microscopic
- e) behaviour

2) Post-mastectomy angiosarcoma

- a) chronic lymphoedema
- b) microscopic
- c) behaviour

3) Kaposi's sarcoma (arguably endothelial in nature)

  a) clinical features
  b) epidemiological associates
    i)   (HIV, genetic)
  c) microscopy
    i)   early
    ii) late
    iii) nodular
  d) behaviour

(October 1985, Paper 1, Question 5)

References

1   Enzinger, F.M., Weiss, S.W. Benign tumors and tumorlike lesions of blood
    vessels,   haemangioendothelioma: vascular   tumors   of   intermediate
    malignancy and malignant vascular tumors. In: Soft Tissue Tumors, 2nd
    edition, p489–580. C.V. Mosby Co, St Louis
2. Robbins, S.L. Cotran, R.S., Kumar, V. Blood vessels. In: Pathologic Basis of
    Disease, 4th edition. p587–593. W.B. Saunders, Philadelphia (1989).
3. Ashley, D.J.B. Tumours of the vascular system. In: Recent Advances in
    Histopathology 13. P.P. Anthony, R.N.M. MacSween (eds.) p95–107. Churchill
    Livingstone, Edinburgh (1987).

Describe the naked eye and histological appearances of Kaposi's sarcoma. Give an account of its nature, behaviour and associations

Cutaneous Kaposi's sarcoma

1) Macroscopic appearances

  a) patch (colour, margin, size)
  b) plaque
  c) nodule

Note tendency of nodules to coalesce and ulcerate in the non-AIDS endemic patients

2) Microscopic appearances

  a) patch
    i)   upper dermis
    ii) proliferation of jagged irregular vascular spaces, avoid normal vessels
    iii) blood endothelial cells
    iv) dissection of collagen by vessels
    v)   paucity of spindle cells in stroma

  b) plaque
      i)   entire dermis +/- subcutaneous tissue
      ii)   greater vascular proliferation
      iii) addition of spindle cells in stroma +/- erythrocyte containing clefts
      iv)   atypia may still be minimal
  c) nodule
      i)   sarcomatous
      ii)   angiomatoid
      iii) mixed

Visceral KS

1) Sites

  a) any (except brain)
  b) especially GIT, lung, lymph node

Microscopic as before

Clinical setting of KS

1) Endemic

  a) Elderly males
      i)   age >50
      ii)   epidemiology
      iii) site
      iv)   behaviour indolent
  b) African
      i)   epidemiology
      ii)   age/sex
      iii) behaviour aggressive
      iv)   metastases – visceral

2) Immunodeficiency-associated

  a) AIDS
      i)   age
      ii)   HIV status
      iii) sites – cutaneous/visceral
      iv)   behaviour aggressive
      v)   metastases – visceral and nodal
  b) allograft recipients
      i)   rare
      ii)   behaviour as AIDS

Nature of KS

1) Histogenesis

  Two possibilities

a) ?vascular endothelial cell – morphological features but
   i)   Factor VIII rAg -ve
   ii) no Weibel-Palade bodies
b) ?lymphatic endothelial cell independent regions, association with lymphoedema, absence in brain

Association with CMV infection

a) antibody studies
b) DNA studies

(October 1984, Paper 2, Question 3)

References

1   Millard, P.R., Chapel, H.M. Immunodeficiency states including AIDS. In: Recent Advances in Histopathology 13. P.P. Anthony, R.N.M. MacSween (eds.) p138–142. Churchill Livingstone, Edinburgh (1987).
2   Enzinger, F.M., Weiss, S.W. Malignant vascular tumors. In: Soft Tissue Tumors, 2nd edition. p561–575. C.V. Mosby Co, St Louis (1988).

Give an account of tumours that may arise in the orbit (including the eye)

Introduction

Intraocular and extraocular tumours
Benign vs malignant
Incidence

Intraocular tumours

Uveal tract

1) Malignant melanoma

a) choroidal
b) types
   i)   spindle cell
   ii) epithelioid
   iii) pure
c) survival
d) prognostic features

2) Leiomyoma

3) Angioma

4) Haemangioendothelioma

Retina

1) *Retinoblastoma*
   a) age incidence
   b) frequency
   c) histological types
      i) undifferentiated
      ii) rosettes
      iii) diffuse infiltrating

2) *Medulloepithelioma*

3) *Astrocytoma*

4) *Haemangioblastoma*

Non-pigmented ciliary epithelium

1) *Medulloepithelioma*

2) *Adenoma/adenocarcinoma*

Pigmented ciliary epithelium

1) *Adenoma/adenocarcinoma (rare)*

Optic disc tumours

1) *Melanocytoma*

2) *Medulloepithelioma*

3) *Astrocytoma*

Secondary deposits

   1) e.g. breast, lung, GIT, ovaries

Orbital tumours

1) *Optic nerve*
   a) astrocytoma
   b) meningioma

2) *Soft tissues*
   a) embryonal rhabdomyosarcoma
   b) cavernous angioma
   c) malignant lymphoma
   d) Schwannoma
   e) histiocytosis X
   f) lipoma and liposarcoma

3) *Lacrimal gland*

    a) adenoid cystic carcinoma
    b) others

4) *Metastatic carcinoma*

(October 1985, Paper 2, Question 1)

References

1   Zimmerman, L.E., Sobin, L.H. Histological Typing of Tumours of the Eye and Its Adnexa. World Health Organisation International Histological Classification of Tumours, No 24, Geneva (1980).

2   Rosai, J. Eye and ocular adnexa. In: Ackerman's Surgical Pathology, 7th edition. p1791–1858. C.V. Mosby Co, St. Louis (1989).

3. Lymphoreticular System

Give an account of the role of the Epstein-Barr virus in the pathogenesis of Burkitt's lymphoma and glandular fever

Introduction

EBV original isolation from African Burkitt lymphoma (BL)
Later isolated glandular fever
Epidemiology – latent infection widespread (serology)

EBV

1) *Herpes virus (DNA)*

2) *Structure*

3) *Replication*

4) *Transmission*

B lymphocytes and EBV

1) *In vitro studies*
   a) transformation
   b) C3d receptor binding EBV (on B cells)
   c) detection of viral genome vs. expression
   d) expression of viral antigens and polyclonal proliferation
   e) EBNA

BL and EBV

1) *Serology*
   a) EBV titres

2) *Genome in tumour cells (All Africa, 50% Europe)*

3) *Prospective studies (serum storage)*
   a) anti capsid Ag = → risk
   b) Ch 8–14 translocations (c-myc activation)

Influence of other factors

1) *Malaria (falciparum)*

2) *Immunodeficiency and nutrition*

3) *Clinical features*
   a) young adults

GF and EBV

1) *Pathology*

- a) lymph nodes
- b) spleen
  - i) T cell response
- c) serological studies.
  - i) IgM
  - ii) IgG
- d) lymphoblastic cells in circulation + T cells

Immunosuppression and EBV infection

1) *Lymphomas*

October 1984, Paper 2, Question 4

Reference

1) Taussig, M.J. Oncogenic DNA viruses. In: Processes in Pathology and Microbiology, 2nd edition. p792–796. Blackwell Scientific Publications, Oxford (1984).

Discuss the structure and function of the spleen in health and disease

Normal structure

1) *Macroscopic*

- a) size
- b) weight
- c) vascular supply

2) *Microscopic*

- a) red pulp
  - i) sinuses
  - ii) pulp cords
- b) white pulp
  - i) periarteriolar lymphoid sheath
  - ii) lymphoid follicles

3) *Blood flow*

- a) arterial supply via arterioles capillaries into
  - i) 'open' system – cords, sinuses, veins
  - ii) 'closed' system – sinuses, veins

(Diagrammatic illustration suggested)

Functions

1) *Phagocytosis rbcs*

2) *Iron recycling*

3) *Platelet pool*

4) *Immune response*

5) *Haemopoiesis (< 1 year)*

Pathological states

Reduced function

1) *Effects*

    a) immunodeficiencies
    b) effects

2) *Causes*

    a) asplenia/hypostasis
    b) atrophy/infarction
    c) splenectomy
    d) coeliac disease

Hyperplasia

1) *Effects*

    a) splenomegaly
    b) reduced haemopoietic elements
    c) marrow hyperplasia

2) *Aetiology*

Congestive splenomegaly

1) *Causes hepatic cirrhosis, portal vein thrombosis*

2) *R cardiac failure*

3) *Pathological appearances*

    a) weight 0.5–5 kg
    b) congestion red pulp and phagocytosis rbcs
    c) haemorrhage/fibrosis
    d) Gamna-Gandy bodies

Infections

1) *Pathological appearances*
   a) malaria
   b) kala-azar
   c) leishmaniasis
   d) others

Storage disorders

1) *Gaucher's*

2) *Niemann-Pick*

3) *Mucopolysaccharides*

4) *Lymphoma/leukaemia*
   a) CML
   b) CLL
   c) ?ALL
   d) Hodgkin's disease
   e) NHL
   f) Myelofibrosis (myeloid metaplasia)

April 1986, Paper 2, Question 2

References

1) Robbins, S.L., Cotran, R.S., Kumar, V. Spleen. In: Pathologic Basis of Disease, 4th edition. p747–753. W.B. Saunders, Philadelphia (1989).
2) Scothorne, R.J. The spleen: structure and function. Histopathology (1985) 9: 663–669.
3) Van Krieken, J.H.J.M. et al. The human spleen: a histological study in splenectomy specimens embedded in methylmethacrylate. Histopathology (1985) 9: 571–586.

Briefly discuss the normal morphology of the spleen, and outline the pathological processes which may affect this organ

There are subtle differences in the wording of this question compared to the previous essay. In this case, the function of the spleen is not a major consideration, and no great detail is required of the morphology (gross and microscopic). A diagram would be of great use in both of these essays to eliminate a lot of the explanation. Outlining the pathological processes would be made in much the same way as in the previous essay, but with the addition of other entities such as congenital cysts, minor infections, etc. as given in the useful table in the first reference above. There is every opportunity to concentrate many facts within this outline since there are so many different processes which affect the spleen, producing characteristic changes. *(October 1985, Paper 2, Question 2)*

Describe briefly and as far as possible explain, the morphological changes in a) the spleen in typhoid fever b) a lymph node following antigenic stimulation c) the thymus in myasthenia gravis

Essentially a 'short notes' type of question, there is a large amount of information which could be compressed into this answer, especially in section b. Equal weighting should be given to each part of the question however. The various appearances can be reviewed from standard texts.

(April 1974, Paper 2, Question 3)

Discuss the role of macrophages in resistance to infection

It would be best to outline the proposed properties and functions of macrophages, and their mechanisms of interactions with other cells (e.g. lymphocytes, neutrophils, etc.), before illustrating these principles with various types of infections producing different tissue responses where the macrophage plays a major role e.g. bacterial, fungal, viral infections producing acute and chronic suppuration, granulomatous inflammation, antigen presentation and antibody production, intracellular parasitisation, etc. This would illustrate all of the roles of the macrophage in a relatively structured and interesting format.

(November 1971, Paper 1, Question 1)

Reference

1) Taussig, M.J. In: Processes in Pathology and Microbiology, 2nd edition. p59–62; 114–117; 163–164. Blackwell Scientific Publications, Oxford (1984).

Discuss the common causes of non-neoplastic lymph node enlargement and describe the histological changes

This question would be best answered by placing the nodal reactive patterns into broad groups rather than taking a large number of known aetiological agents and describing each in turn, which would result in undue repetition, with an unmanageable volume of writing. The main reactive patterns include acute and chronic non-specific follicular hyperplasia, paracortical hyperplasia, necrotising and non-necrotising granulomatous lymphadenitis, combined granulomatous/follicular hyperplasia.

Within the larger groups, the distinctive features associated with each specific condition can be described (e.g. in necrotising granulomatous lymphadenitis, tuberculosis, cat-scratch disease). It is important to define what is meant by 'common' in the question, and therefore it may be debatable whether to include conditions such as syphilis, fungal lymphadenitis, SLE, etc. which are rare at least in the UK. Emphasis should really be placed on the causes related to the frequency with which they lead to lymph node biopsy.

(October 1978, Paper 1, Question 1)

Reference

1) Stansfeld, A.G. Inflammatory and reactive disorders. In: Lymph Node Biopsy and Interpretation. A.G. Stansfeld (ed.) p85–141. Churchill Livingstone, Edinburgh (1985).

Discuss the role of the histopathologist in the diagnosis and management of Hodgkin's disease

One could organise this answer by dividing the histopathologist's contribution into four parts, 1) diagnosis in lymph node biopsy – pathological features and immunohistochemical methods, 2) classification (and relation to prognosis), 3) staging, 4) follow-up – response to treatment and recurrence. Since the question was set, fine needle aspiration cytology has made it possible to diagnose the disease before biopsy, and with a good preparation it is possible to make an informed assessment of the probable type. At the same time, staging laparotomy has become less popular. The bulk of the answer could be concerned with the pathological features in the Rye classification and its relation to prognosis.

(April 1976, Paper 1, Question 1)

Reference

1) Williams, G.T. Hodgkin's disease. In: Lymph Node Biopsy and Interpretation. A.G. Stansfeld (ed.) p196–227. Churchill Livingstone, Edinburgh (1985).

Discuss the histological criteria for distinguishing the different forms of lymphoma

Effectively this question should be answered by choosing the most familiar (or understandable) lymphoma classification, and outlining the general morphological features. Once again, Hodgkin's disease should not be forgotten. It is arguable whether immunocytochemical information should be included in an answer on purely histological criteria. It might be better to discuss the architectural and cytological categories of lymphoma based on normal cell types (e.g. immunoblastic, centroblastic, centrocytic, prolymphocytic, T cell, etc. and their nodal distribution), and outline the criteria for differentiating them.

(May 1973, Paper 1, Question 4)

References

1) Williams, G.T. Hodgkin's disease. In: Lymph Node Biopsy and Interpretation. A.G. Stansfeld (ed.) p196–227. Churchill Livingstone, Edinburgh (1985).
2) Stansfeld, A.G. Non-Hodgkin's lymphomas, high grade lymphomas and peripheral T cell lymphomas. ibid p228–276; 277–299; 300–329.

Compare and contrast the pathology of malignant lymphomas arising in lymph nodes with those that arise elsewhere

A fascinating question which clearly is still topical, although again the advance in knowledge has resulted in complex lymphoma classifications within the nodal group. It would be best to consider the concept of the normal extranodal lymphoid tissue distribution, including mucosa-associated lymphoid tissue, spleen, bone marrow and brain for instance, and then describe the pathology of the lymphoma types at these sites, highlighting the major differences with nodal lymphomas, it would be impossible to attempt any detailed description of intranodal lymphomas. Candidates should remember to include both Hodgkin's disease and non-Hodgkin's lymphomas in any question of this sort.

(November 1970, Paper 2, Question 5)

Reference

1) Isaacson, P.G., Wright, D.H. Extranodal lymphoma. In: Recent Advances in Histopathology 13. P.P. Anthony, R.N.M. MacSween (eds.) Chapter 10, p159–184. Churchill Livingstone, Edinburgh (1987).

Write a descriptive account of extranodal lymphomas

The content is obviously much the same as in the previous question, but the wording implies there should be only brief references to the nodal lymphomas, with no descriptive account necessary.

(April 1971, Paper 1, Question 3)

Describe the classification of the non-Hodgkin's lymphomas and discuss how immunostaining may be of value in their diagnosis

Introduction

1) *Reasons for classification*

   a) morphological diversity
   b) clinicopathological correlations
   c) retrospective analysis

2) *Requirements for classification schemes*

   a) understandable
   b) clinical relevance
   c) reproducible
   d) scientifically accurate

3) *Different systems in use*

    a) Rappaport
    b) Kiel
    c) British National Lymphoma Investigation
    d) Working Formulation

4) *General observation on complex classification*

5) *Recommended classification (updated Kiel)*

	B	T
Low grade	Lymphocytic-CLL, PLL, HCL	CLL, PLL
		Small cerebriform cell – M.F., Sezary
	LP immunocytoma	Lymphoepithelioid
	Plasmacytic	AIL
	Centroblastic/centrocytic – Foll/diff – Diff	T zone
	Centrocytic	Pleomorphic, small cell
High grade	Centroblastic	Pleomorphic, med/large cell
	Immunoblastic	Immunoblastic
	Large cell anaplastic	Large cell anaplastic
	Burkitt	
	Lymphoblastic	Lymphoblastic

6) *Advantages of single classification*

    a) clinical relevance
    b) scientific assessment
    c) functional correlation

7) *Use of immunostaining in diagnosis of NHL*

Paraffin section

    a) lymphoma vs. carcinoma
      i)   LCA (PD7, 2B11)
    b) B cells (MB2, MB1, L26, LN1)
    c) T cells (UCHL1, MT1)
    d) clonal plasmacytoid B cells (Igs, light chains)

Frozen section

    a) clonal B cells
      i)   Igs
      ii) light chains (surf/cytop)
    b) dendritic cells (S100)
      i)   foll/diffuse

    c) large cell anaplastic lymphoma
      i) Ki-1 antigen
    d) Pre B cell
      i) CALLA
    e) T helper/T suppressor
      i) T4:T8
    f) others

Above identify most lymphomas

(October 1986, Paper 2, Question 2)

Reference

1) Stansfeld, A.G. Lymph Node Biopsy and Interpretation. p 44–66; 228–232. Churchill Livingstone, Edinburgh (1985).

Discuss the classification of lymphomas and the role of immuno-histological techniques in establishing and refining the diagnosis

This question also requires a consideration of Hodgkin's disease, which would be very easy to overlook. The range of available immunohistological reagents was much smaller in 1982. In future questions there might be some qualifying statements on the immunohistochemical aspects, such as considering their use in B cell or T cell lymphomas only.   *(October 1982, Paper 1, Question 1)*

What are your views in the present classifications of non-Hodgkin's lymphomas? How far can the classifications be linked with modern immunological concepts and what value have such classifications in prognosis?

This is an earlier version of October 1986, Paper 2, Question 2, but the relationship to cellular phenotype was less well understood at the time.

(November 1975, Paper 1, Question 4)

Describe the current classifications of lymphomas. Which one do you use in routine practice and why?

The first part of this operation may be difficult to answer these days (it would be difficult to describe the Working Formulation in a few lines!), but it is a useful exercise to assess the Kiel classification outlined previously and its advantages, or the classification used within a department where the candidate has trained. A critical approach should be taken.   *(October 1980, Paper 1, Question 2)*

Give an account of the tumours which are thought to arise from histiocytes

This has been a very changeable subject since the time when this question was set, and some entities previously included within this group have been claimed to be of lymphoid or other lineage by immunohistochemical analysis or gene rearrangement studies. Nevertheless, further questions could be envisaged in this field, such as 'Discuss the concept of neoplastic histiocyte proliferations'.

(October 1981, Paper 2, Question 4)

Describe the necropsy findings in an untreated case of myelomatosis and discuss their pathogenesis

This question could really be divided into two parts, the appearances of the tumour itself in the bones and tissues, and their complications such as pathological fracture or neuropathy, and the results of the tumour function, including myeloma kidney and systemic amyloidosis. Some mention could be made of the terminal complications of the disease (e.g. bronchopneumonia) but the major part of the essay should concentrate on the primary effects of the myelomatosis itself. *(November 1977, Paper 1, Question 3)*

Reference

1) Robbins, S.L., Cotran, R.S., Kumar, V. Diseases of white cells, lymph nodes and spleen – plasma cell dyscrasias and related disorders. In: Pathological Basis of Disease, 4th edition. p739–743. W.B. Saunders, Philadelphia (1989).

4. Alimentary Tract

Define what is meant by a 'congenitally short oesophagus'. Describe the histological features and possible complications of this condition

It is now accepted that this is usually an acquired phenomenon due to gastro-oesophageal reflux, but it might be useful to include other entities with which it might be confused, such as heterotopias and hiatus hernia. The bulk of the answer should be concerned with Barrett's oesophagus, including clinical and pathological diagnostic criteria, with the three forms of metaplastic epithelium that may be found, in some detail. Complications include ulceration, stenosis and malignant change.   *(November 1972, Paper 2, Question 2)*

Reference

1) Jass, J.R. The oesophagus. In: Systemic Pathology. Alimentary Tract. B.C. Morson (ed.), Volume 3, p130–148. Churchill Livingstone, Edinburgh (1987).

Discuss the value of biopsy and cytology in the diagnosis of ulceration of the gastric mucosa

This question relates to the differential diagnosis of various gastric ulcers, and introduction should include the various categories of gastric ulceration such as acute and chronic peptic ulceration, dysplasia, early and advanced gastric cancer, gastric lymphoma emphasising the advantages over clinical methods of diagnosis. The requirements for sufficient biopsies and cytological preparations should be discussed.

The pathological features need to be covered in more detail than for the more wide-ranging questions about the value of GIT biopsy, and the particular advantages of having both biopsy and cytology need to be emphasised, both for improvement of overall diagnostic rate, and in particular circumstances where histology may be difficult e.g. deep ulcers covered in slough, or signet ring cells which may be overlooked (usually better seen on cytology). Other difficult diagnostic problems on biopsy may be given emphasis (e.g. in gastric lymphoma).
(April 1981, Paper 1, Question3)

Discuss the pathology of the malabsorption syndrome and the role of the histopathologist in the diagnosis and management of this condition

Introduction

Definition
Clinical features
Systemic effects

General principles

Dysfunctions of

1) Digestion
2) Absorption
3) Transport
4) Combinations of above
5) Unknown

1) Digestive abnormalities

a) pancreatic diseases
   i) biopsy (bx)
b) hepatic biliary disease
   i) bx of liver and CBD
c) bile salt deconjugation
   i) blind loop
   ii) diverticula
   iii) fistula
   iv) gastrectomy
   v) ? role of histopathologist

2) Absorption

a) metabolic
   i) disaccharidase deficiency
   ii) a beta lipoproteinaemia – features
   iii) vitamin B12 deficiency – gastric bx
b) small bowel disease
   i) coeliac disease – role of biopsy
      – diagnostic gluten
      – response to gluten-free diet
      – response to gluten challenge
   ii) Whipple's disease
      – features – LM, EM, immunocytochemical
      – systemic disease
   iii) allergic enteritis
   iv) chronic ulcerative jejunoileitis – bx
   v) Crohn's disease – bx of small and large bowel
   vi) infection
      – tropical source
      – parasites – strongyloidiasis
                  – giardiasis
                  – schistosomiasis
c) bx features

3) Transport

a) lymphatic blockage
   i) lymphangiectasis
   ii) tuberculosis
   iii) lymphoma
b) bx features

4) _Multiple_

   a) gastrectomy

   b) bowel resection

   c) radiation

5) _Unexplained_

   a) hypogammaglobulinaemia – bx

   b) carcinoid syndrome

   c) diabetes mellitus

   d) endocrine dysfunction

(April 1977, Paper 1, Question 3)

Reference

1) Robbins, S.L., Cotran, R.S., Kumar, V. The gastrointestinal tract. In: Pathologic Basis of Disease, 4th edition. Chapter 18, p875–881. W.B. Saunders, Philadelphia (1989).

Describe the structural alterations in the gastrointestinal tract in patients with steatorrhoea

This answer covers much of the ground in the previous plan, but excluding some of the conditions which do not tend to steatorrhoea per se (e.g. Vitamin B12 deficiency, Crohn's disease, radiation enteritis etc.) which essentially result from inadequate emulsification of fats. As well as the primary pathology, the secondary effects of fat malabsorption e.g. lipofuscinosis, vitamin D and K deficiency, etc should also be considered. *(November 1973, Paper 2, Question 4)*

Discuss the value of endoscopic biopsies in the investigation of diseases of the gastrointestinal tract

(April 1980, Paper 1, Question 5)

Discuss the problems of processing and interpreting gastrointestinal biopsies

An example of a subject which has occurred one year, and then repeated in the subsequent year with alterations in the wording which significantly change the direction of the answer. In the 1980 example, all that would be required is an appraisal of the uses of biopsy from the lower oesophagus to the anus, in both neoplastic and non-neoplastic disease. There is clearly a large volume of information to be included, but the phrase 'Discuss the value' indicates emphasis should be paid to those diseases which are effectively diagnosed or monitored by this technique. This later question has a quite different emphasis, which is more concerned with the practical measures necessary in a laboratory – labelling, wrapping and orientation, etc.) and the requirements for adequate assessment (e.g. deeper levels, special stains, etc.). The answer could be enlivened by including various illustrative examples. The major difference is that the earlier question calls for an appraisal of the circumstances where a diagnosis can be made, while the later one is more concerned with the situations where it might not be.

(October 1981, Paper 2, Question 3)

References

1) Talbot, I.C., Price, A.B.P. Biopsy Pathology of Colorectal Disease. p1–3; 373–382. Chapman and Hall, London (1987).
2) Day, D.W., Husain, O.A.N. Biopsy Pathology of the Oesophagus, Stomach and Duodenum. p1–10. Chapman and Hall, London (1986).

Give an account of iatrogenic disorders of the alimentary tract

This is a rather nebulous question which requires careful organisation. The best approach would be to consider each part of the alimentary tract, from the mouth to the anus, and select the lesions which have a characteristic appearance for the most detailed description. As in other examples, repetition of the descriptive changes where there is a common iatrogenic cause (e.g. radiation) should be avoided, except where there are sufficient differences in the tissue response (e.g. oesophagus vs. large bowel). We suggest that you consider the following categories as examples:

Antibiotic therapy (e.g. candidal infection, pseudomembranous colitis), anti-inflammatory drugs (e.g. gastric ulceration), immunosuppressive agents (e.g. fungal infection), radiation (e.g. enteritis), surgery (e.g. reflux, oesophagitis, intestinal obstruction, malabsorption). It would not be very appropriate to include examples resulting from poor technique, but rather the recognised and largely unavoidable complications. This should provide sufficient material for a descriptive essay.   *(November 1973, Paper 2, Question 4)*

Reference

1) Morson, B.C. (ed.) Systemic Pathology. Alimentary Tract. Volume 3. Churchill Livingstone, Edinburgh (1987).

Discuss the mechanisms underlying coeliac disease and its complications

The introduction should include a definition of coeliac disease and the criteria necessary for the diagnosis, including response to gluten withdrawal and challenge. The microscopic features would need to be described in detail before considering the pathogenesis. The generally accepted modern theory involves a hypersensitivity response to alpha gliadin, mainly cell mediated but with a humoral component in addition. The cellular populations in the mucosa should be described in detail. Complications of coeliac disease include the malabsorption syndrome and its numerous possible sequelae. The development of malignant B cell lymphoma of the gut should also be detailed, and brief mention made of the increased incidence of adenocarcinoma.   *(April 1988, Paper 1, Question 3)*

References

1) Morson, B.C. (ed.) Systemic Pathology. Alimentary Tract. Volume 3. p272–274; 284–286. Churchill Livingstone, Edinburgh (1987).
2) Stansfeld, A.G. Lymph Node Biopsy and Interpretation. p372–373. Churchill Livingstone, Edinburgh (1987).
3) Robbins, S.L., Cotran, R.S., Kumar, V. Pathologic Basis of Disease, 4th edition. p876–878. W.B. Saunders, Philadelphia (1989).

Under what circumstances would you make a diagnosis of dysplasia in endoscopic gastrointestinal biopsies? Discuss the clinicopathological significance of such a diagnosis

Endoscopic biopsies include lower oesophagus, stomach, duodenum and periampullary region and colon as the main areas to be discussed. Each area has particular requirements for the diagnosis of dysplasia, the broad definition of which should be included in an introductory paragraph. Many of the points should be covered by the essays (April 1987, Paper 2, Question 4 and November 1972, Paper 1, Question 1). This answer clearly calls for an assessment of the problems of interpreting such biopsies, and this aspect is the major part of October 1981, Paper 2, Question 3, it requires a practical rather than theoretical approach. The clinicopathological significance relates to the role of histopathological assessment in the decision as to what stage surgical intervention will be required.
(April 1986, Paper 2, Question 4)

Discuss the concept of pre-cancerous conditions, with particular reference to the alimentary tract

Introduction

Definition of pre-cancer, relationship to dysplasia
Clinical significance – assessment of dysplasia and reliability
Major sites
   a) oral cavity
   b) oesophagus
   c) stomach
   d) large intestine

Oral cavity

1) Epithelial dysplasias

    a) associations
    b) diagnosis
       i) cytology and biopsy (bx)
    c) management
    d) progression and diagnosis

Oesophagus

1) Squamous dysplasia

    a) aetiology and geographic factors e.g. China
    b) diagnosis
       i) cytology/bx
    c) management

2) Glandular dysplasia

    a) associations e.g. reflux
    b) diagnosis
       i) cytology/bx
    c) management
       i) risk of progression
    d) treatment

Stomach

1) Glandular dysplasia

    a) aetiology and geographic factors
    b) diagnosis
       i) cytology/bx
    c) definition and grading (mild and mod/severe)
    d) significance
       i) relationship to development of carcinoma vs. occult neoplasia
    e) management

Large intestine

1) Precancerous lesions

'Adenoma-carcinoma' sequence

    a) evidence
       i) polyposis syndromes
       ii) site of lesions
       iii) epidemiology
       iv) early cancers
       v) rarity of de novo carcinoma

    b) inflammatory bowel disease
       i)   evidence of association
       ii) diagnostic problems
       iii) management

(November 1972, Paper 1, Question 3)

Reference

1) Morson, B.C. (ed.) Systemic Pathology. Alimentary Tract. Volume 3. Churchill Livingstone, Edinburgh (1987).

Discuss pre-cancerous lesions of the gastrointestinal tract
(April 1987, Paper 2, Question 4)

Describe the morphology and behaviour of intestinal polyps

This would be a difficult question to answer in the time available unless brief and succinct reviews were given. In the light of recent advances in knowledge, it would probably not be as wide ranging. (If set today, in questions such as this, it is easy to overlook the two aspects of the question, morphology and behaviour. Equal weighting should be given to each.)   *(April 1970, Paper 2, Question 1)*

Give an account of the pathology of colorectal polyposis syndromes. How do the pathological findings influence the clinical management?
(April 1985, Paper 2, Question 5)

Discuss the histological classification of polypoid lesions of the colonic mucosa

Introduction

Inherited syndromes/acquired disease
Types of lesion present
Systemic/localised distribution – colonic involvement
Clinical implications – risk of malignancy in generalised polyposis

Types of colonic polyposis

Inherited

1) *Familial adenomatous polyposis*

    a) macroscopic features
       i)   number of polyps (> 100)
       ii) size and distribution incl. extracolonic lesion
       iii) tubular adenomas – morphology
    b) microscopic
       i)   adenomatous polyps
       ii) cryptal changes
       iii) dysplasia
    c) clinical management
       i)   risk of malignancy
       ii) monitoring of disease
       iii) genetic counselling
    d) Gardner syndrome
       i)   polyposis with additional features (e.g. desmoid tumours, jaw cysts, osteomas, etc.)
    e) Turcot syndrome
       i)   polyposis with CNS changes

2) *Juvenile polyposis*

    a) macroscopic features
       i)   number of polyps
       ii) size and distribution
       iii) appearances
       iv) extracolonic lesions
    b) microscopic
       i)   hamartomatous
       ii) descriptive detail
    c) clinical management
       i)   ?risk of malignancy
       ii) counselling

3) *Peutz-Jeghers' syndrome*

    a) macroscopic features
       i)   predominantly small intestinal
       ii) colonic and rectal polyposis occurs
    b) microscopic features
       i)   hamartomatous (c/w juvenile polyps)
    c) clinical management
       i)   risk of malignancy

4) *Others*

    Colonic involvement in systemic disease, e.g. neurofibromatosis or blue rubber bleb naevus syndrome

5) *Multiple colonic adenomatosis*

   a) macroscopic features
      i)   fewer than FAP (<50)
   b) clinical management
      i)   risk of malignancy
      ii) possible genetic inheritance

Acquired

1) *Inflammatory polyposis – inflammatory bowel disease*

   a) macroscopic features
   b) microscopic features
   c) clinical management
      i)   as for U.C. or Crohn's disease
      ii) differential diagnostic problem

2) *Metaplastic polyposis*

3) *Benign lymphoid polyposis*

   a) differential diagnosis problem

4) *Malignant lymphomatous polyposis*

5) *Lipomatous polyposis*

6) *Pneumatosis coli*

References

1) Bussey, H.J.R. Gastrointestinal polyposis syndromes. In: Recent Advances in
    Histopathology 12. P.P. Anthony, R.N.M. MacSween (eds.) p169–177.
    Churchill Livingstone, Edinburgh (1984).
2) Morson, B.C., Dawson, I.M.P. Adenomatosis and the adenoma-carcinoma
    sequence. In: Gastrointestinal Pathology. Chapter 38. Blackwell Scientific
    Publications, Oxford (1979)   *(April 1978, Paper 1, Question 1)*

Give a brief account of how you would investigate a colectomy specimen removed for malignant disease. Discuss the various staging and grading systems used in this disease mentioning their prognostic significance

A question designed to assess the ability to describe the practical approach to dissection of a common surgical specimen. It would be desirable to indicate the common types of partial and total colectomy, and briefly justify the location and number of blocks to be taken in the ideal situation. Other techniques such as macroscopic photography, localisation of lymph nodes or vascular injection might also be included.

Dukes' classification should be discussed in detail, together with the clinical correlation. The American and TNM classifications should be compared, and the recent criteria proposed by Jass et al., (1987) which have emerged since this question was set should be discussed and evaluated.

(October 1983, Paper 1, Question 5)

References

1) Jass, J.R. The large intestine. In: Systemic Pathology. Alimentary Tract. B.C. Morson (ed.) Volume 3. 3rd edition, p365–377. Churchill Livingstone, Edinburgh (1987).
2) Rosai, J. Appendix-guidelines for handling of most common and important surgical specimens. In: Ackerman's Surgical Pathology. Volume 2. 7th edition, appendix A; p1902–1905. C.V. Mosby Co, St Louis (1989).

Give an account of the pathology of ulcerative colitis and discuss its aetiology

A straightforward description of this disease should include macroscopic appearances, microscopic patterns on resection and biopsy specimens, and complications of the disease such as toxic dilatation, dysplasia and malignancy. The aetiology is more difficult, but several theories have been advanced and should be critically evaluated. It is important not to stray into a discussion of the differentiation of ulcerative colitis from Crohn's disease.

(April 1981, Paper 1, Question 1)

Discuss the principal microscopic and macroscopic features that may help you to differentiate between ulcerative colitis and Crohn's disease of the colon

(November 1975, Paper 1, Question 1)

Discuss the problems of differentiating between the lesions of Crohn's disease and ulcerative colitis

These questions should be answered easily by a candidate for the final examination, without the necessity for revision. It may account for the reason why this comparison has not been set since 1975, since it will be a poor discriminator.

(April 1969, Paper 2, Question 4)

Reference

1) Jass, J.R. The large intestine. In: Systemic Pathology. Alimentary Tract. B.C. Morson (ed.) Volume 3. 3rd edition, p334–346. Churchill Livingstone, Edinburgh (1987).

How would you attempt to establish a diagnosis of pseudomembranous colitis? Discuss its pathogenesis

Introduction

Causation – associations with antibiotic therapy and C. difficile
Distinction between PMC, antibiotic-associated diarrhoea, antibiotic-associated colitis

Clinical features

Pathological features

1) *Gross*
   a) mucosal plaques
   b) distribution
   c) morphology

2) *Microscopic*
   a) 'summit' lesion
   b) plaques
   c) mucosal ulceration and submucosal oedema

Diagnosis

1) *Clinical history*

2) *Toxin estimation*
   a) reliability

3) *Sigmoidoscopy*
   a) gross features
   b) rectal biopsy
      i) techniques and limitations
   c) differential diagnostic problems (e.g. IBD, infective colitis)

Pathogenesis

1) *Early theories*
   a) ischaemia
   b) C. difficile
      i) pathogen or commensal?
   c) toxin
      i) cytopathic properties
   d) animal studies

2) *Epidemiology*

    a) susceptibility to C. difficile colonisation
    b) ? changes in gut flora, growth factors, mucosal adhesiveness of organism
    c) ? role of host factors

(October 1980, Paper 2, Question 2)

Reference

1) Price, A.B., Day, D.W. Pseudomembranous and infective colitis. In: Recent Advances in Histopathology 11. Anthony, P.P., MacSween, R.N.M. (eds.) p99–117. Churchill Livingstone, Edinburgh (1981).

Discuss the role of histopathology in the diagnosis and management of infective disorders of the small and large intestine

This question has a fairly broad scope, although the use of histopathology in diagnosis and management means that relevant weight must be given to these specific aspects; hence a detailed description of typhoid would not be appropriate (although some mention of the changes could be made). The role of endoscopic biopsy should be emphasised, both in the small intestine in conditions such as giardiasis, cryptosporidiosis or even putative infections such as tropical sprue, and in the large bowel in pseudomembranous and infective colitis. It may also be useful to subdivide infection into parasitic (e.g. amoebiasis, strongyloides), bacterial (e.g. Whipple's disease, actinomycosis, tuberculosis), fungal (e.g. candida) or viral (e.g. CMV).

(October 1988, Paper 2, Question 4)

References

1) Dawson, I.M.P. The small intestine. In: Systemic Pathology. Alimentary Tract. 3rd edition, Chapter 6. B.C. Morson (ed.) p229–291. Churchill Livingstone, Edinburgh (1987).
2) Jass, J.R. ibid. Chapter 8, p313–395.

Discuss primary lymphoid tumours of the gastrointestinal tract

This subject has been intensively studied in the intervening years since this question was set, and many new entities have emerged with the use of immunohistochemistry and molecular biology (and have sometimes been reclassified more than once). Excellent reviews are available in the given references, and the advantage of the questions beginning 'Discuss.......' is that one's own views, or those of others, can be given and contrasted if required. The question as worded may be very difficult to answer in the set time nowadays, and to be comprehensive should encompass the stomach to the anal region.

(April 1978, Paper 2, Question 5)

References

1) Isaacson, P.G., Wright, D.H. Extranodal lymphoma. In: Recent Advances in Histopathology 13. P.P. Anthony, R.N.M. MacSween (eds.) p159–184. Churchill Livingstone, Edinburgh (1987).
2) Morson, B.C. The stomach, the small intestine, the large intestine. In: Systemic Pathology. Alimentary Tract. Volume 3. 3rd edition, p216–217; 284–286; 382–384. Churchill Livingstone, Edinburgh (1987).

Discuss the differential diagnosis of ulceration of the large intestine

A question which includes a consideration of neoplasia, inflammatory bowel disease, infections and pseudomembranous colitis, ischaemia and less common causes of ulceration such as mucosal prolapse syndrome. The best approach would be a brief description of the clinical, macroscopic and microscopic features of each category, laying emphasis on the distinguishing characteristics of each condition to avoid tedious repetition.   *(April 1976, Paper 2, Question 2)*

Reference

1) Jass, J.R. The large intestine. In: Systemic Pathology. Alimentary Tract. B.C. Morson (ed.) Volume 3. 3rd edition, p325–354. Churchill Livingstone, Edinburgh (1987).

Discuss the value and limitations of hepatic biopsy as a diagnostic tool

Since the time that this question was set, liver biopsy has been an increasingly used technique and the associated descriptions of disease states have become correspondingly more sophisticated. Thus the value has increased greatly and a large number of conditions can be diagnosed on biopsy. It might be an idea to concentrate on those conditions which have pathognomonic features on liver biopsy (e.g. Wilson's disease, storage diseases, etc.) and those where liver biopsy may resolve a clinically based differential diagnosis (e.g. alcoholic liver disease versus chronic hepatitis), contrasted with situations where liver biopsy often fails to provide a diagnosis, either through the nature of the disease or due to technical factors.   *(November 1975, Paper 1, Question 3)*

Discuss the value of liver biopsy in the diagnosis and understanding of hepatic disease

Another question where the accumulated knowledge in the last 20 years means that it would be difficult to compress into an essay format, but again construction of a lengthy notation form overview of the advantages and limitations of liver biopsy can only be of value in revision.   *(April 1969, Paper 1, Question 2)*

Discuss the factors concerned in the accumulation of abnormal amounts of triglyceride in the liver

Introduction

Types of lipid
Morphological changes – steatosis
Accumulations due to imbalance in production, utilisation or mobilisation
Significance of fatty change

Normal lipid metabolism

1) *Lipid derived from*

    a) diet – FFA + chylomicrons

    b) adipose tissue – FFA

2) *FFA in liver cell-esterified*

    a) triglyceride

    b) cholesterol (minor)

    c) phospholipid (minor)

    Acetate in liver forms FFA

3) *Secretion by apoprotein complexing – 'lipoproteins'*

Causes of triglyceride accumulation

1) *Excess FFA*

    a) dietary

    b) starvation

    c) corticosteroids

2) *↑ FA synthesis from acetate*

3) *↑ esterification of FA*

    a) alcohol

4) *↓ lipoprotein synthesis*

    a) malnutrition

    b) ? fatty liver of pregnancy

    c) ? tetracycline

    d) ? Reyes' syndrome

    e) Na valproate

5) *Impaired lipoprotein secretion*

    a) orotic acid

Complex factors

1) *Alcohol*

Effects
a) Extrahepatic FFA mobilisation
b) decreased FA oxidation
c) block in lipoprotein secretion
d) direct damage to endoplasmic reticulum
e) decreased protein synthesis

Result
a) steatosis

(November 1971, Paper 1, Question 4)

Reference

1) Hall, P. de la M. Alcoholic liver disease. In: Pathology of the Liver. R.N.M. MacSween, P.P. Anthony, P.J. Scheuer (eds.) 2nd edition, p281–285. Churchill Livingstone, Edinburgh (1987).

Discuss the relationship of the hepatitis-associated (Australia) antigen to human liver disease

A great deal of information now exists that was not available at the time this question was set, but it essentially covers much the same ground as the following answers (April 1983, Paper 1, Question 1 and November 1977, Paper 1, Question 4).

(April 1971, Paper 2, Question 3)

References

1) Bassendine, M.F. Aspects of Liver Disease. Hepatitis B virus and liver cell carcinoma. In: Recent Advances in Histopathology 12. P.P. Anthony, R.N.M. MacSween (eds.) Churchill Livingstone, Edinburgh (1984).
2) Gerberg, M.A., Thung, S.N. The diagnostic value of immunohistochemical demonstration of hepatitis viral antigens in the liver. Human Pathol. (1987) 18(8): 771–774.

Discuss the pathogenesis of hepatitis

This would today be a very difficult question to answer within the available time. However, it would be a useful revision exercise to extract all the pathogenetic mechanisms (known and hypothetical) for each type of hepatitis, both acute and chronic. By the end of this, you would not only have resulted in an active review of many important diseases, but should certainly ensure familiarity with the distinction between aetiology and pathogenesis!

(April 1970, Paper 1, Question 1)

Give an account of the possible effects on the liver of infection with hepatitis B virus

This essay involves expanding the aspects answered partly in the previous question with additional consideration of acute liver disease, histological features of chronic HBV infection, and more detailed accounts of the association with neoplasia. It would be pertinent to consider the additional consequences of delta agent infection.   *(April 1983, Paper 1, Question 1)*

Describe the pathology and aetiology of chronic active hepatitis. What laboratory tests are useful in the differential diagnosis of this condition?

The best approach would be to describe the major diagnostic features in chronic active hepatitis, the periportal inflammation with piecemeal necrosis, and the progression of the disease, describing the microscopic features in detail. Consider each of the accepted aetiologies of chronic active hepatitis; viral induced, auto-immune, drug induced and cryptogenic, and indicate the additional diagnostic features which may be of use. The laboratory tests include viral antibody studies, autoantibodies, and hypergammaglobulinaemia in true CAH, versus the findings in primary biliary cirrhosis, Wilson's disease, alpha-1-antitrypsin deficiency, sclerosing cholangitis and alcoholism.   *(April 1977, Paper 1, Question 1)*

Reference

1) Bianchi, L., Spichtin, H.P., Gudat, F. Chronic hepatitis. In: Pathology of the Liver. R.N.M. MacSween, P.P. Anthony, P.J. Scheuer (eds.). Chapter 10, p310–341. Churchill Livingstone, Edinburgh (1987).

Discuss the early diagnosis of primary biliary cirrhosis. Give an account of the natural history of the disease

Introduction

1) Primary vs. secondary disease

2) Clinical features

    a) early and late
    b) associated features
    c) biochemical tests
    d) autoantibody production

3) Aetiology

    a) ? AI disease
    b) MHC expression and 'self antigens'

4) *Pathology*

   a) early lesions
      i)   bile ducts 45 to 75 mm
      ii)   segmental distribution
      iii)   epithelial changes
      iv)   inflammatory infiltrate
      v)   granulomas
      vi)   small ductal changes (focal cell loss)
      vii) absence of bile ducts
      viii) parenchymal changes

Natural history

1) *Clinical progression*

   a) asymptomatic
   b) jaundice
   c) portal hypertension
   d) cirrhosis and liver failure

2) *Pathological evolution*

   a) inflammatory extension
      i)   limiting plate
      ii) parenchymal extension
      iii) cholangiocytic metaplasia
      iv) ductular proliferation
      v) portal-portal linkage
   b) cholestasis
      i)   periportal/paraseptal
      ii) hepatocyte changes 'cholate stasis'
      iii) Mallory bodies and copper
      iv) associated protein
   c) fibrosis
      i)   following inflammatory patterns – 'monolobular'
   d) regeneration and cirrhosis
      i)   irregular
      ii) micronodular
   e) portal hypertension
      i)   effects
   f) ?? malignant transformation

(October 1982, Paper 2, Question 2)

Reference

1) Portmann, B.C., MacSween, R.N.M. Diseases of the intrahepatic bile ducts. In: Pathology of the Liver. R.N.M. MacSween, P.P. Anthony, P.J. Scheuer (eds.) p424–436. Churchill Livingstone, Edinburgh (1987).

Discuss the mechanisms by which alcohol may produce damage to the liver

This sort of question is often a problem for histopathologists in examinations. The subject is quite complex (as is usual when the exact mechanism is not entirely clear) and requires a logical approach and good memory. The danger is the natural tendency to drift away from the mechanism (e.g. metabolic disturbance, cytoskeletal derangement, immunological injury, etc.) for each category of histological injury and start to describe the perhaps more familiar territory of histological features instead, when only brief categorisation of the alcoholic-induced injury is required.   *(April 1985, Paper 1, Question 5)*

Describe the histological features found in the liver in alcohol-induced disease

Introduction

Prevalence
Clinical features
Definition of alcoholism

1) *Fatty change*

   a) macrovesicular steatosis

   b) lipogranulomas

   c) cholestasis

2) *Alcoholic hepatitis*

   a) liver cell damage
      i)   ballooning degeneration
      ii) liver cell necrosis
      iii) Mallory body formation
   b) neutrophil infiltrate
   c) pericellular fibrosis (perivenular) – sclerosing hyaline necrosis
   d) fatty change
   e) megamitochondria
   f) cholestasis
   g) bridging hepatic necrosis

   Variable picture from minimal to fully developed disease

3) *Alcoholic cirrhosis*

   a) early micronodular
   b) late macronodular
   c) fibrosis and inflammation in septa
   d) features of alcoholic hepatitis

4) *Hepatocellular carcinoma*

    a) frequency
    b) sex incidence (M>F)

5) *Siderosis*

    a) ? heterozygotes with haemochromatosis
    b) dietary
    c) haemolysis

                                        (October 1981, Paper 1, Question 3)

References

1) Review by an International Group. Alcoholic liver disease: morphological manifestations. Lancet (1981) i: 706–711.
2) Hall, P. de la M. Alcoholic liver disease. In: Pathology of the Liver. R.N.M. MacSween, P.P. Anthony, P.J. Scheuer (eds.) 2nd edition, p281–309. Churchill Livingstone, Edinburgh (1987).

How is cirrhosis of the liver classified? Discuss the aetiology of the various types included in your classification

Some things do not change, this question being equally pertinent today, and lends itself well to a plan-style outline. There is a large amount of information to be included, and the comparison of the aetiological classification versus the morphological one may be awkward to combine, since more than one morphology is produced by the same aetiological agent, so it is better nowadays to base the classification on the aetiology, as provided in the reference.

                                        (November 1969, Paper 2, Question 3)

Reference

1) Millward-Sadler, G.H. Cirrhosis. In: Pathology of the Liver. R.N.M. MacSween, P.P. Anthony, P.J. Scheuer (eds.) 2nd edition, p342–363. Churchill Livingstone, Edinburgh (1987).

How would you try to discover the underlying cause of a granuloma found in a liver biopsy of an adult patient?

Introduction

Definition
Epithelioid vs. lipo-granuloma
Frequency
General appearances

Causes

Infection

1) *Bacterial*

    a) identification
       i) Gram (Actinomyces), Levaditi (typhoid, syphilis),
       ii) serology (Brucella)

2) *Mycobacterial*

    a) identification
       i) stains: Ziehl-Neelsen, Wade-Fite

3) *Fungal*

    a) identification
       i) stains: PAS, Grocott

4) *Viral*

    a) identification
    b) morphological pattern, nuclear features (CMV)

5) *Parasites*

    a) identification
    b) eosinophils, parasite (Toxoplasma, Leishmania & others), ova
       (Schistosoma, Fasciola & others)

6) *Rickettsia*

    a) identification
       i) (Q fever), granuloma morphology

Drugs

1) *Identification*

    a) eosinophils, history/follow up

Vasculitis

1) *Identification*

    a) clinical features

Neoplasia

1) *Identification*

    a) morphology (Hodgkin's disease), history

Foreign body

1) *Identification*

    a) stains – Sudan black (oil), (PVP), – Congo red

    b) birefringence – silica, starch, suture, barium

    c) minerals – EDAX

Miscellaneous

1) *Sarcoidosis*

    a) Kveim test
       i) identification
      ii) morphology

    b) PBC
       i) identification
      ii) morphology
     iii) serology

    c) biliary obstruction
       i) identification – bile pigment

    d) Whipple's disease
       i) portal changes
      ii) identification – stain – PAS

Idiopathic

1) *Frequency*

2) *Diagnosis of exclusion*

(November 1976, Paper 2, Question 3)

Reference

1) MacSween, R.N.M. Liver pathology associated with diseases of other organs. In: Pathology of the Liver. R.N.M. MacSween, P.P. Anthony, P.J. Scheuer (eds.) 2nd edition, p646–688. Churchill Livingstone, Edinburgh (1987).

Give an account of the pathology of: a) veno-occlusive disease of the liver b) pulmonary veno-occlusive disease

These should be straightforward accounts of two rare conditions, which have relatively different appearances despite the similarity of the names. It would be in order to describe the aetiological factors, clinical setting and complications, which would justifiably be included in the 'pathology'. The macroscopic and microscopic features are relatively limited in any case, and would probably not be sufficient to provide a full answer for the majority of candidates.

(October 1984, Paper 2, Question 5)

References

1) Bras, G., Brandt, K.H. Vascular disorders. In: Pathology of the Liver. R.N.M. MacSween, P.P. Anthony, P.J. Scheuer (eds.) 2nd edition, p485–488. Churchill Livingstone, Edinburgh (1987).
2) Dunnill, M.S. Pulmonary vascular disease. In: Pulmonary Pathology. p281–284. Churchill Livingstone, Edinburgh (1982).

Write a brief essay on the pathogenesis of primary tumours and tumour-like lesions of the liver, briefly describing the histological appearances of the conditions you mention

This is a difficult question to answer unless great care is taken to organise the essay into a review of the various hypotheses for some of the entities. In many cases, especially benign lesions, the pathogenesis is unknown, and these should be listed early on in an introductory paragraph, and then lesions which have some proposed pathogenesis concentrated on e.g. liver cell adenoma and pre-neoplastic changes, hepatocellular carcinoma and its relationship to cirrhosis, hepatitis B infection and other factors which may be related to the pathogenesis, bile duct carcinoma and liver parasitic infestation and haemangiosarcoma and vinyl chloride or arsenic. It should be noted that the question refers to pathogenesis, the mechanisms and changes which may lead to a particular disease state. It would be all too easy to start listing the epidemiological and aetiological factors in this question, without considering the way in which these agents may act. Brief descriptions of the conditions mean that no more than one or two paragraphs should be devoted to each pathology, emphasising the changes during pathogenesis rather than long descriptions of the resulting tumour.

(April 1982, Paper 2, Question 5)

Discuss the relation between hepatitis, cirrhosis and tumours of the liver

This question mainly relates to the well defined linkage and progression of some forms of hepatitis to cirrhosis and the complicating development of hepatocellular carcinoma. Other liver tumours are not clearly related to this sequence, and this should be mentioned in the opening paragraph. Consideration should be given to those forms of hepatitis which are often associated with cirrhosis (e.g. Hepatitis B infection, alcoholism, etc.) and those which do not (Hepatitis A, etc.) and how the pathology of these diseases differs. Following on from this, the relationship between Hepatitis B infection and cirrhosis requires illumination (including epidemiological studies). Some speculation on the incidence of malignant change in other forms of cirrhosis, such as alpha-1-antitrypsin deficiency, primary biliary cirrhosis, Wilson's disease, etc. would be of value.

(October 1979, Paper 1, Question 1)

Evaluate critically the factors which may be of importance in the aetiology of primary malignant tumours of the liver

This question has a somewhat broader scope than the preceding one, and in which the major emphasis should be on hepatocellular carcinoma, along with bile duct carcinoma and its association with liver flukes, inflammatory bowel disease and congenital abnormalities, haemangiosarcoma with vinyl chloride monomers, thorotrast and arsenic. Consideration of rarer entities with less well known factors (e.g. bile duct cystadenocarcinoma developing in a cystadenoma) should only be attempted if there is sufficient time, in a fully developed answer the first three groups should provide more than enough material, remembering that factors such as age, sex, genetic diseases, alcohol, carcinogens, hepatitis B virus and cirrhosis should all be included for liver cell carcinoma alone. The word critically means a weighting should be applied to the degree of importance of each aetiological factor.   (October 1978, Paper 2, Question 1)

Reference

1)   Anthony, P.P. Tumours and tumour-like lesions of the liver and biliary tract. In: Pathology of the Liver. R.N.M. MacSween, P.P. Anthony, P.J. Scheuer (eds.). 2nd edition, p574–645. Churchill Livingstone, Edinburgh (1987).

Describe the pathology of liver tumours. What is know of their aetiology and pathogenesis?

The use of the term 'tumour' is unqualified in this question, and thus there is scope for describing benign and malignant neoplasms along with 'tumour-like lesions', the groundwork for which can be laid in a sensibly outlined introduction.
                                                       (October 1988, Paper 2, Question 3)

Discuss the pathology of the intra-hepatic bile ducts

This covers a large spectrum of disease, both congenital and acquired. In order to cover the subject and avoid repetitious detail, choose the major commoner lesions in each group, and then outline the major differential diagnostic features in other conditions. Make sure the emphasis is balanced, avoiding undue emphasis in rare conditions or secondary involvement of bile ducts in hepatic disease. There is clearly no time to go into the fine detail of each disease mentioned so you would have to estimate the balance of the essay fairly closely when compiling the initial plan.   (October 1985, Paper 2, Question 3)

References

1)   Desmet, V.J. Cholestasis. In: Recent Advances in Histopathology 12. P.P. Anthony, R.N.M. MacSween (eds.) Churchill Livingstone, Edinburgh (1984).
2)   Portman, B.C., MacSween, R.N.M. Diseases of the intrahepatic bile ducts. In: Pathology of the Liver. R.N.M. MacSween, P.P. Anthony, P.J. Scheuer (eds.) 2nd edition. Churchill Livingstone, Edinburgh (1987).

Acute pancreatitis: enumerate the causes, describe the pathological features and discuss the pathogenetic mechanisms

Causes

1) Gallstones
2) Alcohol abuse
3) Hypothermia
4) Viral infection
5) Diabetes mellitus
6) Hyperparathyroidism
7) Trauma (surgery)
8) Shock
9) Gastrectomy

Pathological features

1) Macroscopic

2) Microscopic

   a) periductal
   b) perilobular
   c) panlobular

Pathogenetic mechanisms

Periductal necrosis

1) *Gallstones*
   a) common channel theory
   b) duodenal biliary reflex

   Pathogenesis – conversion of primary bile acids to 2° bile acids – role of infection and trypsin

2) *Alcohol*
   a) ductal inflammation

   Pathogenesis – via stone formation

Panlobular necrosis

1) *Hypotensive episodes*
   a) shock
   b) hypothermia
   c) surgery

Perilobular necrosis

1) _Extension of necrosis by vascular compromise_

2) _Combined aetiologies_

3) _Unknown aetiology_
a) diabetes mellitus
b) hyperparathyroidism
c) alcohol

(April 1983, Paper 3, Question 5)

Reference

1) Foulis, A.K. Gastrointestinal pathology. Acute pancreatitis. In: Recent Advances in Histopathology 12. P.P. Anthony, R.N.M. MacSween (eds.) p188–196. Churchill Livingstone, Edinburgh (1984).

5. Cardiovascular and Respiratory Systems

Discuss the contribution of bronchial biopsy and cytology in investigation of diseases of the lungs and bronchi

The most important contribution bronchial cytology and biopsy make is in diagnosis of malignant epithelial tumours. Useful cytological specimens include sputum, bronchial aspiration and washing, bronchial brushing and in certain cases trans-thoracic fine needle aspiration of bronchial and parenchymal lesions. The use of these techniques in detection of neoplastic lesions should be discussed with comments made about advantages and disadvantages of each. Biopsy specimens are especially useful in accurately diagnosing and typing bronchial tumours, again there are some limitations which should be discussed.

Other uses of cytological preparations include diagnosis of infectious disease particularly viral, parasitic and fungal, but the limitations should be highlighted. The assessment of allergic reactions in the respiratory tree can also be made cytologically. An assessment of pneumoconiosis processes may be possible by identifying the dust particles in sputum or localised collection specimens.

Biopsy uses other than malignant disease include benign neoplastic lesions and inflammatory lesions including those of an infectious nature. Transbronchial biopsies are useful to assess interstitial lung disease.

(April 1979, Paper 2, Question 4)

References

1) Churg, A. Lung biopsy handling and diagnostic limitations. In: Pathology of the Lung. W.M. Thurlock (ed.) p67–78. Thieme Medical Publications, London (1988).
2) Farrell, L., Saccommona, G. Diagnostic cytology techniques including fine needle aspiration: practical consideration. In: Pathology of the Lung. W.M. Thurlock (ed.) p105–146, Thieme Medical Publications, London (1988).

What are the mechanisms that normally present pulmonary infection? Discuss the pathogenesis of bacterial viral and fungal pneumonia in relationship to these mechanisms

Defence mechanisms

Inhaled pathogens and particulate matter

Proximal

1) *Mechanical*
    a) nasal passages
    b) mucociliary clearance proximal airways

2) Immunological mucosal defence

    a) humoral (IgA, IgE)
    b) cellular reactions
       i)   early – polymorphs, phagocytes
       ii) later – cell-mediated immunity

Distal

1) *Macrophage clearance*

2) *Mucosal and interstitial immunological defence mechanisms*

Pathogenesis of pneumonia

Bacterial

1) *Interference with normal clearing mechanisms*

    a) cough reflex
       i)   coma
       ii) anaesthesia
       iii) drugs
       iv) chest pain
       v)   neuromuscular disorders
    b) injury to mucociliary apparatus
       i)   tobacco smoke
       ii) viral diseases
       iii) inhalation of hot or corrosive gases
       iv) immobile cilia syndrome
    c) bactericidal or phagocytic action of alveolar macrophages
       i)   alcohol
       ii) tobacco smoke
       iii) anoxia
       iv) oxygen toxicity
    d) pulmonary congestion and oedema – especially important in bronchopneumonia

2) *Decreased systemic immunity*

    a) chronic diseases
    b) immunological deficiencies
       i)   congenital
       ii) acquired
    c) immunosuppressive therapy
    d) leucopenia – usually virulent organisms

Viral and fungal

Decreased immunological defence, which favours these opportunistic organisms

1) *Immunocompromisation*

   a) congenital
   b) acquired
      i)   iatrogenic (immunosuppressive therapy)
      ii) AIDS
      iii) associated with chronic disease states and disseminated malignancy
                                                    (April 1969, Paper 1, Question 3)

Reference

1) Dunnill, M.S. Pulmonary defence mechanisms. In: Pulmonary Pathology. p1–16. Churchill Livingstone, Edinburgh (1982).

Describe the various sorts of cells lining the pulmonary alveoli. How may they be altered in disease?

This question is restricted to alveolar lining cells, the type I and type II pneumocytes, the morphological, immunohistochemical and ultrastructural features of which should be described. (Neuroendocrine cells are not considered to form part of the alveolar lining.) It is generally considered that type II pneumocytes give rise to type I cells, acting as a stem cell compartment. As the type I pneumocytes are so vulnerable to injury their loss is a feature of any cause of diffuse alveolar damage (shock lung). Thus, type II hyperplasia is a non-specific reparative response to injury to type I cells. The features of diffuse alveolar damage thus need to be well described in this answer. Type II pneumocyte hyperplasia is also seen in more chronic disease states, in association with interstitial damage and disorganisation. Mention should be made of some examples such as usual interstitial pneumonia, desquamative interstitial pneumonia, alveolar proteinosis and extrinsic allergic alveolitis for instance, but it is important not to digress into descriptions of the bronchiolar and vascular changes associated with such diseases. The replacement of normal alveolar lining cells by neoplastic glandular cells in bronchioloalveolar carcinoma at the growing edge of adenocarcinomas could also be mentioned. This question is relatively stringent in its requirements and poses considerable difficulties for those who did not have particularly detailed knowledge about this subject.

(November 1977, Paper 1, Question 1)

Reference

1) Spencer, H.S. The anatomy of the lung, and various headings. In: Pathology of the Lung, 4th edition. p37–48; 726–730; 536–541; 788–798. Pergamon Press, Oxford (1985).

List the types of pulmonary emphysema. Discuss their pathogenesis

The list of the various types should include a brief explanation of the terms used but no more. This question requires a detailed consideration of the pathogenesis and it would be important not to digress into morphometry, pathological features, etc. It is the sort of question where there is not a great deal of factual information to be extracted for the average candidate to comfortably complete a 45 minute answer. *(April 1975, Paper 1, Question 4)*

References

1) Dunnill, M.S. Emphysema. In: Pulmonary Pathology. p81–112. Churchill Livingstone, Edinburgh (1982).
2) Spencer, H.S. Emphysema. In: Pathology of the Lung, 4th edition. p557–594. Pergamon Press, Oxford (1985).

How is emphysema classified and what morphometric methods are available to quantify it? Discuss the aetiology and pathogenesis

This is a fairly precise question which lends itself well to an essay plan. It should start with a definition of the term emphysema and classification into the well-recognised types with a brief explanation relating to the anatomy of the pulmonary lobule (in which diagrammatic representations may be helpful). Morphometric analysis is straightforward but the methods of lung preparation should be described in addition. The aetiology and pathogenesis, including a consideration of the role of neutrophils and anti-proteases (alpha-1-antitrypsin), have been covered in other questions. *(November 1976, Paper 2, Question 5)*

Describe the post-mortem examination of the respiratory tract in a case of chronic obstructive airways disease. How may the findings explain the patients' symptoms and signs

Introduction

Definition COAD (NB Bronchiectasis and asthma included in US but not in UK) Association of chronic bronchitis and emphysema

Emphysema

Definition

1) *Macroscopic*

   a) dissection and fixation of lungs
      i)   formal saline (under pressure)
      ii) formal vapour
   b) morphometric analysis
      i)   Gough-Wentworth slices
      ii) subgross techniques

    c) features
       i)   centrilobular
      ii) panlobular
     iii) periseptal
     iv) bullae

2) *Microscopic*

    a) features of emphysema
    b) secondary pulmonary hypertension (hypoxic type)
    c) morphometric analysis

3) *Clinicopathological correlation*

    a) panlobular
       i)   'pink puffer' – normal O_2 $\downarrow$ CO_2
      ii) $\downarrow$ alveolar surface area
     iii) V/P
     iv) $\downarrow$ elasticity leads to $\uparrow$ expiration phase
    b) centrilobular
       i)   'blue bloater' – $\downarrow$ O_2 $\uparrow$ CO_2
      ii) n alveolar surface area
     iii) $\downarrow$ alveolar ventilation
     iv) ? role of peribronchial fibrosis
    c) mixed

Chronic bronchitis

Clinical definition

1) *Macroscopic*

2) *Microscopic*

    a) goblet cell hyperplasia
    b) bronchial gland hyperplasia
    c) inflammatory pattern in bronchi/bronchioles

3) *Clinicopathological correlation – features due to*

    a) Mucous gland hypertrophy
    b) Mucus plugs
    c) Peribronchial fibrosis – cough due to
       i)   mucus over-production
      ii) ? mucosal inflammation – inflammatory mediators

(April 1988, Paper 1, Question 4)

Reference

1) Dunnill, M.S. Chronic bronchitis and emphysema. In: Pulmonary Pathology, p33–49; 81–112. Churchill Livingstone, Edinburgh (1982).

Discuss the pathogenesis and pathology of bronchiectasis

This is an example of a subject which appeared in two consecutive years, where alterations in the wording completely altered the approach to and content of the answer. In this case, after the introduction where bronchiectasis should be defined, the pathogenesis is considered under collapse of the lung parenchyma and infection. The various aetiological factors which lead to these pathways could be introduced, including obstructive lesions (bronchial tumours, mucus, foreign bodies, etc.) congenital diseases which predispose to infection (e.g. Kartagener's syndrome, immunodeficiency states, cystic fibrosis, etc.), but it is important not to become obsessed with the aetiological factors at the expense of the common pathogenetic mechanisms. The pathological features could be discussed under the classification outlined in the preceding essay plan. It is important not to digress into description of the association aetiological agents rather than concentrating on the pathology of bronchiectasis in general.   (October 1983, Paper 2, Question 1)

References

1) Dunnill, M.S. Bronchiectasis. In: Pulmonary Pathology. p67–80, Churchill Livingstone, Edinburgh (1982).
2) Robbins, S.L., Cotran, R.S., Kumar, V. Bronchiectasis. In: Pathologic Basis of Disease, 4th edition. p777–779. WB Saunders, Philadelphia (1989).

How would you classify the different types of bronchiectasis and what are the pathological consequences of this condition?

Introduction

Definition
Associations
Clinical features

Classification

Congenital – Williams-Campbell syndrome
Acquired – Whitwell

Pathological features of each group

1) Saccular

    a) lower lobes (L>R)

    b) distal to 3/4 segmental branches

    c) macroscopic features

2) Atelectasis

    a) R middle commonest

    b) all segmental branches

    c) usually obstruction (e.g. ca, lymph nodes, etc.)

3) *Follicular*

    a) lymphoid infiltrate and follicles
    b) otherwise resembles saccular type

Pathological consequences

1) *Infection*

    a) recurrent bronchopneumonia
    b) pulmonary abscess/emphysema
    c) infective endocarditis
    d) 'metastatic' abscess

2) *Pulmonary fibrosis*

3) *Mucosal ulceration*

    a) squamous metaplasia
    b) haemorrhage

4) *Pulmonary hypertension*

    a) hypoxic
    b) obstructive (fibrotic)

5) *Hypertrophic osteoarthropathy*

6) *Amyloidosis*

    a) reactive systemic

(April 1984, Paper 2, Question 1)

Reference

1) Dunnill, M.S. Bronchiectasis. In: Pulmonary Pathology. p67–80. Churchill Livingstone, Edinburgh (1982).

What are the causes of pulmonary hypertension? Describe the pathological changes which are seen in the lungs

Introduction

Pulmonary circulation
Definition of pulmonary hypertension
Clinical features

Major causes

1) *Increased blood flow*

   a) pre tricuspid shunt
      i)   ASD
      ii) TAPVD
   b) post tricuspid shunt
      i)   VSD (cong)
      ii) PDA
      iii) Transposition

2) *Pulmonary venous congestion*

   a) severe LVF
   b) mitral valve stenosis/regurgitation
   c) L atrial myxoma
   d) pulmonary venous compression
   e) pulmonary veno-occlusive disease

3) *Pulmonary arterial obstruction*

   a) recurrent thromboembolism
   b) emboli (e.g. tumour, particulate material in drug abuse, schistosomal ova)

4) *Alveolar hypoxia*

   a) high altitude
   b) upper airway obstruction
   c) lower airway obstruction (chronic asthma, chronic bronchitis)
   d) obesity (Pickwickian syndrome)

5) *Destruction of distal capillary bed*

   a) interstitial lung disease
   b) emphysema

6) *Idiopathic*

   a) primary pulmonary HT

7) *Miscellaneous*

   a) hepatic disease/portal HT
   b) collagen vascular disease
   c) drugs

Pathological changes

1) *Macroscopic*

   a) pulmonary atheroma
   b) focal interstitial haemorrhage
   c) changes of underlying disease

2) *Microscopic*

   a) Reversible changes
      Grade I   – hypertrophy muscular pulmonary arteries
                – muscularisation of arterioles (<100µm vessels)
      Grade II – I and internal cellular proliferation in small arteries (smooth
                muscle)
      Grade III – II and lamellar fibrosis
                – obliterative lesions in muscular arteries
   b) Irreversible changes
      Old grades IV – VI

3) *Dilatation lesions*

   a) associations
      i)   primary pulmonary HT
      ii) congenital heart disease
      iii) hepatic cirrhosis
   b) pathological features
      i)   venous-like branches
      ii) plexiform lesions
      iii) angiomatoid lesions

4) *Late sequelae*

   a) fibrinoid vasculosis/necrosis
   b) interstitial haemorrhage/fibrosis

(April 1983, Paper 2, Question 4)

References

1) Dunnill, M.S. Pulmonary pathology. In: Pulmonary Vascular Disease. Chapter 14, p245–292. Churchill Livingstone, Edinburgh (1982).
2) Spencer, H.S. Chronic pulmonary hypertension. In: Pathology of the Lung, 4th edition, p631–704. Pergamon Press, Oxford (1985).

Discuss the causes of pulmonary hypertension, describe the histopathological features of the lungs in this condition
(April 1977, Paper 1, Question 5)

What pathological changes may be induced in the pulmonary arterial tree by diseases of the heart and lungs. How may these changes influence the clinical course of the predisposing disease?

This question requires a description of the pathological changes of pulmonary hypertension (see April 1983, Paper 2, Question 4). The changes of pulmonary hypertension induce a compensatory hypertrophy of the right ventricle, which may result in terminal right sided cardiac failure. In cases where cardiac shunts have resulted in pulmonary hypertension, the shunt may ultimately reverse with increased load on both ventricles which speeds the path to failure. Brief comments may be made about the exact changes induced by the pulmonary hypertension for the separate aetiological groups.   *(April 1972, Paper 1, Question 1)*

Discuss the aetiology of chronic pulmonary hypertension and describe the pathological changes that may be found in the lungs

As there are so many causes of pulmonary hypertension, it is doubtful whether any candidate could attempt to provide a comprehensive list, but all three questions on this subject allow for some selective expansion of various aspects, and particular attention might be paid to be differences between the changes found in chronic hypoxia, in severe pulmonary venous hypertension (e.g. tight mitral stenosis), and in the rather restricted group of conditions leading to plexogenic pulmonary arteriopathy, areas which cause particular confusion. Note also that while the Heath and Edwards Grades 1–3 still reflect increasing severity of disease, Grades 4 and 5 are not found in all conditions and Grade 6 (necrotising arteries) indicates severe and/or prolonged disease which is irreversible and so the changes in these grades are not necessarily sequential.
                                                (April 1976, Paper 2, Question 5)

References

1) Dunnill, M.S. Pulmonary vascular disease. In: Pulmonary Pathology. Chapter 14. Churchill Livingstone, Edinburgh (1982).
2) Spencer, H.S. Chronic pulmonary hypertension. In: Pathology of the Lung. 4th edition. p631–704. Pergamon Press, Oxford (1985).

Describe the histological features and pathogenesis of the plexiform lesion in the lung. In what conditions does it occur? What are its prognostic implications when found in a lung biopsy specimen

This is a much more specific question on pulmonary hypertension, and requires a detailed consideration of the conditions associated with this lesion, usually post-tricuspid shunts in congenital heart disease, primary pulmonary hypertension and pulmonary hypertension associated with cirrhosis. It is useful to describe the associated changes of pulmonary hypertension (as outlined previously) is that the pathogenesis of the plexiform lesion, a cellular intimal proliferation, can be explained.   *(April 1987, Paper 2, Question 1)*

References

1) Spencer, H.S. Chronic pulmonary hypertension. In: Pathology of the Lung. 4th edition. p631–704. Pergamon Press, Oxford (1985).

Discuss the criteria for a pathological diagnosis of cor pulmonale. Describe the changes in the pulmonary vasculature and how you would assess their severity at autopsy

The introduction to such an answer requires a definition of the term cor pulmonale, and its clinical setting. The criteria for the pathological diagnosis should be outlined, and in particular the practical measures necessary in the accurate measurement of right ventricular weight. The effects of right ventricular failure should also be mentioned (e.g. in the liver) The question does not call for a discussion of the numerous causes of cor pulmonale, but there needs to be some consideration of the various causes of pulmonary hypertension, both hypoxic and primary vascular types. The assessment at autopsy includes both macroscopic and microscopic features.   *(October 1980, Paper 2, Question 3)*

Reference

1) Dunnill, M.S. Pulmonary vascular disease. In: Pulmonary Pathology. p245–292. Churchill Livingstone, Edinburgh (1982).

Give a concise account of those diseases of lung parenchyma which are brought about by occupation

The bulk of the answer should be concerned with those diseases caused by dust inhalation and noxious fumes. The ducts could be divided into the inorganic (e.g. silicosis (acute and chronic), coal-miner's pneumoconiosis, asbestosis and berylliosis among others) and organic (extrinsic allergic alveolitis, e.g. farmer's lung, bagassosis). Noxious fumes include cadmium, bauxite and gases Development of bronchial carcinoma (e.g. in uranium mining or asbestosis) does not strictly fall within the bounds of a parenchymal disease, but pulmonary adenocarcinoma in asbestosis would be a justifiable inclusion. Likewise mesothelioma is not a parenchymal disease, and only brief mention should be made. Note that the question indicates that all of the occupation diseases require consideration, instead of describing one in detail from each group and mentioning the main differences in the remainder.   *(October 1979, Paper 1, Question 3)*

Reference

1) Spencer, H. The pneumoconioses and other occupational lung diseases. In: Pathology of the Lung, 4th edition. Chapter 11, p413–450. Pergamon Press, Oxford (1985).

What is meant by extrinsic allergic alveolitis? Give an account of the pathology of this condition

Introduction

EAA (Hypersensitivity pneumonitis)

Provoking antigens a) thermophilic actinomycetes (e.g. farmer's lung)
                    b) moulds (e.g. suberosis)
                    c) animal proteins (e.g. bird fancier's lung)

Clinical features

Relapsing acute condition on exposure
Chronic interstitial disease

Pathological features

1) *Acute*

   a) unknown

2) *Subacute*

   a) miliary nodules
      i)   epithelioid granulomas
      ii)   bronchiolar damage and obstruction
      iii) foamy intra-alveolar macrophages
      iv)   interstitial inflammatory infiltration
      v)   crystalline intracellular inclusions

3) *Chronic*

   a) fibrosis and obliterated airspaces
   b) 'honeycomb' lung
   c) diffuse interstitial fibrosis
   d) few subacute changes
   e) pulmonary vascular disease

Pathogenesis

1) *Antigen in wall of bronchioles*

2) *IgG in plasma cells*

3) *C3 in histiocytes*

   a) ? complement activation via alternative pathway unlike type III
      hypersensitivity
   b) ? type IV reaction – T lymphocytes in alveoli
   c) ? granulomatous disease resulting from lymphokine release

(May 1973, Paper 2, Question 5)

References

1) Dunnill, H.S. Extrinsic allergic alveolitis. In: Pulmonary Pathology. p113–124.
    Churchill Livingstone, Edinburgh (1982).
2) Spencer, H.S. The pneumoconioses and other occupational lung diseases. In:
    Pathology of the Lung, 4th edition. p497–510. Pergamon Press, Oxford (1985).

Describe the changes found in the lung in fibrosing alveolitis and extrinsic allergic alveolitis. What mechanisms may be involved in the causation of these diseases?

Most of the information is contained within the two preceding essay plans. The mechanisms involved in both diseases appear to have a very similar immunological basis, at least in the light of current knowledge, although extrinsic allergic alveolitis has a more acute course in general than the insidious progress of fibrosing alveolitis.   *(April 1975, Page 2, Question 2))*

Describe the gross and microscopic features of pulmonary fibrosing alveolitis and discuss the pathogenic mechanisms

Introduction

Definition of terms
Variants (DIP, VIP, LIP, etc)

Macroscopic features

1) *Early*

   a) parenchymal fibrous thickening

2) *Late*

   a) bilateral shrunken, firm lungs
   b) bosselated pleural surface
   c) loss of normal pattern with enlarged airspaces bound by fibrous tissue – 'honeycomb' lung

Microscopic features

Patchy process, both inter and intra-lobular

1) *Early*

   a) ? diffuse alveolar damage or interstitial disease

2) *Established*

   a) interstitial fibrosis
   b) chronic inflammation
   c) smooth muscle hyperplasia
   d) metaplastic changes
       i)   type II pneumocyte hyperplasia
       ii) bronchiolar-type columnar
   e) hyaline membranes +/- alveolar macrophages
   f) pulmonary hypertensive vascular changes

Pathogenesis

1) *Aetiology*

a) unknown

2) *Genetic influences (M>F)*

3) *Immunological factors*

a) increased circulating immune complexes
b) cryoglobulinaemia
c) IgG (granular) in septal wall
d) associations
   i)   RA
   ii) SLE
   iii) systemic sclerosis

4) *Complexed antigen unknown*

5) *Broncho-alveolar lavage – increased neutrophil count*

6) *Possible sequence*

a) intrapulmonary accumulation of immune complexes
b) macrophage activation
c) neutrophil chemotaxis
d) protease release
e) death of type I pneumocytes
f) structural damage and regenerative changes

(November 1976, Page 2, Question 4)

References

1) Robbins, S.L., Cotran, R.S., Kumar, V. The respiratory system. In: Pathologic Basis of Disease, 4th edition. p789–793. W.B. Saunders, Philadelphia (1989).
2) Dunnill, M.S. Pulmonary fibrosis. In: Pulmonary Pathology. p216–244. Churchill Livingstone, Edinburgh (1982).

Discuss the pathogenic mechanisms involved in diffuse pulmonary fibrosis

Diffuse pulmonary fibrosis is a non-specific reaction to injury of the lung and is associated with a wide range of diseases and injurious agents. The pathogenic mechanisms are poorly understood, however the best method to cover what is known is to use a classification of interstitial fibrosis and consider the mechanisms for each. The idiopathic group (usual interstitial pneumonia or fibrosing alveolitis) has been considered in the answers previously on this subject (see November 1976, Paper 2, Question 4). Those pulmonary interstitial fibroses where aetiological factors are known, and pathogenic mechanisms may be better understood, include drug reactions (especially chemotherapeutic agents), diffuse pulmonary infections (viruses, mycoplasma), industrial or environmental inhalants (especially asbestos) and the interstitial changes seen in collagen-vascular diseases. Comments can be made about each of these in turn, using them to highlight possible pathogenic mechanisms. It is important to only consider states resulting in diffuse pulmonary fibrosis, and although there is a temptation to include the pneumoconiosis group, apart from pulmonary asbestosis these diseases tend to result in parenchymal nodules of varying size, thus the changes are not diffuse. Extrinsic allergic alveolitis may result in a diffuse interstitial fibrosis and can be considered in the environmental inhalant group.

(April 1980, Paper 2, Question 3)

Describe the pathological features of adult shock lung syndrome and discuss their pathogenesis

Introduction

1) *Definition*

   a) non-specific but predictable sequence of events
   b) aetiologies

Pathological changes

1) *Acute exudative phase (up to 7 days)*

   Early
   a) oedema – interstitial/alveolar
   b) alveolar haemorrhage/fibrin deposition

   Intermediate
   a) 'hyaline' membrane (pneumocyte necrosis/fibrin)
   b) interstitial infiltrate – lymphocytes, plasma cells, macrophages
   c) capillary/small arterial thrombi

   Late
   a) type II pneumocyte hyperplasia
   b) squamous metaplasia of regenerative bronchiolar epithelium

2) *Organising phase (7–14 days)*

   Early
   a) loose interstitial fibrosis
   b) macrophage digestion of hyaline membrane
   c) florid type II pneumocyte hyperplasia
   d) focal alveolar fibrosis

Late
a) interstitial expansion by fibrosis
b) distortion of air spaces
c) progression to chronic phase or
d) resolution

Pathogenesis

Toxic injury to pneumocytes and/or capillary endothelium

1) *Aetiological agents*

   a) infection – virus, mycoplasma
   b) inhaled gases– oxygen, nitrogen, sulphur dioxide, smoke, or other noxious fumes
   c) drugs – narcotics, paraquat, chemotherapy
   d) 'shock' states – septicaemia, injury etc.
   e) miscellaneous – radiation, high altitude, uraemia, aspiration pneumonitis

2) *Mechanisms*

   a) superoxide radicals
      i) oxygen toxicity
      ii) paraquat
   b) neutrophil aggregation in capillaries

Postulated sequence:– complement activation (sepsis, bacterial toxin, bypass surgery, etc.) → leucocyte aggregation/activation → free radical generation and enzymes → vascular permeability → interstitial oedema → protease digestion of interstitium → pneumocyte death and fibrin formation.

Also microthrombosis due to kinin activation/prostaglandin release.

(April 1985, Paper 1, Question 2)

References

1) Dunnill, M.S. Pulmonary oedema and shock lung. In: Pulmonary Pathology. p17–32. Churchill Livingstone, Edinburgh (1982).
2) Robbins, S.L., Cotran, R.S., Kumar, V. The respiratory system. In: Pathologic Basis of Disease, 4th edition. p760–762. W.B. Saunders, Philadelphia (1989).

Describe the various lesions which may be produced in the lungs by therapy including drugs, and by other toxic chemical substances of a non-particulate nature

This question primarily calls for a consideration of diffuse alveolar damage (shock lung) and the more chronic process of diffuse pulmonary interstitial fibrosis, despite the initial impression that there might be a wide spectrum of diseases to consider. Both are associated with drugs, (including chemotherapeutic agents, antibiotics, penicillamine) medical radiation and gas inhalation (both therapeutic, e.g. oxygen, or toxic, e.g. sulphur dioxide). The pathological features are described in the preceding two answers.   *(November 1973, Paper 1, Question 1)*

Describe the possible effects on the lungs of exposure to asbestos. What are the medicolegal complications?

In the introduction the point should be made that the pleura do not strictly form part of the lungs, and a decision has to be made about whether to include these effects in the answer. Most authorities would accept that the pleura would be considered a part of the lungs, just as the bronchi would be also. The types of asbestos should be described, and then descriptions made of the various pathologies, including pulmonary fibrosis, and bronchial carcinoma, pleural plaques, pleural effusion and malignant mesothelioma. The medicolegal implications result from the compensation payable to victims and dependents, and are affected by the diagnostic acumen of the pathologist, especially in the assessment of interstitial fibrosis. The role of the Pneumoconiosis Medical Panel should also be considered.   *(April 1988, Paper 2, Question 1)*

Reference

1) Gibbs, A.R. Industrial lung disease. In: Recent Advances in Histopathology 13. P.P. Anthony, R.N.M. MacSween (eds.) p109–117. Churchill Livingstone, Edinburgh (1987).

What detailed and logical arguments could you use to convince a sceptical scientist of a causal relationship between smoking and lung disease?

Since 1971 there has been overwhelming evidence for this linkage from epidemiological and experimental studies, and it is unlikely that the sceptical scientist still exists.   *(November 1971, Paper 1, Question 2)*

'While many pulmonary cancers consist predominantly, sometimes exclusively, of growth of a particular type, it must be emphasised that there is only one entity, carcinoma of the lung' (Willis, 1960). Discuss this statement with reference to aetiology, pathogenesis and classification of lung cancer.

Behind this question lies a paper in the Journal of Pathology (Gatter et al., 1986) suggesting that, because careful examination of lung carcinomas reveals evidence of differentiation along most of the lineages represented in pulmonary malignancy, these tumours arise from a pluripotential stem cell. Thus there is 'only one entity' but showing cell lineage representation in differing amounts.

Introduction

Observation confined to carcinomas
Classifications – morphological (WHO)
Histogenesis – definition – relation to differentiation
Differentiation – definition – relation to morphology

Classification (WHO)

Squamous cell carcinoma

1) *Microscopic*

   a) 1 or more features of squamous differentiation

2) *Aetiology*

   a) tobacco
   b) radiation

3) *Pathogenesis*

   a) squamous metaplasia carcinogens in tobacco

4) *Behaviour*

Adenocarcinoma

1) *Microscopic*

   a) glandular differentiation +/- mucin production
   b) ? scar cancer
   c) peripheral vs. hilar

2) *Aetiology*

   a) tobacco
   b) pulmonary scarring – diffuse and ? focal

3) *Pathogenesis*

   a) scarring may increase epithelial turnover
   b) susceptible to carcinogenesis

4) *Behaviour*

   a) solid vs. bronchioloalveolar

Small cell (oat cell) carcinoma

1) *Microscopic*

   a) oat cell, intermediate, mixed, ultrastructure

2) *Functional characteristics*

3) *Aetiology*

   a) tobacco
   b) radiation

4) *Behaviour*

Large cell carcinoma

1) *Distinction from above groups*

Others

1) *Evidence for single entity*

   a) mixed carcinomas and tumour heterogeneity (LM)
   b) ultrastructural heterogeneity
   c) the ideal evidence would be a cloned cell line(s) with ability to differentiate along any lineage!

2) *Evidence against*

   a) differences in behaviour – clinical and metastatic pattern
   b) chemotherapeutic responses
   c) lack of pluripotential cloned cell line

(April 1986, Paper 1, Question 4)

References

1) Lamb, D. Lung cancer and its classification. In: Recent Advances in Histopathology 13. P.P. Anthony, R.N.M. MacSween (eds.) p45–59 (1987).
2) Gatter, K.C. et al. Human lung tumours: a correlation of antigenic profile with histological type. Histopathology (1985) 9: 805–823.

Write an essay on small cell (oat cell) carcinoma of the lung

Introduction

Definition of terms
Incidence
Relation to other lung carcinomas

Aetiology

1) *Tobacco*

2) *Radiation*

Clinical features

1) Pulmonary carcinoma presentation

2) Spread

3) Prognosis

4) Ectopic hormone

   a) ACTH – Cushing's
   b) ADH – hyponatraemia
   c) 5HT – carcinoid syndrome

Macroscopic

1) Site

   a) bronchial wall

2) Size, colour, infiltration

3) Spread

   a) local
   b) nodal

Microscopic

1) Cellular

   a) nuclear
   b) cytoplasmic
   c) classification – oat, intermediate, mixed

2) Stroma

   a) vasculature
   b) haematoxyphilic fibre staining ('Azzopardi' effect)

3) Special stains

   a) argyrophilia (rare)
   b) immunostaining
       i)   chromogranin
       ii)   ACTH
       iii) Cytokeratin
       iv) LCA (negative)
       v)   others

4) Cytological diagnosis

   5) *Ultrastructure*
- a) neuroendocrine granules
- b) paranuclear intermediate filaments
- c) lack of desmosomes

Differential diagnosis

1) *Atypical carcinoid*

2) *Poorly differentiated squamous carcinoma*

3) *Lymphoma*

4) *Mixed pulmonary carcinoma*

Spread

1) *Local*

2) *Nodal*

3) *Dissemination*
- a) liver – sinusoidal infiltration
- b) brain
- c) adrenal (>50%)
- d) bone marrow – osteoblastic/fibroblastic response

(April 1985, Paper 2, Question 2)

Reference

1) Spencer, H. Carcinoma of the lung. In: Pathology of the Lung, 4th edition. p837–932. Pergamon Press, Oxford (1985).

Give an account of the changes that you would expect to find in the heart and systemic vasculature at necropsy in a case of coarctation of the aorta

It would first be advisable to clarify the major differences between so-called 'infantile' and 'adult' forms of coarctation, a situation where diagrammatic comparison would definitely enhance the answer. In the main part of the answer, it would be reasonable to assume that the case was untreated, or succumbed to known complications such as infective 'endocarditis'. As well as the effects on the heart and pressure effects on vessels, it is important to remember to include associated congenital defects such as berry aneurysms, other forms of congenital heart disease and association such as Turner's syndrome. In the more protracted distal (postductal) forms, aortic aneurysmal dilatation and dissection may develop, as well as atherosclerosis, complications which all require description.

Some comment should also be made on the vessels distal to the coarctation, with a brief description of the microscopic structure of the coarctation.

(April 1987, Paper 2, Question 3)

References

1) Robbins, S.L., Cotran, R.S., Kumar, V. The heart -- congenital heart disease. In: Pathologic Basis of Disease, 4th edition. p618–626. W.B. Saunders, Philadelphia (1989).
2) Berry C.L. Congenital heart disease. In: Paediatric Pathology, p63–123. Springer-Verlag, Berlin (1989).

Describe the effects of sustained systemic hypertension on blood vessels

This answer requires a definition of hypertension with some general epidemiological and clinical features to provide a broad introduction. The remainder of such an essay would be very straightforward and logical, to consider the macroscopic and microscopic features affecting large elastic arteries, large and small muscular arteries, and arterioles in turn. Although atherosclerosis should be considered and described, it would be important not to digress too much into this subject. Malignant (accelerated) hypertension should also be described in detail, as it affects the smaller calibre vessels in particular.

(May 1973, Paper 2, Question 1)

Reference

1) Robbins, S.L., Cotran, R.S., Kumar, V. The kidney. In: Pathologic Basis of Disease, 4th edition. p1062–1069. W.B. Saunders, Philadelphia (1989).

Discuss the pathogenesis of atherosclerosis

Introduction

Definition
Epidemiology, historical and current concepts
Clinical and experimental observations
'Response to injury' hypothesis

Pathological observations

1) Atheroma

   a) macroscopic
   b) microscopic
      i) fibrolipid plaque

2) *'Precursor' lesions*
  a) fatty streak
  b) features against precursor status
      i)   ubiquitous occurrence
      ii) distribution and location
      iii) lipid content – cholesterol oleate vs. linoleate
  c) unknown role
  d) gelatinous lesion
      i)   pathology
      ii) composition – LBL and fibrinogen – little cholesterol

Historical theories

1) *Insudation (Virchow)*

2) *Encrustation (Rokitansky)*
  a) endothelial injury

'Risk factors' and endothelial injury

1) *Smoking*

2) *Hypertension*

3) *Diabetes mellitus*

4) *Hyperlipidaemia*

Role of plasma lipids

1) *High risk*
  a) LDL and VLDL

2) *Low risk*
  a) HDL

3) *Familial/epidemiological studies and risk*

Pathogenesis

1) *Endothelial injury and platelet deposition*

2) *Release of PGDF*
  a) platelets
  b) activated macrophages

3) *Migration of smooth muscle cells*

4) *Insudation of plasma lipids*

Progression

1) *Persistent endothelial injury*

2) *Hyperlipidaemic states*

Complications

1) *Ulceration and thrombosis*

2) *Ischaemia, embolism*

Monoclonal theory of Benditt

1) *G6PD 'clonality'*

2) *Recent evidence ? oligoclonal*

(October 1982, Paper 1, Question 4)

References

1) Ross, R. The pathogenesis of atherosclerosis – an update. New Engl. J. Med. (1986) 314: 488–499.
2) Martinet, Y., et al. Activated human monocytes express the c-sis proto-oncogene and release a mediator showing PDGF-like activity. Nature (1986) 519: 158–160.
3) Taussig, M.J. Processes in Pathology and Microbiology. 2nd edition. p649–672. Blackwell Scientific Publications, Oxford (1984).

Describe current views in the pathogenesis of atherosclerosis
(October 1980, Paper 1, Question 1)

Discuss the current views on the relationship between lipids and atherosclerosis

This essay would provide an opportunity to go into more detail on the pathological and epidemiological data, as well as outlining the pathogenetic mechanisms. There is still a large amount of factual information to be compressed into this essay, which should be kept as succinct and relevant as possible.

(April 1971, Paper 1, Question 2)

The geographical variations in the incidence of a disease may be of significance. Discuss this statement in relation to ischaemic heart disease

One of the more uncommon type of questions which is largely based on epidemiology, but nevertheless relevant as pathologists have a major responsibility in the assessment of the prevalence and severity of ischaemic heart disease by ensuring detailed necropsy information is available and more importantly in the accurate death certification from which this may be assessed. In the specific answer much of the detailed pathological information is presented in the previous questions on atherosclerosis, but in this case it should be presented in the light of the social and epidemiological data available, such as differences in smoking habits, diet, possible genetic differences, etc. This information is largely derived from national studies (e.g. Scotland vs. England, Japan vs. US) and from intensive population studies, such as the Framingham experiment. It may be difficult for some pathologists to concentrate sufficient information in this sort of answer, unless they have experience of integrating epidemiological and pathological data.   *(November 1988, Paper 1, Question 3)*

References

1) Kaunel, W.B., Thom, T.J. Implication of the declining mortality rate of cardiovascular disease in the USA. In: Recent Advances in Cardiology, Volume 10 p49–69. D.J. Rowlands (ed.) Churchill Livingstone (1987).
2) Stebbens, W.E. An appraisal of the epidemic rise of coronary heart disease and its decline. Lancet (1987) i: 606–611.

Discuss the aetiology and pathology of aneurysms

Introduction

Definition
Sites
Incidence and aetiologies

Aorta and major vessels

1) Atherosclerotic

    a) aetiological factors
    b) haemodynamic effects
    c) pathology
       i)   gross
       ii) microscopic
       iii) complications

2) Luetic

    a) aetiology (tertiary syphilis)
    b) pathology
       i)   gross
       ii) microscopic
       iii) complications

3) _Dissecting_

   a) aetiology (trauma, atherosclerosis, cystic medial degeneration, hypertension)
   b) gross
   c) microscopic

Cerebral arteries

1) _'Berry' aneurysm_

   a) gross
   b) microscopic
   c) complications

Other sites

1) _Infective_

   a) localised suppuration
   b) embolic

2) _Vasculitis_

   a) PAN
   b) Kawasaki disease (coronary)

3) _Rarely_

   a) post radiation
   b) surgery
   c) neoplastic invasion

                                        (November 1970, Paper 2, Question 1)

Reference

1) Robbins, S.L., Cotran, R.S., Kumar, V. Blood vessels. In: Pathologic Basis of Disease, 4th edition. p579–585. W.B. Saunders, Philadelphia (1989).

Describe how you would examine the atrioventricular bundle. What changes may be found in the bundle in heart block?

This question requires the candidate to be familiar with a method of examining the cardiac conduction system, from the atrioventricular node to the bundle branches. A good method is described in the reference.

One way is to take a block of tissue including low interatrial septum and upper interventricular septum at autopsy. This is divided horizontally below the tricuspid valve ring. The upper block is sectioned vertically, while the lower is sectioned horizontally. This will require hand processing. Every 30 sections are then examined, keeping the intervening sections to examine if required. The upper block will contain the AV node and proximal atrioventricular bundle, while the lower block features the more distal bundle and its branches. It is much easier to answer this question with personal experience. The changes which may be found in heart block are manifold. The main ones include idiopathic bundle branch fibrosis (three types A, B and C) ischaemic destruction of bundle (usually associated with a large septal myocardial infarct), myocarditis, heavy calcification of mitral and/or aortic valve rings, syphilitic gumma, fibrosis occurring in association with connective tissue diseases, amyloidosis, haemochromatosis, 'interatrial mesothelioma', metastatic carcinoma, lymphoma/leukaemia tissue infiltrates and fibrosis in cardiomyopathy. These can all be briefly described. However, this is regarded as a particularly difficult examination question for the average candidate.   *(April 1972, Paper 2, Question 2)*

Reference

1) Lamb, D. Examination of the conducting system. In: Pathology of the Heart. A. Pomerance, M.J. Davies (eds.) p26–31. Blackwell Scientific Publications, Oxford (1975).

Discuss the changing pattern of infective endocarditis
April 1970, Paper 2, Question 2

Give an account of the changing pattern of infective endocarditis

It is important to point out that much of the change relates to Western countries, where there has been a shift from the young adult with rheumatic heart disease to older adults with normal or slightly abnormal valves, with reduced distinction between acute and subacute endocarditis. Another factor has been the emergence of unusual forms of endocarditis with increasing foreign travel and immunosuppressive treatment regimes.   *(April 1980, Paper 1, Question 4)*

Reference

1) Pomerance, A. Infective and non-bacterial thrombotic endocarditis. In: Pathology of the Heart. A. Pomerance, M.J. Davies (eds.) p343–366. Blackwell Scientific Publications, Oxford (1975).

Discuss the aetiology and pathology of conditions causing functional disturbance of the mitral valve

This question could either be approached from the point of view of the pathologies leading to stenosis, regurgitation, or both, or from an anatomical point of view, such as abnormalities of the valve leaflet, chordae tendinae, papillary muscles, mitral valve annulus or generalised cardiac disease. From a practical point of view the first approach is probably simpler, and it would be possible to divide each section into possible causes, congenital and acquired. It would be a mistake to concentrate purely on diseases of the valve only, such as rheumatic heart disease or mucoid degeneration, without including the many disorders of the endocardium (e.g. endocardial fibroelastosis) or myocardium (e.g. ischaemic rupture of papillary muscle, cardiomyopathies, etc.) which can interfere with normal function. It is important to place the correct emphasis on each condition according to its relative frequency and morbidity in clinical practice (e.g. overemphasising congenital fibroelastosis at the expense of rheumatic heart disease).   *(October 1984, Paper 1, Question 3)*

Reference

1)   Davies, M.J. Non-rheumatic disorders of the heart valves. In: Recent Advances in Histopathology 10. p139–158. Churchill Livingstone, Edinburgh (1978).

Give an account of the changing patterns in the United Kingdom of the pathology of mitral incompetence

It is best to define what is understood by mitral incompetence (generally regurgitation) prior to a general overview of the disease prevalence in the population. Note that the question does not ask for detailed description of the pathology (which can be mentioned briefly however), but for the patterns of disease, i.e. aetiology and to a lesser extent pathogenesis. The major shifts have been in rheumatic heart disease and a lesser rise in ischaemic heart disease and its complications, and a rise in infective endocarditis due to several factors which all require detailing. Those conditions which have remained relatively static should also be mentioned (e.g. floppy valve, congenital heart disease, etc.). This is a deceptively difficult question to answer in as much as there remains a great temptation to digress into detailed pathological description.
(April 1982, Paper 1, Question 5)

Reference

1)   Davies, M.J. Non-rheumatic disorders of the heart valves. In: Recent Advances in Histopathology 10. p139–158. Churchill Livingstone, Edinburgh (1978).

Write an account of the non-rheumatic lesions of the aortic valve

This essay requires an introduction which covers the prevalence of these disorders in the population, and a consideration of the clinical features including sudden death. It would be best to describe the major congenital abnormalities first, then consider the acquired disorders in various age groups, including a description of aetiology, pathogenesis and complication as well as the pathological features. Disorders such as aortic root dilatation, which are technically part of the functioning valve, could also be included.   *(October 1982, Paper 2, Question 3)*

Write an essay on tricuspid valve disease of the heart

The main feature of tricuspid valve disease is that it is much less common than diseases involving the mitral and aortic valves, much of this difference relates to the lower pressures in the right side of the heart. Congenital abnormalities of the tricuspid valve should be considered first, and then the rare diseases which primarily involve the tricuspid valve. Carcinoid heart disease and infective endocarditis in intravenous drug abusers are the two main disease processes. Libman-Sacks endocarditis seen in patients with systemic lupus erythematosus, rheumatic heart disease, non-bacterial thrombotic and infective endocarditis and mucoid degeneration are all conditions which occur in association with similar and sometimes more severe changes in the mitral valve. Tricuspid valve involvement in the rare restrictive cardiomyopathies, endomyocardial fibrosis, Loeffler's syndrome and endocardial fibroelastosis would also be included in a comprehensive answer.   *(November 1972, Page 2, Question 5)*

References

1) Pomerance, A. Chronic, rheumatic and other inflammatory valve disease; and rarities and miscellaneous endocardial abnormalities. In: Pathology of the Heart. A. Pomerance, M.J. Davies (eds.) p313–4; 504–7. Blackwell Scientific Publications, Oxford (1975).
2) Robbins, S.L., Cotran, R.S., Kumar, V. The heart. In: Pathologic Basis of Disease, 4th edition. p626–640. W.B. Saunders, Philadelphia (1989).

Describe critically the examination of the heart in cases of sudden death

This question requires an introduction defining the meaning of sudden death, and a consideration of the major cases where the heart is primarily involved. The word critically is included to indicate that a flexible approach is necessary to enable the demonstration of the various causes which may be obscured if a standard protocol is followed without due regard to clues which may be gathered during the course of the examination. It is therefore probably best to list the cause as primary cardiac sudden death, and then describe how the changes may be manifest at each stage of the examination, and how it might alter the direction of the dissection. The main stages are: a) in situ and pericardial inspection, b) external examination, c) valve inspection, d) right atrium and ventricle, e) coronary circulation, f) left atrium, g) left ventricle, h) conducting system.   *(April 1986, Paper 1, Question 3)*

Reference

1) Davies, M.J., Anderson, R.H. Pathology of the conducting system. In: Pathology of the Heart. A. Pomerance, M.J. Davies (eds.) p404–406. Blackwell Scientific Publications, Oxford (1975).

Describe the pathology of subendocardial myocardial necrosis and discuss its pathogenesis

The introduction to this essay must define precisely what is meant by the term subendocardial myocardial necrosis, and its major associations. Pathological considerations also include the clinical features and conditions which may predispose to left ventricular hypertrophy. The macroscopic appearances with detailed description of the acute and chronic forms, macroscopic demonstration of the necrosis, together with the microscopic appearances and evolution of the lesion all require description along with the complications that may occur such as papillary muscle rupture, thrombus formation, etc. In respect of the pathogenesis, the normal high metabolic demand of the subendocardial myocytes needs to be emphasised and that they are compromised in hypertrophic states, hypercirculation for any cause, or susceptibility to metabolic disturbance and how vascular compromise may tip the balance. This should provide material for a relatively circumscribed essay. Much of the detail would already be familiar to a pathologist who has performed necropsies on patients with sudden death.

(October 1983, Paper 2, Question 2)

Reference

1) Davies, M.J. Pathology of ischaemic heart disease. In: Recent Advances in Histopathology 13. P.P. Anthony, R.N.M. MacSween (eds.) p185–201. Churchill Livingstone, Edinburgh (1987).

Discuss the pathology of the cardiomyopathies
(April 1978, Paper 2, Question 4)

Classify the cardiomyopathies and describe the pathology of the heart in each case
(October 1988, Paper 2, Question 5)

Discuss the classification and pathology of cardiomyopathies

Introduction

Definition
Primary vs. secondary (specific)
Incidence

Primary

Congestive (dilated)

1) **LV dilatation** (myocardial failure)

   Macroscopic

   a) endocardium
      i) thrombi
   b) myocardium
      i) flabby, thin
      ii) fibrosis

   Microscopic

   a) endocardium
      i) smooth muscle
      ii) hypertrophy
   b) myocardium
      i) degenerative change

   Secondary effects

   a) LV failure
   b) emboli

Hypertrophic

1) **LV compliance decreased**

   Macroscopic

   a) LV thickening symmetrical/asymmetrical endocardial fibrosis (Ant. M.V. leaflet)

   Microscopic

   a) fibre changes and degeneration

   EM

   a) myofibrillary disarray

Restrictive

1) **Endocardial fibroelastosis**

   Clinical

   a) congenital abnormalities

   Macroscopic

   a) porcelain fibrosis

   Microscopic

   a) hyaline collagen deposition

2) *Endomyocardial fibrosis*

Clinical

Macroscopic

a) RV > LV
b) Apex > base

Microscopic

a) fibrosis, eosinophils (Loeffler's syndrome)

Secondary

1) *Toxic*

   a) alcohol
   b) cobalt
   c) catecholamines
   d) Co
   e) Li
   f) As
   g) anthracyclines
   h) cyclophosphamide

2) *Metabolic*

   a) hypo- and hyperkalaemia
   b) hypo- and hyperthyroidism
   c) nutritional deficiencies
       i)   Vitamin B1
   d) haemochromatosis

3) *Infiltrative*

   a) sarcoidosis
   b) amyloid
   c) tumour

4) *Neuromuscular*

   a) Friedreich's ataxia
   b) muscular dystrophy
   c) congenital atrophies

5) *Storage disorders*

   a) Fabry's
   b) Pompe's diseases

(October 1980, Paper 2, Question 1)

Reference

1) Davies, M.J. The cardiomyopathies: a review of terminology, pathology and pathogenesis. Histopathology (1984) 8: 363–393.

Discuss classification and pathology of the primary cardiomyopathies

This question is very similar but the causes of secondary cardiomyopathy do not need consideration. It is important not to overlook these when questions are set on cardiomyopathy without specification.   *(April 1976, Paper 2, Question 3)*

Define right ventricular hypertrophy and discuss its pathogenesis

This is a similar question, but includes all causes of pulmonary hypertension including shunts, vascular disease and pressure effects due to left heart failure as well as the previously cited causes of pulmonary hypertension. It might be better to discuss the diagnosis of right ventricular hypertrophy in detail, and then take one or two examples of each group to illustrate the different pathogenetic mechanisms.   *(April 1971, Paper 2, Question 4)*

What is a cardiac myxoma? How may it give rise to clinical signs and symptoms?

This requires a straightforward pathological description of this entity, to include macroscopic, microscopic, histochemical, immunohistochemical and ultrastructural features, with speculation on the histogenesis. The complications of cardiac myxoma are well defined and largely predictable. This type of question could be answered with relative ease by a candidate who has reached the required standard for the examination.   *(November 1974, Paper 1, Question 2)*

References

1) Davies, M.J. Tumours of the heart and pericardium. In: Pathology of the Heart. A. Pomerance, M.J. Davies (eds.) p428–433. Blackwell Scientific Publications, Oxford (1975).
2) Landon, G. et al. Cardiac myxoma. An immunocytochemical study using endothelial, histiocytic and smooth muscle markers. Arch. Pathol. Lab. Med. (1986) 110: 116–120.

6. Endocrine System

Discuss the aetiology and pathology of Cushing's syndrome
(April 1979, Paper 1, Question 3)

Describe the macroscopic and microscopic changes which may be found in the adrenals in patients with Cushing's syndrome. What bearing may the changes have in the treatment of the case?
(November 1971, Paper 2, Question 2)

Discuss the pathological basis of Cushing's syndrome
(April 1970, Paper 2, Question 3)

Give a detailed description of the changes that may be found in the adrenal glands in Cushing's syndrome. Discuss the changes that may occur in the other tissues and organs

These essays are substantially the same in terms of basic content, but each requires a different emphasis. The earliest question requires only the primary adrenal causes to be considered, but secondary changes from an ectopic source of ACTH need to be mentioned. The effect on other tissues in Cushing's syndrome is wide ranging and requires careful planning.

In the 1970 question, division should be made on the basis of abnormal stimulation of the adrenal glands by ACTH, from pituitary, ectopic and iatrogenic sources, and adrenal causes including hyperplasia and neoplasia.

The 1971 question requires a discussion on the aetiology and pathogenesis of the changes as this information is required for appropriate treatment.

The 1979 question requires a discussion rather than a description and problems in diagnosis and histological assessment should be considered.
(November 1969, Paper 2, Question 1)

Give an account of the structure and behaviour of tumours arising in the adrenal medulla and the sympathetic nervous system

The 'structure' in this question presumably relates more to the microscopic and the ultrastructural features than the macroscopic appearance. Phaeochromocytoma, neuroblastoma and ganglioneuroma are the main tumours to be considered, and their systemic effects as well as benign or malignant behaviour should be described. The sympathetic nervous system may give rise to similar extra-adrenal tumours, and their principal sites and behaviour should be summarised in one or two paragraphs. In addition, it would be appropriate to include description of paragangliomas arising in the carotid body and other sites, comparing and contrasting features with phaeochromocytoma.
(November 1973, Paper 1, Question 4)

References

1) Robbins, S.L., Cotran, R.S., Kumar, V. Adrenal medulla. In: Pathologic Basis of Disease, 4th edition. p1262–1267. W.B. Saunders, Philadelphia (1989).
2) Enzinger, F.M., Weiss, S.W. Tumors of the sympathetic nervous system and paraganglioma. In: Soft Tissue Tumors, 2nd edition. p816–860. C.V. Mosby Co, St Louis (1988).

Write a short essay on the pathology of the carotid bodies

While most pathologists should be familiar with the neoplasms which arise from the carotid bodies, the normal structure and the alterations encountered in cases of chronic hypoxia, systemic hypertension and pulmonary hypertension are less well known, and the information is not provided to any major degree in the more basic pathology texts. The question requires some consideration of these states. The information is provided in the first reference in fairly detailed form, but otherwise a lecture in a symposium or teaching course including non-neoplastic disease of the carotid body may be the only way to acquire this knowledge for the average candidate.   *(April 1981, Paper 1, Question 2)*

References

1) Heath, D., Smith, P. The Pathology of the Carotid Body and Sinus. Edward Arnold, London (1985).
2) Enzinger, F.W., Weiss, S.W. Paraganglioma. In: Soft Tissue Tumors, 2nd edition. p836–860. C.V. Mosby Co, St. Louis (1988).

Give an account of the structure and behaviour of tumours arising in the adrenal medulla and the sympathetic nervous system

This essay requires a concentration on phaeochromocytoma as well as neuro-blastoma and ganglioneuroma, with less detailed mention of the paragangliomas described in the preceding answer. (Although the latter might be argued to arise from the parasympathetic rather than ortho-sympathetic system, they could still be justifiably included. Subtle distinctions such as this would not cause a candidate to be marked down, especially if they had discussed and qualified the terminology in an introduction.) Other entities such as myelolipoma could be mentioned, but secondary carcinoma should not be discussed, as the question requires only those lesions arising in the adrenal gland.

(November 1973, Paper 1, Question 4)

Reference

1) Rosai, J. Adrenal gland and other paraganglia. In: Ackerman's Surgical Pathology. Volume 1, 7th edition. Chapter 16, p789–818. C.V. Mosby Co, St. Louis (1989).

Give an account of the histological and ultrastructural features of the chemodectoma. How does this tumour behave? What tumours with the same microscopic appearance occur elsewhere in the body

Introduction

Syn. carotid body paraganglioma
Sites of paraganglia
Function of paraganglion cells
General features

Histological appearances

1) *Benign*

   a) capsule
   b) zellballen
   c) nuclear features inc. pleomorphism
   d) cytoplasm (spindle cell change)

2) *Malignant?*

   a) irregular cell clusters
   b) mitotic activity
   c) necrosis

3) *Special stains*

   a) grimelius
   b) formalin-induced fluorescence

4) *Ultrastructure of*

   a) chief cell
   b) dark and light cells
   c) cell junctions
   d) dense core granules 100–200µm

5) *Clinical behaviour*

   a) local recurrence
   b) metastasis (<10%)
      i) lymph nodes
      ii) lung and bone

6) *Other tumours*

    a) phaeochromocytoma of adrenal gland

    b) glomus jugulare tumour

    c) vagal paraganglioma

    d) mediastinal paraganglioma

    e) retroperitoneal paraganglioma

    f) others e.g. larynx, orbit, bladder

(April 1986, Paper 2, Question 1)

Reference

1) Enzinger, F.W., Weiss, S.W. Paraganglioma. In: Soft Tissue Tumors. 2nd edition. p836–860. C.V. Mosby Co, St. Louis (1988).

Discuss the concept of the diffuse endocrine system and the neoplasms that can arise from it

(November 1977, Paper 2, Question 3)

What are APUD cells? How may they be identified? Give a short account of the tumours ('apudomas') which can arise from these cells

The second of these two questions was clearly related to the publication of the first reference. Since that time there has been considerable discussion in the literature as to the proposed 'neural crest' origin of these cells, but this issue is to some extent peripheral to the concerns of a diagnostic pathologist, and certainly in relation to the content of these answers. So also is the expanding body of knowledge on various peptides (and combination of peptides), which may prove confusing for the average trainee trying to keep up with the literature. It is much better to read the simpler review articles on the subject, so that the problem of 'not seeing the wood for the trees' is avoided!   *(October 1978, Paper 2, Question 4)*

References

1) Gould, R.P. The APUD cell system. In: Recent Advances in Histopathology 10. P.P. Anthony, N. Woolf (eds.) p1–22. Churchill Livingstone, Edinburgh (1978).

2) Dawson, I.M.P. Diffuse endocrine and neuroendocrine cell tumours. In: Recent Advances in Histopathology 12. p111–128. Churchill Livingstone, Edinburgh (1984).

3) Polak, J.M., Bloom, S.R. Pathology of peptide-producing neuroendocrine tumours. Br. J. Hosp. Med. (1985) 33: 78–88.

Give an account of inflammatory and inflammatory-like diseases of the thyroid gland

The conditions which could be described in these answers include acute thyroiditis, and more chronic diseases such as primary thyrotoxicosis (which could be included as a form of 'auto-immune' disease), Hashimoto's disease, granulomatous (De Quervain's) thyroiditis, lymphocytic and chronic atrophic thyroiditis. Riedel's thyroiditis could also justifiably be included (especially as an 'inflammatory-like disease') even though it is probably a form of fibromatosis (or even sclerosing carcinoma).   *(October 1985, Paper 2, Question 4)*

References

1) Robbins, S.L., Cotran, R.S., Kumar, V. Thyroid gland. In: Pathologic Basis of Disease. 4th edition. p1220–1227. W.B. Saunders, Philadelphia (1989).
2) Rosai, J. Thyroid gland. In: Ackerman's Surgical Pathology. Volume 1. 7th edition. Chapter 1, p391–448. C.V. Mosby Co, St Louis (1989).

Write an essay on inflammatory lesions of the thyroid gland
(November 1977, Paper 1, Question 5)

Discuss the pathology of the clinically solitary thyroid nodule

Introduction

Definition – discrete palpable mass in thyroid
Prevalence
Significance

Pathological categories

Colloid ('involutional') nodule

1) *Macroscopic features*

2) *Microscopic*

Adenoma

1) *Macroscopic features*

2) *Microscopic*
   a) follicular
   b) foetal
   c) trabecular/embryonal
   d) oxyphil
   e) ?atypical adenoma

Cysts

1) *Degenerative*

2) *Developmental*

Carcinoma

1) *Follicular*

  a) well differentiated
      i)   macroscopic
      ii)   microscopic
      iii) variants
      iv)   clear cell ca
      v)   oxyphil
  b) poorly differentiated

2) *Papillary*

  a) macroscopic
      i)   unifocal and multifocal
  b) microscopic
  c) variants

3) *Medullary*

  a) localised
      i) macroscopic
      ii) microscopic
  b) multifocal
      i) genetic association (MEA)
      ii) C cell hyperplasia

4) *Undifferentiated*

  a) macroscopic
  b) microscopic
      i)   small cell ca
      ii)   giant cell ca

(October 1982, Paper 2, Question 5)

References

1) Brown, C.L. The solitary thyroid nodule. In: Recent Advances in Histopathology 11. P.P. Anthony, R.N.M. MacSween (eds.) p203–212. Churchill Livingstone, Edinburgh (1981)
2) Robbins, S.L., Cotran, R.S., Kumar, V. Thyroid gland. In: Pathologic Basis of Disease, 4th edition. p1227–1242. W.B. Saunders, Philadelphia (1989).

Write an essay on thyroid cancer

(April 1976, Paper 1, Question 4)

Give a classification of malignant tumours of the thyroid and describe briefly the behaviour of each type of tumour

This answer requires an expansion of the relevant section from the previous plan, and should provide relatively little problem for the average candidate, since most of these entities are regularly encountered in diagnostic practice, and are frequently discussed in the literature. There are several good accounts of thyroid malignancies but there is more than enough detail in the given reference.

(April 1969, Paper 2, Question 3)

Reference

1) Rosai, J. Thyroid gland. In: Ackerman's Surgical Pathology, Volume 1. 7th edition, Chapter 9, p391–448. C.V. Mosby Co, St. Louis (1989).

Give an account of malignant thyroid neoplasms and relate this to their clinical behaviour

(April 1980, Paper 2, Question 1)

7. Renal Pathology

Describe the alterations that may be found in the kidney in a) polyarteritis nodosa b) scleroderma c) renal artery stenosis

This is really a 'short notes' type of question, although the wording indicates that formal sentence construction is required. Each section therefore constitutes a small essay, and in view of the relatively brief nature of each section all that is really required as a plan is a few key words and notes under each heading, especially as each of these subjects is circumscribed and straightforward.

(April 1980, Paper 2, Question 2))

What correlation is found between renal function tests and morphological appearances of renal biopsies

A difficult question to answer, there being great potential to digress without a structured plan and it is essential to try to be concise as well as thorough. Normal function is obviously dependent on the presence of sufficient nephrons being able to carry out their role, and thus one simple scheme might be to take various components of the nephron in turn. Abnormalities at each level could then be highlighted and their functional significance considered. A possible sequence to consider would be vascular supply; muscular arteries, arterioles, glomerular capillaries, efferent arterioles, vasa recta and renal veins; glomeruli; capillary walls, mesangial support, tubules, collecting ducts and finally interstitium. Each of the above can be briefly considered in the light of various pathological abnormalities and their effects on functional tests at the clinical level.

No specific references are provided, as the information to answer this question has to be derived from a number of sources. This has been a particular feature of the questions in this section, and there is a particular emphasis on broad overviews on several subjects in renal pathology. While this is usually straight-forward for candidates who have wide-ranging practical experience, other candidates may find difficulty in coordinating and comparing all of these entities within an examination – these points should be borne in mind when revising renal pathology, when extra effort should be made to compare and contrast different diseases. *(May 1973, Paper 1, Question 3)*

Discuss the value of renal biopsy in the diagnosis and prognosis of renal disease

This question is so wide-ranging the problem arises from selecting those conditions which could be discussed under this heading. Perhaps the best way is to select those diseases whose prompt and accurate diagnosis would significantly alter the clinical management to the benefit of patients, illustrating the particular features which are most important. Examples could include biopsy diagnosis in the nephrotic syndrome, in glomerulonephritis or in management of allograft rejection, there are clearly many areas which could be covered. This is another example where a 'global' knowledge of renal pathology is required to answer the question. *(November 1977, Paper 2, Question 4)*

How would you handle the investigation of a renal biopsy specimen in the laboratory? What techniques would you use and what information would you hope to derive from them?

Essentially a question directed to the candidate experienced in diagnostic work, it also illustrates the importance of considering more than just interpretation of stained sections. The handling of a biopsy is critical, and methods for the division of biopsies for processing, cryostat sectioning for immunofluorescence and electron microscopy, all of which should ideally contain glomeruli, require description. Fixation and storage methods should be considered, and the range of special staining techniques (including methanemine silver, toluidine blue, PAS and trichrome stains all have applications), along with immunohistochemical studies and the range of abnormalities present in the commoner forms of glomerulonephritis could be described. In addition, other diseases such as amyloidosis can also be considered and the range of stains detailed. Electron microscopic analysis could also be reviewed, and selected diseases which have a characteristic appearance described. The range of options in such an answer is very wide, and it would be difficult to provide a balanced answer without a carefully thought out plan. No reference is given because this answer more or less encompasses the whole of renal biopsy pathology.

(April 1987, Paper 2, Question 5)

Discuss the pathology of renal diseases occurring in pregnancy

A difficult question if the problems of renal disease in pregnancy have not been specifically considered prior to the examination! There are two broad groups of renal disease in pregnancy – those specific to pregnancy, and those which occur in other circumstances but are predisposed to by pregnancy. The former can be discussed first and include pre-eclampsia/eclampsia, idiopathic post-partum acute renal failure, cortical necrosis and fatty liver with acute renal failure. Details of these conditions can be obtained from the reference below. Those diseases predisposed to but not specific for pregnancy include urinary tract infection/ acute pyelonephritis and essential hypertension.

(October 1977, Paper 2, Question 1)

Reference

1)   Heptinstall, R.H. Renal diseases in pregnancy. In: Pathology of the Kidney, 3rd edition. p963–991. Little, Brown & Co, Boston (1983).

Discuss the possible autopsy findings in a patient who has died from chronic pyelonephritis

Renal

1) *Macroscopic features*

   a) kidneys reduced in size (except when secondary to distal obstruction –
      PN and hydronephrosis)
   b) pathognomonic change – irregular coarse discrete corticomedullary scars
      overlying distorted calyx
   c) predilection for poles
   d) unscarred areas normal or secondary hypertensive changes

2) *Microscopic features*

   a) tubules
      i)   atrophic shrinkage
      ii) atrophic dilated +/- colloid casts 'thyroidisation'
   b) interstitium
      i)   fibrosis, inflammation – variable predominantly chronic
   c) glomeruli
      i)   variable from essentially normal – periglomerular fibrosis – global
           sclerosis – loss with incorporation into fibrotic scar
   d) pelvicalyceal region
      i)   chronic inflammatory and submucosal fibrosis
   e) non-scarred regions
      i)   variety of changes including ischaemic, hypertensive and
           hyperfiltration changes
   f) vasculature
      i)   changes secondary to hypertension

   No specific ultrastructural or immunofluorescent changes

Systemic

1) *CVS*

   a) pericardium
      i)   fibrous pericarditis, pericardial effusion
   b) heart
      i)   LVH
      ii) LVF changes
      iii) myocardial calcification (secondary to hyperparathyroidism)
      iv) oxalate deposition (including conducting system)
   c) systemic arteries
      i)   hypertensive changes
      ii) medial calcification
      iii) oxalate deposition
      iv) accelerated atherosclerosis

Respiratory system

1) *Pleura*

   a) fibrinous pleurisy
   b) effusion

2) _Lungs_

   a) heavy, features of uraemic pneumonitis

Skeletal system

1) _Renal osteodystrophy (including changes of secondary hyperparathyroidism)_

Endocrine

1) _Secondary hyperparathyroidism_

   a) diffuse parathyroid hyperplasia

2) _Tertiary hyperparathyroidism_

   a) exaggerated changes in gland (functional autonomy)

Alimentary tract

1) _Mucosal inflammatory changes +/- ulceration and haemorrhage at all levels_

2) _Pancreatic duct dilatation_

3) _Ascites +/- uraemic fibrinous peritonitis_

Central nervous system

1) _Cerebral haemorrhage secondary to hypertension and vascular changes_

2) _Changes of terminal infection may involve any system, especially respiratory_

3) _Other changes, microscopic only e.g. hypoplastic bone marrow_
                                                        (April 1981, Paper 2, Question 2)

References

1) Robbins, S.L., Cotran, R.S., Kumar, V. The kidney. In: Pathologic Basis of Disease, 4th edition. p1015–1017; 1055–1057. W.B. Saunders, Philadelphia (1989).
2) Kashgarian, M., Rosai, J. The urinary tract. In: Ackerman's Surgical Pathology, Volume 1, 7th edition. p819–922. C.V. Mosby Co, St Louis (1989).

Discuss the aetiology and pathogenesis of chronic pyelonephritis

The introduction should include an adequate definition of chronic pyelonephritis, primarily that it is a chronic tubulointerstitial disorder in which renal scarring is associated with pathological involvement of calyces and pelvis. Emphasis is placed on bacterial infection associated with vesicoureteric reflux or obstruction distal to the pelvis which is considered to play the major role in the development of chronic pyelonephritis. Thus pathogenically there are two major causes of chronic PN – chronic obstructive PN and the more common chronic reflux associated PN. In chronic obstructive PN a haematogenous route of infection is favoured, as the obstructed kidney is much more vulnerable to circulating organisms that are potentially pathogenic than the normal kidney. Chronic reflux associated PN is thought to be associated with ascending infection. The importance of vesicoureteric reflux in childhood should be described in detail, along with the significance of compound refluxing renal papillae leading to intra-renal reflux.   *(November 1972, Paper 2, Question 1)*

References

1) Heptinstall, R.H. Urinary tract infection, reflux and pyelonephritis. In: Pathology of the Kidney, 3rd edition. p1257–1304. Little Brown & Co, Boston (1983).
2) Risdon, R.A. Cystic disease of the kidney and reflux nephropathy. In: Recent Advances in Histopathology 11. R.N.M. MacSween, P.P. Anthony (eds.) Churchill Livingstone, Edinburgh (1981).

Discuss the pathology and pathogenesis of interstitial nephritis

This may be a difficult question for those candidates who have not worked within a Department receiving biopsies from a renal specialist unit, as the possible aetiological factors are quite wide ranging. It would be best to define acute and chronic interstitial nephritis and discuss the gross and microscopic changes in both, including the nature of the interstitial changes (and their consequences) and the composition of the cellular infiltrate. Since there are a large number of aetiological and associated conditions, it would be best to list the main aetiologies in each (e.g. the acute group includes infection, drugs and toxins, glomerulonephritis, SLE, transplantation and the chronic group includes infection, obstructive uropathy, ischaemia, papillary necrosis, radiation injury, sarcoidosis and several others). The major differences in pathogenesis between the groups should be emphasised to avoid repetition of the common features.

(October 1983, Paper 2, Question 3)

Reference

1) Risdon, R.A., Turner, D.R. Interstitial nephritis. In: Atlas of Renal Pathology. p35–39. J.B. Lippincott Co, Philadelphia (1980).

Discuss how therapeutic agents may induce kidney disease and how they can modify lesions of pre-existing disorders

A very broad question which covers many fields. The renal diseases induced by therapeutic agents include acute tubular necrosis (e.g. antibacterials, anaesthetic agents), interstitial nephritis (e.g. antibiotic or diuretics), analgesic nephropathy, nephrocalcinosis (Vitamin D), radiation nephritis, urate nephropathy (e.g. treatment of leukaemias), and glomerulonephritis (e.g. gold salts, penicillamine). Therapeutic agents modifying renal disease include antibiotics in pyelonephritis and ureteric reflux, steroids in some forms of glomerulonephritis, antibiotics in post-streptococcal glomerulonephritis and cytotoxic drugs in crescentic glomerulonephritis and lupus nephritis, or antihypertensive agents in hypertensive disease. There are several other examples which could be considered. It is difficult to provide specific references to these broad categories of disease, which are drawn from many sources in the major renal texts.

(April 1969, Paper 2, Question 1)

Describe the changes found in necrosis of the renal papillae. Discuss the aetiology and pathogenesis of this condition

Renal papillary necrosis occurs in two main settings, analgesic abuse and acute pyelonephritis, and since the changes are sufficiently distinctive in each case they could be described separately. For analgesic nephropathy, the macroscopic appearances should be given in detail, along with the microscopic features, in both early and late stages. As expected, superimposed suppurative changes are important in the pyelonephrotic cases.

As regards aetiology and pathogenesis, there is experimental and epidemiological evidence for analgesias leading to renal papillary necrosis, thought to be due to acetaminophen binding to cellular proteins and depleting renal glutathione, which normally prevents oxidative damage, exacerbated by interference with prostaglandin synthesis by aspirin. In pyelonephritis and obstructive uropathy, pressure effects and interference with local vascularity are proposed, and these hypotheses should be discussed and criticised as appropriate.

(April 1975, Paper 2, Question 4)

Reference

1) Robbins, S.L., Cotran R.S., Kumar, V. The kidney-tubulointerstitial diseases. In: Pathologic Basis of Disease, 4th edition. p1051–1061. W.B. Saunders, Philadelphia (1989).

Discuss the nature of the relationship between stenosis of the renal artery and arterial hypertension

This is one of the most thoroughly investigated mechanisms of hypertension, although the explanation is far from complete and can't be applied to every case of renal artery stenosis. The answer should concentrate on the relationship and not provide a lengthy description of the various lesions which can produce the stenotic lesion. A brief mention of the pathological lesions producing renal artery stenosis would be all that is required. In discussing the relationship between stenosis and hypertension the pioneering experiments of Goldblatt should be highlighted. This leads on to a description of the renin angiotensin system which best explains the development of arterial hypertension after renal artery stenosis including the means by which stenosis leads to increased renin release by the juxtaglomerular apparatus in the kidney rendered relatively ischaemic by the stenosis. A line diagram of the renin angiotensin system may help in this answer.

In concluding this discussion it should be noted that only 50% of patients with long term arterial hypertension secondary to renal arterial stenosis have elevated renin levels. This implies that there are additional mechanisms, which may include sodium retention, altered peripheral vascular reactivity to vasopressor substances and changes in prostaglandin and kinin systems. There is no need to discuss morphological changes in the kidney secondary to renal artery stenosis, as these have not been requested.   *(November 1969, Paper 2, Question 5)*

References

1) Robbins, S.L., Cotran, R.S., Kumar, V. The kidney. In: Pathologic Basis of Disease, 4th edition. p1062–1069. W.B. Saunders, Philadelphia (1989).
2) Heptinstall, R.H. Hypertension – III secondary forms. In: Pathology of the Kidney, 3rd edition. p248–267. Little, Brown & Co, Boston (1983).

Discuss the pathogenesis and pathology of immune complex nephritis

Introduction

Explanation of terms used
Experimental models vs. human disease

Experimental nephritis

1) In situ immune complex formation

   a) anti GBM
      i) nephrotoxic (Masugi) heterologous anti GBM antisera injection heterologous/autologous phases
      ii) AI (Steblay)
   b) Other fixed Ag
      i) Heymann nephritis
   c) 'Planted' antigens
      i) endogenous
      ii) exogenous

2) Circulating immune complex

   Localisation due to physicochemical/haemodynamic factors

   a) acute serum sickness
   b) chronic serum sickness

Human disease

1) Goodpasture's syndrome

   a) ?nephrotoxic

2) *Membranous GN*

   a) ?chronic serum sickness

3) *Lupus nephritis*

   a) various

4) *Acute proliferative*

   a) ?acute serum sickness

(October 1982, Paper 1, Question 3)

References

1) Heptinstall, R.H. Immunologic mechanisms in glomerular disease. In: Pathology of the Kidney, 3rd edition. p301–386. Little, Brown & Co., Boston (1983).
2) Robbins, S.L., Cotran, R.S., Kumar, V. The kidney. In: Pathologic Basis of Disease, 4th edition. p1022–1042. W.B. Saunders, Philadelphia (1989).

Describe the various forms of glomerulonephritis that may be found in the nephrotic syndrome. Indicate the clinical course of the various types

Introduction

Nephrotic syndrome NS – proteinuria (>3.5 g/day), hypoalbuminaemia, oedema, hyperlipaemia, lipiduria

Frequency – adults vs. children

GN associated with NS

Proliferative

Acute diffuse (rare)

Crescentic (rare)

Mesangial proliferation

Focal

Histological features

1) *Clinical*

   a) response to Px
   b) Focal sclerosing glomerulosclerosis (FSGS) in 50–70%
      i)   crescentic
      ii) prognosis

Membranous

Histological features *(EM + immunocytochemistry)*

1) *Clinical*
    a) children 10 YSR 90%
    b) adult 20% remission
              25% partial remission
              15% relapsing
              50% die within 15 years

Mesangiocapillary

Histological features *(EM + immunocytochemistry)* *(type I and type II)*

1) *Clinical*
    a) type I
        i)   persistent NS 40%
        ii) 10 YSR
        iii) proteinuria
        iv) 85% 10 YSR
    b) type II
        i)   worse prognosis

FSGS

Histological features *(+EM)*

1) *Clinical*
    a) remission 37%
    b) relapsing 14%
    c) chronic renal failure 50%

Minimal change

Histological features *(EM)*

1) *Clinical*
    a) remission 7–40%
    b) relapsing 60%

2) *Other causes of NS with GN picture*
    a) SLE, HSP
    b) drugs e.g. penicillamine, Au
    c) infection e.g. syphilis, malaria, SBE
    d) miscellaneous e.g. transplantation glomerulopathy, sarcoid

(April 1972, Page 2, Question 1)

Reference

1) Turner, D.R. Glomerulonephritis. In: Recent Advances in Histopathology 10. P.P. Anthony, N. Woolf (eds.) p240–259. Churchill Livingstone, Edinburgh (1978)

Discuss the renal changes and discuss the aetiology of focal glomerulonephritis. What factors determine prognosis?

Classification

Focal and segmental proliferative glomerulonephritis (FSPGN)
Focal and segmental glomerulosclerosis (FSGS)
Focal global sclerosis

FSPGN

1) Primary (IgA and non IgA)

2) Secondary part of systemic disorders: SLE; PAN; HSP; bacterial endocarditis; shunt nephritis; Wegener's granulomatosis; Goodpasture's syndrome

1) *Morphology*

Similar for 1° and 2°

a) changes focal (only some glomeruli) and segmental (only part of glomerulus)
b) +/- mesangial
c) segmental cellular proliferation +/- necrosis
d) +/- small crescents anatomically related to segmental damage
e) 'mature' lesions solidified +/- adherence to Bowman's capsule
f) tubules, interstitium and blood vessels, minor changes – focal tubular atrophy/interstitial fibrosis

2) *Immunofluorescence*

a) 1°
   i) IgA nephropathy – diffuse (all glomeruli) mesangial IgA +/- lesser mesangial IgG, C3
   ii) non IgA nephropathy – diffuse mesangial C3 +/- other Igs
b) 2°
   i) depends on disease, e.g. SLE vs. Goodpasture's
c) TEM variable depending on specific disease and stage

3) *Aetiology*

Immunological mechanisms almost certainly involved in most cases

4) *IgA nephropathy*

   a) IgA production deposits, some alteration in normal regulation and primary environmental stimulus e.g. virus
   b) alternative pathway complement activations in mesangium
   c) ? mesangial overload leading to focal and sequential lesions at sites of overload

5) *SLE*

   a) deposition of circulating complexes, complement activation, variety of possible lesions depend on
      i) level of complexes
      ii) local activation mediators of inflammation

FSGS

1) *Morphology*

   a) early glomeruli
      i) most normal
      ii) juxtamedullary glomeruli – segmental solidification of one or more lobules especially perilobular +/- hyalinosis
   b) later glomeruli
      i) segmental solidification +/- global sclerosis, hyalinosis and foam cells
   c) tubules
      i) focal atrophy
   d) interstitium
      i) focal fibrosis
   e) advanced
      i) global glomerular sclerosis, esp. juxtamedullary region. Extensive tubular atrophy and accompanying interstitial fibrosis

2) *Immunofluorescence*

   a) diffuse mesangial IgM, G and C3
   b) sclerotic areas secondary entrapment of IgM and C3

3) *TEM*

   a) segmental sclerosis, overlying epithelial swelling podocyte effacement and separation
   b) subendothelial hyalinosis

Prognosis

1) % of glomeruli showing sclerotic lesions at initial biopsy significant, if >20% then high probability of terminal RF
2) Individuals with associated diffuse mesangial hypercellularity progress more rapidly
3) Allograft recurrence

Aetiology

Unclear – disputed claim FSGS phase of minimal change disease
(April 1978, Paper 1, Question 4)

References

1) Turner, D.R. Glomerulonephritis. In: Recent Advances in Histopathology 10. P.P. Anthony, N. Woolf (eds.) p249–254. Churchill Livingstone, Edinburgh (1978).
2) Heptinstall, R.H. Focal glomerulonephritis. In: Pathology of the Kidney. 3rd edition, p557–600. Little, Brown & Co, Boston (1983).

Give an account of the changes that may be found in the kidney in systemic lupus erythematosus

Introduction

Clinical features of renal involvement frequency and severity

Pathological features

1) Gross

   a) granular, contracted

   b) cortical infarction and haemorrhages in accelerated HT

   c) superimposed pyelonephritis

2) Microscopic

   a) glomeruli (lupus nephritis)
      i)   normal
      ii) mesangial (5–10%)
      iii) focal proliferative (33%)
      iv) diffuse proliferative (50%)
      v) membranous (10%)

    additional features
      i)   hyaline (fibrin) thrombi
      ii) tubuloreticular structures
      iii) fingerprint deposits
      iv) haematoxylin bodies
      v) wire looping
   b) tubules
      i)   hyaline droplets (proteinuria)
      ii) haematoxylin bodies in lumina
      iii) tubular atrophy
   c) interstitium
      i)   fibrosis with tubular atrophy
      ii) inflammatory infiltrate

d) vessels
  i) vasculitis
  ii) HT changes – benign
                  – accelerated
  iii) renal vein thrombosis (membranous GN with nephrotic syndrome)
                                    (October 1982, Paper2, Question 2)

Reference

1) Robbins, S.L., Cotran, R.S., Kumar, V. Diseases of immunity. In: Pathologic
    Basis of Disease, 4th edition. p197–200. W.B. Saunders, Philadelphia (1989).

Discuss the mechanisms underlying the rejection of transplanted kidneys

Introduction

Clinical features
Types of rejection

Mechanisms

1) Sensitisation

  a) MHC Ags
  b) blood group Ags
  c) minor HC Ags

2) Source of Ag

  a) subcellular, into host RE cells
  b) donor lymphoid/haemopoietic cells
  c) allograft endothelium

3) Effector mechanisms

  a) cell mediated
     i)   macrophages (Ag presentation)
     ii) T helper (Abs, lymphokines)
     iii) T cytotoxic

Types of rejection

1) Hyperacute

  a) pre-existing host Ab to
     i) donor endothelium
     ii) MHC Ag
  b) effect
     i) activation of clotting cascade
     ii) ischaemic necrosis

2) _Acute_ *(two forms)*

    a) interstitial cellular
        i)   T cytotoxic cells
        ii) Ab-mediated cytotoxicity
    b) vascular
        i)   Ab deposition
        ii) complement activation
        iii) T cytotoxic resection to endothelium

3) _Chronic_

    a) arterial intimal changes
        i)   repeated acute damage
        ii) continuous platelet/fibrin deposition
    b) glomerular changes
        i)   subendothelial Ig
        ii) plasma protein

(April 1985, Paper 1, Question 1)

References

1) Heptinstall, R.H. Renal transplantation. In: Pathology of the Kidney. p1455–1511. Little, Brown and Co, Boston (1983).
2) Robbins, S.L., Cotran, R.S., Kumar, V. Diseases of immunity – transplant rejection. In: Pathologic Basis of Disease, 4th edition. p183–187. W.B. Saunders, Philadelphia (1989).

Describe the changes in the kidney when rejection follows renal transplantation and discuss the significance of the features you describe

(November 1973, Paper 1, Question 3)

Write a critical account of the pathogenesis and pathological features of rejection of a transplanted kidney

This answer requires morphological changes to be discussed in addition to the mechanism. If the question is approached considering in turn hyperacute, acute and chronic rejection and describing morphological changes, and the underlying mechanisms in less detail, then a full coverage can easily be provided.

(April 1969, Paper 1, Question 1)

Discuss the significance of the changes that may be found in a human allograft

This question can be answered using kidney allografts to illustrate the answer, as in the preceding examples.

(May 1973, Paper 2, Question 3)

Discuss the changes which have occurred in the blood vessels of transplanted organs and discuss their significances

This question can also be answered using kidney allografts as the main consideration. The vascular changes characterising hyperacute, acute vascular and chronic rejection should be described. These changes are of prime pathogenic importance in kidney rejection and their pathogenesis should be outlined.

(April 1970, Paper 1, Question 5)

Discuss the role of the mesangium in health and disease

An interesting question which highlighted the importance of this area which had been relatively neglected in conventional teaching until recently. The morphology, function and biochemical activity should occupy about a third of the essay, with the remainder considering the changes in various types of glomerulonephritis, including mesangial proliferative, mesangiocapillary, focal and diffuse proliferative types, together with diabetic glomerulosclerosis and amyloidosis. It is important to avoid a digression into the 'extramesangial' features as far as possible.   *(November 1975, Paper 2, Question 3)*

Reference

1) Michael, A.F. The glomerular mesangium. Contr. Nephrol. (1984) 40: 7–16.

Describe the changes in renal blood vessels and glomeruli in diabetes mellitus and discuss their pathogenesis

Glomerular changes

1) *Histopathology (+ histochemistry, EM)*

2) *Glomerulosclerosis*
    a) nodular
    b) diffuse

3) *Fibrin caps*

4) *Capsular drops*

5) *Thickened GBM*

Arterial changes

1) *Large vessels*
    a) atheroma
    b) intimal fibrosis

Pathology + EM

1) *Small vessels*

    a) hyalinosis (afferent & efferent arterioles)

Pathogenesis of glomerulosclerosis

1) *Animal studies*

    a) injection glycosylated proteins produce changes

    b) mesangial changes – response to protein accumulation

    c) glomeruli increased content of PGE2 and prostacyclin

    d) cultured diabetic mesangial cells produce more prostacyclin, fibronectin, collagen I, II, IV, V.

Pathogenesis of thickened GBM

    a) seen within months of onset of insulin-dependent DM

    b) ↑ glycosylated hydroxylysine-rich subunits

    c) ? influence on cross-linking

    d) inhibits packing of structural proteins

    e) reduces proteolytic turnover

    f) normal ageing of collagen ↑ in diabetics

Pathogenesis of large vessel changes

    a) cultured medial cells – ↑ proliferation in diabetic serum

    b) also in presence of GH

    c) hyperglycaemic serum

        i)   cytopathic to endothelial cells

        ii) reduces PG secretion

(November 1969, Paper 2, Question 4)

References

1) Morley A.R. Invited review: Renal vascular disease in diabetes mellitus. Histopathology (1988) 12: 343–359.
2) Robbins, S.L., Cotran, R.S., Kumar, V. The kidney. In: Pathologic Basis of Disease, 4th edition. p1043–1047. W.B. Saunders, Philadelphia (1989).

Discuss the pathology of the renal complications of diabetes mellitus

(November 1970, Paper 1, Question 2)

Discuss the pathology of the kidney in diabetes mellitus

(April 1979, Paper 1, Question 1)

Describe the changes which may be found in the kidney in diabetes mellitus and discuss their pathogenesis

These three questions have a much broader scope, and are to some extent less satisfactory, because there is a vast amount of information which could be covered in addition, so the answer should be compiled in small sections, probably covering each component of the kidney to be affected, so that blood vessels and glomeruli are involved as in the previous essay (in less detail), tubular changes, interstitial nephritis and acute pyelonephritis with renal papillary necrosis. An essay plan can be formulated along these lines.

(October 1986, Paper 2, Question 3)

Discuss the pathogenesis of acute renal failure

Definition ARF

Reduction in daily urine production to less than 400 ml

Causes – six groups

1) *Acute tubular necrosis* *(two forms) (Oliver)*

   a) ischaemic (tubulorrhectic) complicated shock states
   b) nephrotoxic – direct damage to tubular cells
   c) pathogenetic mechanisms –
      i)   failure of glomerular filtration due to decreased renal perfusion
      ii) loss of tubular integrity
      iii) tubular obstruction (interstitial oedema or intratubular casts)
      iv) glomerular capillary changes – short circuit outer capillaries or decrease capillary wall permeability

   More than one of the above may occur in each case

2) *Renal infarction*

   a) arterial
      i)   embolism (heart, atherosclerotic aorta)
      ii) proximal disease of renal artery
      iii) cortical necrosis
      iv) trauma or surgical ligation of renal artery
   b) venous
      i)   renal vein thrombosis

3) *Organic occlusion of small renal vessels*

   Malignant hypertension, microangiopathic polyarteritis, scleroderma, haemolytic uraemic syndrome, idiopathic post-partum acute renal failure, sickle cell disease.

4) _Severe forms of glomerulonephritis_

5) _Severe infections_
   a) acute PN
   b) DIC in septicaemia

6) _Obstruction to outflow_
   a) intraluminal causes
      i) neoplasms, calculi, blood clots, sloughed renal papillae
   b) extraluminal causes
      i) prostatic hyperplasia, neoplastic compression, retroperitoneal fibrosis
      (April 1974, Paper 2, Question 5)

Reference

1) Heptinstall, R.H. Acute renal failure. In: Pathology of the Kidney, 3rd edition. p1069–1133. Little, Brown and Co, Boston (1983).

Write an account of the histopathology of acute renal failure. Discuss the aetiology and pathogenesis of this condition and relate histopathological change to pathophysiology

This question is very similar to April 1974, Paper 2, Question 5 but is more specific and directs the candidate to headings for the essay plan. It appears slightly ambiguous asking for histopathology of acute renal failure (ARF) which could be either renal changes, systemic changes or both. The second sentence in the question concentrates on the different renal changes causing acute renal failure, these cannot be easily discussed without reference to histopathological changes. Therefore an outline similar to that provided for April 1974, Paper 2, Question 5 is appropriate. Each group of causes of ARF should be discussed providing brief details of histopathological change, aetiology and pathogenesis. At the conclusion, a brief note can be made about systemic changes in acute renal failure, these will include oedema – especially pulmonary, sterile fibrinous pericarditis, uraemic colitis and other possibilities e.g. secondary changes after vomiting (aspiration pneumonitis), changes secondary to pruritus scratching, and changes associated with liver failure often seen in severe renal failure.

(April 1976, Paper 1, Question 2)

Give an account of renal neoplasms and their effects

Benign

Rare 5% of all renal tumours

1) *Mesoblastic nephroma*

    a) congenital (c.f. Wilm's)
    b) gross – solid yellow to grey
    c) resembles fibroid
    d) microscopic – cellular spindled
    e) entrapped tubules and glomeruli
    f) no capsule

2) *Angiomyolipoma*

    a) 1/3 patients tuberous sclerosis, also with lymphangiomyomatosis
    b) macro, yellow with haemorrhage and frequent extrarenal growth
    c) micro, extrarenal lymph nodes may be involved

3) *Multicystic nephroma*

    a) clinical – urinary obstruction by daughter lobules
    b) gross – sharply defined lesion
    c) microscopic – cyst wall of smooth muscle
    d) stroma (striated muscle cells)

4) *Adenoma*

    a) frequency
    b) significance
    c) association with dialysis kidney
    d) gross
    e) microscopic
    f) behaviour

5) *Juxtaglomerular cell tumour*

    a) renin secreting
    b) microscopic
    c) EM

Malignant

1) *Wilm's tumour*

    a) infants, occasionally congenital
    b) associations
    c) gross
    d) microscopic

Bone metastasising renal tumour of childhood = clear cell sarcoma
– c.f. Wilm's
– prognosis

2) *Renal cell carcinoma*

   a) gross
   b) microscopic – clear cell, tubulopapillary, sarcomatoid
   c) spread
   d) prognosis
   e) effects
   f) local
      i)   pain
      ii)   mass
      iii) haematuria
   g) systemic
      i)   fever
      ii)   malaise
      iii)   weakness
      iv)   weight loss
      v)   amyloidosis
      vi)   anaemia
      vii) polyneuromyopathy
      viii) leukaemoid reaction and eosinophilia
      ix)   endocrine – Cushing's
                     – feminisation
                     – hypertension
                     – hypercalcaemia
                     – polycythaemia
   h) metastatic

NB RCC most common recipient of metastasis from one cancer into another
(April 1983, Paper 2, Question 1)

References

1) Kashgarian, M., Rosai, J. Urinary tract. In: Ackerman's Surgical Pathology. J. Rosai (ed.) 7th edition. p819–922. C.V. Mosby Co, St. Louis (1989).
2) Beckwith, J.B. Wilm's tumour and other renal tumours of childhood. Human Pathol. (1983) 14: 481–492.

Discuss the pathological features, classification and possible causation of epithelial tumours of the urinary bladder

Classification and pathological features (Mostofi – WHO)

Benign

1) *Transitional cell papilloma* *(exophytic/inverted)*

2) *Squamous cell papilloma*

3) *'Nephrogenic' adenoma*

Malignant

1) *Transitional cell carcinoma*

    a) papillary

    b) flat
        i) non-invasive
        ii) invasive
        iii) grading (1–3)
        iv) behaviour

    c) variants
        i) squamous and glandular metaplasia

2) *Squamous cell carcinoma* – *associated features (e.g. calculus, schistosomiasis etc.)*

3) *Adenocarcinoma*

    a) ? metaplasia

    b) ? urachal origin

4) *Undifferentiated carcinoma*

Causation

    a) aniline dyes
        i) beta-naphthylamine and biphenyls
        ii) risk in dye, rubber and other workers

    b) schistosomiasis
        i) ? local effect – usually squamous
        ii) also in bladder calculi

    c) tobacco

    d) tryptophane

(April 1974, Paper 1, Question 1)

References

1) Robbins, S.L., Cotran, R.S., Kumar, V. The lower urinary tract. In: Pathologic Basis of Disease, 4th edition. p1090–1094. W.B. Saunders, Philadelphia (1989).
2) Kashgarian, M., Rosai, J. Bladder and urethra. In: Ackerman's Surgical Pathology. Volume 1, 7th edition. p898–922. C.V. Mosby Co, St Louis (1989).

Give a classification of bladder tumours and discuss its value in prognosis

The previous plan would include a description of the classifications of epithelial tumours of urinary bladder, and the WHO classification referenced in this answer is comprehensive in this respect. This classification is used by most diagnosticians and although proposed in 1972 is still the best to use in your answer. The prognosis of malignant bladder tumours depends on the type of tumour (e.g.

squamous cell carcinoma is much worse than transitional cell carcinoma). Other factors to emphasise in the answer include the grade of tumour (i.e. degree of differentiation), depth of invasion of bladder wall (and a detailed description of the various stages) and the presence or absence of disease spread beyond bladder-direct spread and lymphatic/haematogenous metastases. In transitional cell tumours the separation of non-invasive from invasive carcinomas, papillary vs. flat and the grade must be emphasised as all have great prognostic significance.

(November 1969, Paper 2, Question 2)

Reference

1) Mostofi, F.F. et al. Histological typing of urinary bladder tumours. In: Classification of Tumours 19. WHO Geneva (1972).

8. Central Nervous System

Describe the likely pathological findings in a patient with dementia

Introduction

Definition
Clinical features
Incidence

Pathology

Alzheimer's disease

1) *Macroscopic*

    a) weight reduction

    b) 'shrinkage' especially hippocampus

2) *Microscopic*

    a) neurofibrillary tangles
      i) LM
      ii) EM

Other diseases with neurofibrillary tangles – Down's syndrome, boxing, Steele-Richardson-Olszewski syndrome

    b) senile plaques
      i) LM – early
              – late
      ii) EM
    c) Hirano bodies
    d) neural processes

Pick's disease

1) *Macroscopic*

2) *'Knife-edge' gyral atrophy*

3) *Microscopic*

4) *Pick bodies*

Cerebrovascular disease

Difficulty in categorisation
Association with hypertension (Binswanger's disease)

1) *Microscopic*

    a) diffuse gliosis

    b) loss of myelinated fibres

    c) +/- focal infarcts

    d) vascular changes

Creutzfeldt-Jakob Disease

1) *Spongiform encephalopathy*

2) *Incidence and aetiology*

3) *Microscopic*

    a) spongiform change

    b) astrocytosis

    c) nerve cell degeneration and loss

Cerebral injury/anoxia

1) *Microscopic*

    a) focal or diffuse gliosis

    b) maximal in vascular boundary zones

    c) ischaemic cell change

(April 1984, Paper 2, Question 5)

References

1) Janota, I. Pathology of dementia. In: Recent Advances in Histopathology 11. P.P. Anthony, R.N.M. MacSween (eds.) p49–63. Churchill Livingstone, Edinburgh (1981).

2) Adams, J.H., Graham, D.I. Diffuse brain damage in non-missile head injury. In: Recent Advances in Histopathology 12. P.P. Anthony, R.N.M. MacSween (eds.) p241–257. Churchill Livingstone, Edinburgh (1984).

Describe the naked eye and microscopical changes that may be found post mortem in virus infections of the nervous system and mention what investigations would be helpful in establishing the diagnosis in each case

Introduction

Incidence

Tropism

Latency

Diagnosis – brain biopsy, immunohistology, viral probes, serology

General features of viral infection

1) *Perivascular infiltrate*

2) *Glial nodules*

3) *Inclusion bodies*
   a) Cowdry A
   b) Cowdry B
   c) Negri

4) *Neuronophagia*

Causes of viral encephalitis

1) Childhood infection – measles, mumps, rubella, varicella zoster
2) Respiratory viruses
3) Enteroviruses
4) CMV, herpes zoster, herpes simplex, arboviruses

Specific features of some viruses

1) *Herpes simplex*
   a) adult
      i)   localisation
      ii) microscopic features
      iii) resolution
   b) neonatal
      i)   global
   c) meningitis
   d) herpes labialis
      i)   localisation
      ii) histology

2) *Herpes zoster*
   a) localisation
      i)   brain
      ii) spinal cord
   b) histology

3) *Poliomyelitis*
   a) acute
      i)   macroscopic
   b) chronic
      ii) microscopic

4) *Rabies*

   a) localisation

   b) microscopic

5) *Slow viruses*

   a) subacute sclerosing panencephalitis
      i)   gross
      ii) microscopic
      iii) EM and immunohistology
   b) progressive multifocal leucoencephalopathy
      i)   associations
      ii) gross
      iii) microscopic
      iv) EM
   c) ?Jakob-Creutzfeldt disease – microscopic
      i)   EM

(November 1973, Paper 2, Question 2)

Reference

1) Morris, J.H. The nervous system – viral diseases. In: Pathologic Basis of Disease. S.L. Robbins, R.S. Cotran, V. Kumar (eds.) 4th edition. p1382–1388. W.B. Saunders, Philadelphia (1989).

What are the pathological effects of viruses on the nervous system?

(April 1983, Paper 2, Question 3)

Describe the pathological changes that may occur in the brain after infection by

1)   Toxoplasma gondii
2)   Cryptococcus neoformans
3)   Mycobacterium tuberculosis

There is abundant information which can be introduced into each of these categories, and would probably best be laid out by short side headings with concentrated information. It is important to include congenital disease in these conditions, and the effect of immunosuppression on disease patterns.

(November 1976, Paper 1, Question 5)

Describe the changes that occur in the central nervous system in demyelinating diseases and discuss the causes and mechanisms that are implicated

It is important to define what the term 'demyelinating diseases' actually refers to. Demyelination may occur in other conditions where there is white matter degeneration (such as motor neurone disease, subacute combined degeneration of the cord etc.), but the demyelinating diseases primarily include multiple sclerosis and its variants (see following paragraphs for pathogenetic considerations); acute disseminated encephalomyelitis as a hypersensitivity autoimmune phenomenon along with necrotising haemorrhagic leucoencephalitis (primary vasculitis), leucodystrophies (unborn errors in myelin metabolism) and progressive multi-focal leucoencephalopathy (viral infection). There are other rare conditions such as central pontine myelinolysis or Marchiafava-Bignami disease in alcoholics which might be mentioned. Thus, there is a lot of ground to be covered in this answer. One example from each group should be chosen to illustrate the changes both macroscopic and microscopic, since they are individually distinctive, before considering pathogenesis.   *(April 1981, Paper 1, Question 5)*

References

1) McDonald, W.I. The pathogenesis of multiple sclerosis: the Bradshaw lecture 1986. Journal Royal Coll. Phys. London (1987) 21(4): 287–294.
2) Robbins, S.L., Cotran, R.S., Kumar, V. In: Pathologic Basis of Disease, 4th edition. p1422–1426. W.B. Saunders, Philadelphia (1989).

Describe the pathology of multiple sclerosis and discuss its pathogenesis

This would be a straightforward account, considering the gross and microscopic changes in the various stages of the disease, including immunohistochemical studies on the lymphoid populations. The various theories of pathogenesis can be considered in some depth, including currently topic aspects of primary venulitis or relation to human immunodeficiency virus infection. In the earlier question, the aetiological factors are considered in relation to the pathogenetic mechanisms.
(April 1977, Paper 2, Question 2)

Reference

1) McDonald, W.I. The pathogenesis of multiple sclerosis: the Bradshaw Lecture 1986. Journal Royal Coll. Phys. London (1987) 21(4): 287–294.

Describe the lesions in the central nervous system in multiple (disseminated) sclerosis. Discuss modern concepts in aetiology
(November 1970, Paper 2, Question 4)

Give a critical review of the theories of the aetiology of multiple (disseminated) sclerosis

This question is somewhat more difficult to answer, as the aetiological agents are unknown, and thus the pathogenetic hypotheses still have to be considered in depth. It would be justifiable to discuss these as before, pointing out the support each hypothesis lends for a particular aetiological agent. Questions phrased in this fashion are responsible for much of the failure to appreciate the distinctions between aetiology and pathogenesis in the minds of examination candidates.

(November 1976, Paper 1, Question 2)

Discuss the aetiology and pathogenesis of the lesions found in Alzheimer's disease

Description of lesions

1) *Macroscopic*

    a) weight down

    b) cortical atrophy – frontal temporal, posterior parietal

2) *Microscopic*

    a) neuronal loss
       i)   neocortical large pyramidal cells of layers III and V
       ii) hippocampal pyramidal cells in Sommer's sector
       iii) parahippocampal cortical stellate neurones of lamina II
       iv) nucleus basalis of Meynert (quantitative study)
       v)   locus ceruleus

    b) results of neuronal loss
       i)   neurofibrillary tangles (NFT)
       ii) senile plaques (SP)
       iii) granulovacuolar degeneration
       iv) Hirano bodies

Aetiology

Unknown

1) *Possibilities*

    a) toxic environmental agent
       i)   virus
       ii) aluminium
       iii) others

    b) hereditary factors

    c) Down's syndrome – ?gene location

Pathogenesis

1) *Down's syndrome studies*

    a) SP – amyloid protein precedes peripheral plaque neurites

    b) NFT – in all damaged cell types
          – ? reactive to toxic change

Aluminium levels in diet and within affected brains ? toxic

Interference with nerve function by NFTs by
  a) crowding out of cell organelles
  or
  b) interruption axoplasmic flow

Significance of granulovacuolar degeneration and Hirano bodies unclear
(April 1987, Paper 1, Question 5)

References

1) Mann, D.M.A. The neuropathology of dementia. Bull. Royal Coll. Pathol. (1988) 64: 8–10.
2) Glenner, G.G. Current topics – on causative theories in Alzheimer's disease. Human Pathol. (1985) 16: 433–435.

What changes may be found at necropsy in a subject who died with a significant increase in intracranial pressure?

Introduction

Clinical features
Definition (CSF > 15 mm Hg)

General features

1) Herniation

  a) subfalcine herniation
  b) uncinate or tentorial herniation
  c) cerebellar tonsils ('coning')
  d) contralateral damage

2) Compression effects on brain and ventricles

Secondary effects

Vascular compression
Pontine haemorrhages
e.g. Posterior occipital artery occlusion and calcarine infarction

Causes of raised intracranial pressure

1) Tumours – intra and extracerebral

  Macroscopic features

  a) meningioma
  b) glioma
  c) lymphoma
  d) secondary carcinoma

2) *Cerebral abscess*

3) *Intracerebral haemorrhage*

4) *Extracerebral haemorrhage*

5) *Cerebral oedema*
   a) infections
   b) lead encephalopathy
   c) trauma

6) *Adult hydrocephalus*
   a) neoplasms
   b) inflammation

(April 1986, Paper 2, Question 2)

Reference

1) Morris, J.H. The nervous system. In: Pathologic Basis of Disease. S.L. Robbins, R.S. Cotran, V. Kumar (eds.) 4th edition. p1388; 1389. W.B. Saunders, Philadelphia (1989).

Describe in detail the effects on the intracranial contents of an expanding lesion in the left cerebral hemisphere
(April 1972, Paper 1, Question 3)

Describe the findings at necropsy in a subject who died with greatly raised intracranial pressure due to a rapidly-expanding lesion of the left cerebral hemisphere

Similar questions but which need more detailed consideration of circumscribed, rapidly expanding lesions, predominantly haemorrhagic or perhaps infective.
(October 1979, Paper 2, Question 3)

Reference

1) Morris, J.H. The nervous system. In: Pathologic Basis of Disease. S.L. Robbins, R.S. Cotran, V. Kumar (eds.) 4th edition. p1388; 1389. W.B. Saunders, Philadelphia (1989).

A man of 60 develops a right hemiplegia and some impairment of consciousness over 2–3 days. What are the likely causes? Describe the pathology of one of these

A question along similar lines to the preceding ones, with the addition of cerebrovascular disease, cerebral infarction being the most likely cause. In view of

the familiarity of most pathologists with these appearances, it is suggested that
this be developed for the final part of the question.

(November 1974, Paper, 2, Question 4)

Discuss the pathogenesis of intracranial haemorrhage and describe the relevant post-mortem appearances

Introduction

1) *Classification*

    a) cerebral
    b) subarachnoid
    c) subdural
    d) mixed

Cerebral

1) *Pathogenesis*

    a) hypertension
    b) trauma
    c) aneurysm
    d) vascular malformation
    e) bleeding diathesis

2) *Macroscopic features*

    a) location
    b) early
       i) secondary effects of intracranial expansion
       ii) location in trauma
    c) late
       i) changes in hypertensive disease

3) *Microscopic features*

Subarachnoid

1) *Pathogenesis*

    a) Berry aneurysms
       i)   location
       ii) structure
       iii) cause of rupture – HT
                                – trauma
    b) hypertensive
    c) 'mycotic' aneurysms

2) *Macroscopic features*

   a) early
   b) late

3) *Microscopic features*

   a) aneurysm structure

Extradural

1) *Pathogenesis*

   a) trauma to middle meningeal artery

2) *Macroscopic features*

Subdural

1) *Pathogenesis*

   Acute
   a) bridging vein tear

2) *Macroscopic features*

   Chronic
   a) clinical features

3) *Microscopic features*

Mixed

1) *Tumours*

2) *Arteriovenous malformations*

(October 1983, Paper 1, Question 1)

Reference

1) Morris, J.H. The nervous system – intracranial haemorrhage. In: Pathologic Basis of Disease. S.L. Robbins, R.S. Cotran, V. Kumar (eds.) 4th edition. p1405–1411. W.B. Saunders, Philadelphia (1989).

Discuss the aetiology and pathogenesis of strokes

This is the type of question which all pathologists should be able to answer adequately without any revision, since it is an important cause of morbidity and mortality. For the same reasons, such questions tend to be poor discriminators, which may account for their non-appearance in subsequent examinations.

(May 1973, Paper 1, Question 1)

A patient suffered several transient cerebral ischaemic attacks before death. Describe how you could demonstrate the cause of the attacks at post mortem laying special emphasis on the methods of examination of the cerebral circulation

Introduction

Definition of TIA
Clinical features
Association with cerebral infarction

Pathogenesis

1) Atherosclerosis

    a) emboli
    b) flow reduction

2) Thrombosis in atherosclerosis

3) Emboli

    a) heart (SABE, atria in AF, ventricles, MI)
    b) bone marrow (trauma)
    c) sites of lodgement
       i)   middle cerebral (90%)
       ii) others

4) Pathology

    a) lacuna stroke
       i)   motor paresis
       ii) sensory paresis
    b) cerebral haemorrhage – macroscopic
    c) embolic infarct – macroscopic appearance

Vascular dissection

1) Aorta

    a) orifices of carotid and vertebral arteries

2) Carotid arteries

    Sites
    a) bifurcation
    b) carotid sinus

3) Vertebral arteries

    a) anatomy
    b) method of dissection

Removal of brain

Vascular supply to brain

(October 1986, Paper 1, Question 3)

Reference

1) Morris, J.H. The nervous system – vascular disease. In: Pathologic Basis of Disease. S.L. Robbins, R.S. Cotran, V. Kumar (eds.) 4th edition. p1402–1411. W.B. Saunders, Philadelphia (1989).

Discuss the factors which determine the distribution of infarcts of the brain

It would be important to avoid the temptation to go into macroscopic and microscopic features in the evolution of cerebral infarction, as the question clearly calls for an account of the vascular pathology, including local arterial disease, (e.g. atherosclerosis, thrombosis) abnormality in the supply to the cerebral vessels (carotid, vertebral or aortic disease), cerebral infarction secondary to cardiac disease, and embolic phenomena. A description of the arterial supply to the brain would be of great value, including an outline of collateral supply, and a diagram may help in this respect. Infarction due to venous occlusion also deserves consideration, and is easily overlooked.   *(April 1969, Paper 2, Question 2)*

Reference

1) Morris, J.H. The nervous system – vascular disease. In: Pathologic Basis of Disease. S.L. Robbins, R.S. Cotran, V. Kumar (eds.) 4th edition. p1402–1411. W.B. Saunders, Philadelphia (1989).

Describe and discuss the morbid anatomical changes in the brain that may be produced by chronic hypoxia

Hypoxia is a term embracing several states which impair the consumption of oxygen by the brain, namely stagnant hypoxia (with ischaemia) pure hypoxia (seldom occurring naturally except at birth and at high altitude), anaemic hypoxia, and hypoglycaemia (lack of glucose impairs uptake of oxygen by neurons). By approaching the answer in this manner most candidates should be able to formulate a reasonable answer, but this is regarded as one of the more difficult questions which have been set.   *(November 1972, Paper 2, Question 4)*

Reference

1) Blackwood, W., Corsellis, J. Cerebral hypoxia. In: Greenfield's Neuropathology. W. Blackwood (ed.) p43–85. Edward Arnold, London (1976).

Describe the changes which occur in the central nervous system, and elsewhere, in syringomyelia, and speculate as to how the changes may be caused

A very interesting question, requiring more than usual thought in its preparation. Initially this seems to be a narrow, rather specialised pathology, but the secondary effects due to the dissociated sensory loss and motor weakness may be wideranging. A diagram illustrating the distribution of the lesions in a cross section of a spinal cord could be included. There is ample scope for speculation on mechanisms in 'primary' and 'secondary' syringomyelia. Having said this, it would probably be better to avoid this type of question if easier options are available.   *(October 1978, Paper 2, Question 5)*

Give an account of the primary tumours located in the posterior cranial fossa in children and adults

A fairly straightforward question especially for candidates who have completed a neuropathology attachment. One way of approaching this is to consider the anatomical contents of the posterior fossa, i.e. cerebellum, pons and medulla, choroid, nerves (including the auditory nerve) meninges, blood vessels, and then describe the most important tumours arising from them in each group. Where there is some overlap (e.g. adult medulloblastomas), only describe the major differences rather than duplicating the common features. Tumours that require description include in children, astrocytoma, ependymoma, medullobastoma and haemangioblastoma, and in adults ependymoma, astrocytoma, glioma, choroid plexus papilloma, neurilemmoma and meningioma.

(October 1986, Paper 2, Question 5)

Reference

1) Rosai, J. Neuromuscular system – tumors. In: Ackerman's Surgical Pathology. Volume 2, 7th edition, p1724–1771. C.V. Mosby Co, St Louis (1989).

9. Osteoarticular Pathology

Discuss genetic diseases of bone

It is probably best to approach this by briefly explaining the difference between congenital disease of bone, which often has an environmental influence (e.g. spina bifida, congenital syphilis, etc.) and those which have a defined genetic and hereditary component. Then explain the different types of disease, including clinical features, mode of transmission, pathological abnormalities and complications and pathogenesis if known. Suggested entities are osteogenesis imperfecta, achondroplasia, osteopetrosis, osteochondromatosis, enchondromatosis. Also involvement of the bones as a major feature in hereditary disorders such as storage diseases or Maffuci's syndrome should be considered, without expanding on the extraskeletal manifestations. Polymorphisms closely linked to the gene for some disorders, e.g. osteogenesis imperfecta are available for diagnosis, and should also be mentioned briefly.   *(April 1980, Paper 2, Question 5)*

Reference

1) Robbins, S.L., Cotran, R.S., Kumar, V. The musculoskeletal system. In: Pathologic Basis of Disease, 4th edition. p1315–1345. W.B. Saunders, Philadelphia (1989)

Describe the possible macroscopic and microscopic findings in an autopsy on a 60 year old woman who had refused further investigation or treatment after repeated findings of hypercalcaemia and hypophosphataemia over a period of four months before death

Hypercalcaemia (and consequent hypophosphataemia) may result from several conditions, of which malignancy is probably the commonest cause. Tumours include myelomatosis and secondaries from breast or lung cancers for example, and a brief comparison of the findings in such cases may be made. Although some tumours elaborate calcium mobilising substances without skeletal metastases, these should not be discussed in great detail as it is not something which can be surmised from the macroscopic or microscopic findings, except from a negative aspect. Hyperparathyroidism should be discussed in detail, including both the various features of the parathyroid glands, in primary hyperparathyroidism, and the effects on the bones and kidneys. The period of four months cited in the question may indicate that the gross changes (osteitis fibrosa cystica) would probably not be apparent, but microscopic diagnosis may be made. Renal changes in primary (calculus formation, nephrocalcinosis) and tertiary hyperparathyroidism (primary renal disease) may be described. Mention should be made of multiple endocrine neoplasia syndromes. Other causes of hypercalcaemia could be discussed such as milk alkali syndrome, sarcoidosis, etc, but again it should be noted that the mechanisms are not required, only relevant pathological features. This is the type of question where very close attention must be paid to the wording.   *(April 1974, Paper 1, Question 3)*

Reference

1)   Robbins, S.L., Cotran, R.S., Kumar, V. The endocrine system. In: Pathologic Basis of Disease, 4th edition. p1243;1244. W.B. Saunders, Philadelphia (1989).

Describe the various changes that may be found in the bones in chronic renal failure including patients on haemodialysis. Discuss the pathogenesis of the various lesions

Introduction

Types of bone disease in CRF
Incidence
Symptomatology

Osteitis fibrosa

1)   *Accelerated bone resorption*

2)   *Paratrabecular marrow fibrosis*

3)   *Osteocytic osteolysis*

4)   *Increased bone function with osteoid and woven bone*

   Quantitative measurements
   a) excessive osteoid covered trabeculae
   b) normal seam width
   c) normal mineralisation rate

Osteomalacia

1)   *Increased extent of osteoid seams* (undecalcified bone)

2)   *Reduced mineralisation front* (toluidine blue)

   Quantitative measurements
   a) increased osteoid seam thickness
   b) reduced mineralisation rate (double tetracycline labelling)

Osteosclerosis

Increased mineralised woven bone

Osteoporosis

Rare – in steroid therapy or elderly

Pathogenesis

1) *Hypocalcaemia* due to

    a) renal retention of PO4
    b) intestinal malabsorption of Ca2+ in CRF
    c) ? defective Vit D3 suppression of parathyroids compensatory ↑ in PTH

2) *Osteomalacia* due to

    a) ? defective 1α hydroxylation of 25DHCC
    b) systemic acidosis in CRF alters Vit D metabolism
    c) hypophosphataemia in Fanconi syndrome, renal tubular acidosis, etc.

Haemodialysis

1) *Osteitis fibrosa and osteomalacia*

Pathogenesis

    a) PO4 binding resin
    b) dialysis
    c) anticonvulsants
    d) unknown

2) *Dialysis and osteomalacia*

    a) symptoms
    b) osteomalacia with little osteitis fibrosa
    c) inactive osteoid seams, ↓ mineralisation front
    d) normal alkaline phosphatase

Pathogenesis

    a) aluminium toxicity
    b) bone measurements, animal toxicity
    c) reduction after deionisation

(October 1982, Paper 2, Question 1)

Reference

1) Ellis, H.A. Metabolic bone disease. In: Recent Advances in Histopathology 11. P.P. Anthony, R.N.M. MacSween (eds.) p185–202. Churchill Livingstone, Edinburgh (1981).

What lesions of bone may be found in chronic renal failure? Discuss their pathogenesis

(November 1973, Paper 1, Question 2)

Describe the macroscopic and microscopic changes which may develop in bone secondary to renal disease

There is abundant material to write on in this answer ranging from the clinical and radiological features of renal osteodystrophy and its pathological consequences, to the microscopic features best described in the earlier stages on bone biopsy, including osteomalacia, secondary hyperparathyroidism and osteosclerosis, with a detailed description of morphometric analysis (including dynamic measurements such as tetracycline labelling). A discussion on dialysis osteomalacia should also be included.   *(April 1972, Paper 1, Question 4)*

Describe the macroscopic and microscopic changes in bone affected by Paget's disease (osteitis deformans). What are the complications of this disease?

(April 1971, Paper 2, Question 2)

Write an essay on Paget's disease of bone

(NB Good writing style and paragraph construction required)

Introduction

Osteitis deformans
General features
Pathological definition – remodelling of bone in a coarser mould
Incidence and epidemiology

Clinical features

1) Sites

Monostotic/polyostotic

2) Symptoms
   a) asymptomatic
   b) deformity
   c) arthritis
   d) pain
   e) fractures
   f) nerve compression (optic, auditory, vertebral, etc.)
   g) heart failure

3) Investigations
   a) ↑ alkaline phosphatase, normal calcium, phosphorus, and PTH
   b) radiographic features – osteolytic, mixed, sclerotic

4) *General pathology*

   a) sites – pelvis > skull > femur > spine > tibia > humerus > jaw
   b) loss of corticomedullary distinction and enlargement
   c) consistency – early – porous late – sclerotic
   d) deformity

5) *Microscopic*

   a) osteolytic phase
      i) disorganised osteoclastic activity
      ii) morphology of osteoclasts
   b) osteoblastic response
      i) stromal vascularisation
      ii) haphazard matrix deposition
      iii) 'mosaic' reversal lines with osteoid persistence at margins
      iv) subperiosteal
   c) sclerotic phase
      i) ↓ osteoclasis
      ii) osteoblastic activity leads to bone thickening

Complications

1) *Pathological fractures*

2) *Haemodynamic changes*

   a) bone hypervascularity
   b) arteriovenous shunting
   c) osteogenic sarcoma
      i) incidence 1%
      ii) distribution
      iii) pathology
      iv) behaviour

Aetiology

1) *Previous theories*

   a) inborn error of connective tissue
   b) autoimmune disorder

2) *Recent? 'slow' viral infection*

   a) tubular viral structures in osteoclasts on EM
   b) immunocytochemistry
   Absence of antibody response or isolation of virus

(April 1983, Paper 1, Question 4)

Reference

1) Ellis, H.A. Metabolic bone disease. In: Recent Advances in Histopathology 11. P.P. Anthony, R.N.M. MacSween (eds.) p185–202. Churchill Livingstone, Edinburgh (1981).

Discuss the mechanisms involved in the pathogenesis of osteomalacia and outline the histopathological techniques used in its assessment

Introduction

Vitamin D deficiency in adults
Clinical features
General functions of Vitamin D

Metabolism of Vitamin D

1) *Skin*

    a) 7DHC converted to D3 (UV light)

2) *Diet*

    a) D3 (animal products)

3) *Absorption*

    a) small bowel
    b) transported to liver
    c) 25 hydroxylation
    d) 1α hydroxylation
    e) 1,25 (OH)2D3 in kidney

4) *Receptors*

    a) small intestine villus cells for 1,25 (OH)2D3
    b) osteoblasts
    c) renal tubular cells

5) *Actions of Vitamin D*

    a) intestinal absorption of calcium
    b) mobilises calcium and phosphorus at bone interface with PTH
    c) renal tubular resorption

Factors involved in deficiency

1) *Vitamin D3 lack*

    a) dietary insufficiency
    b) insufficiency of UV light
    c) malabsorption – various causes

2) *Chronic renal failure*

    a) failure of 1α hydroxylation
    b) acidosis

3) *Hypophosphataemia*

    a) renal tubular acidosis

    b) Fanconi syndrome

4) *Hereditary disease*

    a) Vitamin D dependent rickets

5) *Drug induced*

    a) anticonvulsants

Assessment of osteomalacia

1) *Bone biopsy*

    a) undecalcified sections – surface osteoid estimation
       i) percentage of surface of osteoid seams (n<30%)
       ii) thickness of polarised seams (n<3 'bright lines')
       iii) total bone mass
    b) decalcified sections
       i) mineralisation fronts (Toluidine blue)
       ii) mineralisation rate (double tetracycline labelling)
       iii) osteoclast concentration
       iv) osteoblast activity

(April 1982, Paper 1, Question 4)

References

1) Ellis, H.A. Metabolic bone disease. In: Recent Advances in Histopathology 11. P.P. Anthony, R.N.M. MacSween (eds.) p185–202. Churchill Livingstone, Edinburgh (1981).
2) Eastwood, J.B. Quantitative bone histology in 38 patients with advanced renal failure. J. Clin. Pathol. (1982) 35: 125–134.

Describe the effects of Vitamin D deficiency on the skeletal system

This should include an outline of Vitamin D metabolism and osteomalacia as outlined in the previous question, together with a substantial section on rickets.

(May 1973, Paper 2, Question 2)

Describe the methods available for measurement of the relative amount of osteoid in a bone biopsy. Discuss the value of such quantititation in the diagnosis of metabolic bone disease

(October 1980, Paper 2, Question 5)

Discuss the uses and limitations of biopsy in the diagnosis of metabolic disease of bone, and give an account of the histological techniques you would employ to obtain as much information as possible from a sample

The latter question involves expanding the outline of the morphometric and dynamic measurements, and relating this to the findings in the major forms of metabolic bone disease; osteomalacia, osteoporosis, chronic renal failure and hyperparathyroidism.

The 1978 essay pre-dates the widespread use of double-labelling techniques for dynamic measurements, and thus some of the limitations are overcome. Others include sampling error, complex situations such as renal failure with its multifactorial effects, and the possibility of misleading results from fracture sites, etc. Otherwise the outline is very similar to the previous plan (April 1982, Paper 1, Question 4).   *(October 1978, Paper 2, Question 2)*

Give an account of the causes of hyperparathyroidism. What corresponding bone changes may be present?

The causes of hyperparathyroidism should include a discussion of primary (adenoma, hyperplasia, carcinoma), secondary (chronic renal failure, malabsorption, hypercalcitoninaemia) and tertiary forms.

The bone changes need to be clearly discussed with respect to the increase in number of both osteoclasts and osteoblasts in hyperparathyroidism. Abundant osteoclasts result in numerous resorption lacunae, (erosion of phalangeal tufts) and formation of brown tumours (diaphysis, ribs, jaw). A mention of the early sensitive and specific sign of paratrabecular fibrosis is required. Hyperosteoidosis is a feature of hyperparathyroidism and needs to be differentiated from osteomalacia using tetracycline labelling (include a comment on the relevant aspects of bone morphometry, as discussed in the previous examples).
(April 1988, Paper 2, Question 2)

Reference

1) Revell, P.A. Metabolic bone disease. In: Pathology of Bone. p113–146. Springer-Verlag, Berlin (1985).

An elderly woman with backache is found to have a collapsed lumbar vertebra and diffuse decrease in bone density of the spine. List the possible underlying causes, indicating their relative probability and explain how laboratory investigations could help in reaching a diagnosis

Essentially a question about osteomalacia and osteoporosis in another form, the underlying causes are wide ranging. The laboratory investigations not only include the biochemical and histological evaluation of metabolic bone disease, but in the investigation of the underlying causes such as malabsorption syndrome, renal disease, Cushing's syndrome, etc. It is important to understand that the underlying causes relate more to the metabolic bone disease than other factors which may lead to collapsed vertebrae e.g. myeloma or secondary carcinoma – these would be unlikely to produce a picture of diffuse decrease in spinal bone density.   *(April 1976, Paper 1, Question 5)*

Describe the structural changes in the bones in osteoporosis, and discuss its causation

There is relatively little information which can be provided on the exact aetiology of osteoporosis, but some of the metabolic alteration and associations could be discussed. The structural alterations are relatively straightforward, but this type of essay might prove quite difficult to answer in the examination situation because of the relatively restricted amount of information which could be provided, certainly by the average pathologist.   *(November 1971, Paper 2, Question 1)*

Describe briefly the normal mechanism of bone formation and destruction. How may the processes be altered in disease?

The answer involves a discussion of normal bone metabolism and turnover as already outlined, but the second part of the answer could essentially involve all forms of metabolic bone disease, perhaps with the effects of secondary carcinoma or even primary bone tumours as well. However, the wording of the question is quite subtle, in that it is the alteration of the processes, and not the pathological consequences that requires description. It could either be approached by describing the altered mechanism in each disease state, or taking each individual component (e.g. osteoclast, osteoblast, fibroblast, etc.) and illustrate how their function may alter in response to such disease. This would require considerable thought to be given in advance of the examination; it would be difficult to organise an approach like this during it.   *(November 1977, Paper 1, Question 2)*

Discuss the differential diagnosis of cysts in bone

Introduction

Meaning of 'cyst'
Radiological versus pathological cysts

1) *Simple cyst*
   a) sites
   b) clinical and radiographic features
   c) gross pathology
   d) histopathological appearances

2) *Ganglion cyst*

   a) sites

   b) radiological appearance

   c) histological appearance

3) *Epidermoid cysts*

   a) sites

   b) radiological features

   c) histological appearance (middle ear infection)

4) *Joint disease*

   a) osteoarthritis

      i)   macroscopic

      ii)   microscopic

   b) rheumatoid disease

      i)   inflammatory

      ii)   degenerative

   c) villonodular synovitis

      i)   microscopic

5) *Aneurysmal bone cyst*

   a) sites

   b) clinical features

   c) radiological changes

   d) gross pathology

   e) microscopic

6) *Hydatid disease*

   a) sites

   b) radiological features

7) *Jaw cysts*

   a) radicular cyst

   b) follicular cyst

   c) fissural cysts

   d) odontogenic cysts

(October 1985, Paper 1, Question 2)

Reference

1) Dahlin,D.C. Unni, K.K. Conditions that simulate primary neoplasms of bone, and odontogenic and related tumours. In: Bone Tumours. 4th edition, p356–440. Charles C. Thomas, Illinois (1986).

Write an essay on benign tumours of bone

It would clearly be impossible to cover all of the benign bone tumours with any depth, unless emphasis was given to the commoner ones and those which require particularly careful evaluation (e.g. giant cell tumour). Headings and discussion of each entity could be made separately, but it might be preferable to use a formal essay style, perhaps to compare aspects of the differential diagnosis of benign bone tumours. Entities to consider are chondroma, chondroblastoma, chondro-myxoid fibroma, osteoma, osteoid osteoma, osteoblastoma, giant cell tumour, non-ossifying fibroma, with brief mention of others such as haemangioma, neurofibroma, etc.   *(October 1978, Paper 1, Question 5)*

Reference

1) Dahlin, D.C., Unni, K.K. Chapters 2–13. In: Bone Tumours. 4th edition, p18–192. Charles C. Thomas, Illinois (1986).

Discuss the application of synovial biopsy to diagnosis

This question may have been prompted by the appearance of the cited reference. Some candidates may require a broader range of knowledge in order to make a comprehensive, balanced answer, as the article in question only seeks to cover certain selected aspects in detail. The commoner diagnostic problems, especially acute and chronic synovitis, are mentioned briefly but would require considerable elaboration for an adequate review. An alternative approach would be to use some introductory paragraphs to explain the non-specific features in many inflammatory processes, and concentrate on the more characteristic features which would enable a specific diagnosis to be made, as outlined in Table 6.1 of the reference. It is important for candidates to recognise that answers to questions using wording such as 'Discuss' allow considerable flexibility, providing the omission of certain topics is acknowledged and briefly justified.

(November 1988, Paper 1, Question 2)

Reference

1) Revell, P.A. The synovial biopsy. In: Recent Advances in Histopathology 13, Chapter 6, p79–93. Churchill Livingstone (1987).

Discuss the pathogenesis of rheumatoid disease
(October 1986, Paper 2, Question 1)

Discuss the aetiology of rheumatoid disease

These two questions illustrate the necessity of understanding the distinction between aetiology and pathogenesis, although there is a tendency for the two to become confused when the aetiology, i.e. cause, is not certain. The pathogenesis deals with the mechanisms which lead to the tissue damage, and in this sort of disease, the aetiology, although to be considered, would play a relatively minor part in the overall answer. *(October 1984, Paper 1, Question 4)*

Reference

1) Robbins, S.L., Cotran, R.S., Kumar, V. Joints and related structures. In: Pathologic Basis of Disease, 4th edition. p1349–1354, W.B. Saunders, Philadelphia (1989).

Describe the post-mortem findings in a woman who died of rheumatoid arthritis. Indicate the significance of the lesions to the disease as a whole

This answer should be fairly straightforward, with both articular lesions and systemic associations requiring description, concentrating on the macroscopic appearances. The extra-articular complications are more likely to account for the demise of the patient, and should be assessed accordingly.

(April 1970, Paper 2, Question 4)

Discuss the non-articular lesions associated with rheumatoid arthritis

Since the type of rheumatoid arthritis is not stated, both juvenile and adult forms could be considered. The approach should be on a systematic basis, discussing lymphoreticular changes, rheumatoid nodules, cardiac, pulmonary and vascular changes, including immunopathology when appropriate. It is suggested that the more tenuous associations (e.g. complications of therapy) are avoided as far as possible.

(April 1972, Paper 2, Question 5)

10. Reproductive System

Discuss the impact that the widespread use of synthetic oestrogens and progesterone has had on the practice of gynaecological pathology

At first glance this is not an easy question, but with a little reflection most surgical histopathologists would have encountered many examples of tissue changes connected with these agents. There are two ways to approach this answer, either by describing the general category of usage (e.g. contraception, dysfunctional uterine bleeding, management of carcinoma, etc.) or the changes induced by each particular agent (or combination) and its effect on normal and pathological states. It is important to firstly describe in detail the effect on normal tissues (endometrium and cervix predominantly), and their effects on pathological conditions, (e.g. endometrial hyperplasia, endometrial carcinoma) together with some consequences of such therapy, in particular the diethylstilboestrol syndrome, and potential effects on other tissues such as breast and liver (which could justifiably be included). In order to answer this question adequately, it is important to relate the difference that not only the effect of these agents has had on the pathology of submitted specimens, but what changes there have been in nature and numbers of material sent for examination in order to monitor the effects of treatment, requiring somewhat broader scope than mere descriptive pathology.

(November 1974, Paper 1, Question 4)

References

1) Buckley, C.H. Pathology of contraception and of hormonal therapy. In: Obstetrical and Gynaecological Pathology. H. Fox (ed.) Volume 2. Chapter 20, p839–873. Churchill Livingstone, Edinburgh (1987).
2) Campbell, J.S. et al. Iatrogenic disease of the female genital tract. ibid p882–888.

Describe the tissue changes that have been attributed to oral contraceptive therapy

(May 1973, Paper 2, Question 4)

What adverse effects may result from orally administered oestrogens?

These two questions share much common ground, but it should be noted that the second does not restrict itself to contraception since it includes oestrogens taken orally in later life for the purpose of hormone replacement and also for the treatment of prostatic carcinoma. The term 'tissue changes' in the first question strictly includes the desired action of oral contraceptives (both combined and progestagen-only types) on the reproductive system, as well as possible systemic effects (e.g. venous thrombosis or atherosclerosis) while the second question does not require a discussion of the primary action. The reference given contains a good discussion of effects on the endometrium, cervix, vagina, ovary, cardiovascular system, breast and liver.   *(April 1978, Paper 2, Question 3)*

Reference

1) Buckley, C.H. The pathology of contraception. In: Obstetrical and Gynaecological Pathology. H. Fox (ed.) 3rd edition. p847–889. Churchill Livingstone, Edinburgh (1987).

Write an essay on neoplasia of the uterine cervix

Introduction

Spectrum of diseases
Incidence of ca cervix vs. other tumours
Clinical features and diagnosis

CIN

1) Squamous

    a) classification and nomenclature

    b) pathological features

    c) cytological diagnosis

    d) pathogenesis
        i)   epidemiology and incidence
        ii) viral infection
            – HPV
            – HSV

    e) management
        i)   role of pathologist
        ii) role of cytologist

2) Glandular

    a) pathological features

    b) cytology

    c) relationship to squamous CIN

Invasive carcinoma

1) Squamous

    a) relationship to CIN

    b) microinvasive disease
        i)   definition
        ii) diagnosis
        iii) prognosis

    c) larger tumours
        i)   classification
        ii) spread
        iii) prognosis

2) *Adenocarcinoma*
   a) classification and pathology
   b) behaviour
   c) spread
   d) rare variants
      i) ciliated (serous)
      ii) mucinous
      iii) carcinoid
      iv) oat cell carcinoma
   e) Peutz-Jeghers' disease (adenoma malignum)
   f) management

Mesenchymal tumours

Benign

1) *Leiomyoma*

   a) pathological features

Malignant

1) *Sarcoma botryoid*

   a) pathological features

2) *Mixed Müllerian tumours*

3) *Müllerian adenosarcoma*

4) *Lymphoma*

5) *Leiomyosarcoma*

(October 1986, Paper 2, Question 4)

References

1) Anderson, M.C. Premalignant and malignant disease of the cervix. In: Obstetrical and Gynaecological Pathology. H. Fox (ed.) 3rd edition. p255–301. Churchill Livingstone, Edinburgh (1987).
2) Brescia, R.J. et al. The role of human papilloma viruses in the pathogenesis and histologic classification of precancerous lesions of the cervix. Human Pathol. (1986) 17: 552–558.

'Carcinoma of the cervix is a disease that is eradicable from the community'. Discuss this statement

This essay requires a structured plan more than most, as with questions which have a scope as broad as this one there is a danger of producing an imbalanced and partly irrelevant discourse, a concentration on quantity rather than quality. The answer should be divided into two parts, the first considering the premise that the pre-invasive and early stages of carcinoma of the cervix are detectable by exfoliative cytology, and treatable by various means. In addition, the significance of minor degrees of cervical dysplasia should be considered. The second part of the answer should consider the reasons for the present inability to eradicate the disease, including social and logistical factors (e.g. efficiency of recall systems) and technical aspects (e.g. screening failures). The subject is topical at present and highly likely to be set again. There are frequent reviews in pathology and general medical journals (e.g. *British Medical Journal* and *The Lancet*) on aspects of this subject which are usually worth reading, and assessments of the efficiency of the national computer recall system will emerge in the next few years.

(November 1976, Paper 2, Question 2)

References

1) Reid, B.L. Causation of cervical carcinoma. In: Clinics in Obstetrics and Gynaecology. A. Singer (ed.) Chapter 1, p1–18. W.B. Saunders, Philadelphia (1985).
2) Hudson, E.A. The place of the cytological smear test. ibid. p33–52.

Discuss the role of viruses in the aetiology of disorders of the cervix uteri

The previous essay included some reference to the role of viruses, but there is now so much information in the literature, with abundant review articles, that most modern pathologists would be able to write a detailed essay on this subject. The issue is still contentious, however, and a balanced view should be taken to encompass the role of herpes viruses as well as human papillomavirus. The epidemiological evidence together with oncogenic properties of these viruses should be discussed, along with the pathological evidence (e.g. morphological, immunocytochemical, in situ hybridisation), for their associations. It is relevant that Koch's postulates have still not been fulfilled in respect of virus-associated carcinomas, but the theoretical basis for this is complicated, to say the least.

(April 1987, Paper 1, Question 3)

Reference

1) Anderson, M.C. Premalignant and malignant diseases of the cervix – viruses. In: Obstetrical and Gynaecological Pathology. H. Fox (ed.) 3rd edition. p261–265. Churchill Livingstone, Edinburgh (1987).

Write an account of trophoblastic tumours

A question which is somewhat difficult to answer because of the vagueness of the term 'tumour'; is a partial or even complete hydatidiform mole to be regarded as a tumour in the neoplastic sense, or within a broader context? This is one situation where an introductory paragraph would be used to clearly define the understanding of the term and justify the inclusion of these entities. It is fairly obvious that atypical and typical choriocarcinomas should be described in detail, together with the differential diagnosis from a normal placental implanted site ('syncytial endometritis'). It would probably not be justifiable to include chorio-carcinomatous differentiation in teratomas of the testis, but this might be mentioned in passing, or in desparation. *(April 1979, Paper 2, Question 1)*

Reference

1) Elston, C.W. Gestational trophoblastic disease. In: Obstetrical and Gynaecological Pathology. H. Fox (ed.) 3rd edition. p1045–1078. Churchill Livingstone, Edinburgh (1987).

Give an account of the pathology, including the pathogenesis of hydatidiform mole

A more circumscribed question which is relatively straightforward to answer. A more detailed account of the pathogenesis is required, and a comprehensive account may be found in the previous references.

(November 1975, Paper 2, Question 2)

How would you differentiate between the various types of endometrial hyperplasia?

It is probably best to approach this answer by describing the various forms into hyperplasia with or without cytological and architectural atypia, defining the point at which frank carcinoma can be diagnosed. This should be an easy question for any working histopathologist providing a structured framework is used.

(April 1974, Paper 1, Question 2)

Reference

1) Hendrickson, M.R., Kempson, R.L. Endometrial hyperplasia, metaplasia and carcinoma. In: Obstetrical and Gynaecological Pathology. H. Fox (ed.) 3rd edition. p354–361. Churchill Livingstone, Edinburgh (1987).

Give an account of malignant neoplasms of the uterus other than carcinomas

This question lends itself very well to being answered in small sections concerning each entity, and is best divided into tumours of proposed endometrial origin, and those from the myometrium and uterine wall. The former group include the mixed Müllerian tumours, such as malignant mixed Müllerian tumour, of which a detailed account should be made with mention of the rarer variants such as adenosarcoma. Endometrial stromal sarcoma, low grade and high grade require consideration. Choriocarcinoma, both typical and 'atypical' (placental site trophoblastic tumour), although not strictly of uterine origin, should be included in your account, and could be easily overlooked.

Sarcoma botryoides of the cervix could be covered briefly, but the major emphasis in non-endometrial malignancies should be given to leiomyosarcomas and the various criteria for diagnosis in the well differentiated forms. Brief descriptions could be made of tumours such as haemangiopericytoma or other sarcomas which rarely affect the uterus, and possibly lymphoma although it is probably not a primary site.   *(October 1979, Paper 2, Question 5)*

References

1) Kempson, R.L., Hendrickson, M.R. Pure mesenchymal neoplasms of the uterine corpus. In: Obstetrical and Gynaecological Pathology. H. Fox (ed.) 3rd edition. p 411–456. Churchill Livingstone, Edinburgh (1987).
2) Honore, L.H. Mixed Müllerian tumours of the uterus. ibid p457–478.

Discuss the primary malignant tumours of the uterus

There are so many entities involved in answering this question that there would be little time for anything other than a brief discussion. One device might be to exclude tumours of the uterine cervix, explaining the reasons in an introductory paragraph. Discussion could then be confined to endometrial carcinoma and other entities considered in the answer to October 1979, Paper 2, Question 5, or problems such as the distinction between epithelial hyperplasia and neoplasia in the endometrium, or on the criteria for diagnosis of malignancy in smooth muscle tumours. This would have to be a selective essay which could be adapted to suit each individual's areas of greatest interest or knowledge.

(November 1970, Paper 2, Question 2)

Give an account of the histopathology of ovarian carcinoma and relate this to its biological behaviour

A very straightforward essay which includes a consideration of serous, mucinous, endometrial, clear cell and undifferentiated carcinomas. Germ cell tumours such as yolk sac tumour and choriocarcinoma could reasonably be included, together with metastatic carcinoma and a brief reference to carcinomas in cystic teratomas. A reasonable proportion of the essay should be devoted to a consideration of 'borderline' tumours including criteria for diagnosis, and behaviour.

(April 1975, Paper 1, Question 5)

References

1) Russell, P. Common epithelial tumours of the ovary. In: Obstetrical and Gynaecological Pathology. H. Fox (ed.) 3rd edition. p556–622. Churchill Livingstone, Edinburgh (1987).
2) Nogales, F. Germ cell tumours of the ovary. ibid p637–675.

Describe the pathology of fibrocystic disease of the breast (excluding sclerosing adenosis) and discuss its aetiology and significance

The most authoritative discussion of this subject is to be found in this reference, but adequate though less comprehensive coverage can be found in general texts of pathology. The subject is bedevilled by an excess of terminology, and further confused by transatlantic differences (e.g. papillomatosis vs. epitheliosis). Fibrocystic disease (or better, cystic disease) should be strictly defined according to the guidelines provided in the reference.   *(April 1986, Paper 1, Question 5)*

Reference

1) Azzopardi, J.G. Terminology, plus cystic disease and duct ectasia. In: Problems in Breast Pathology. p23–38; 57–91. W.B. Saunders, Philadelphia (1979).

Discuss the pathological appearances which may be seen in testicular swellings

Introduction

Testis and epididymis
Clinical features
Pre-operative investigations
Role of biopsy

Acquired diseases

Inflammation

1) *Generalised infection*
   a) viral
      i)   mumps
           – pathological features
      ii) coxsackie
      iii) other
   b) bacterial
      i)   TB
           – pathological features
      ii) syphilis
           – pathological features
      iii) others

2) *Localised infection*

    a) bacterial
        i)   gonorrhoea
            – pathological features
            – non-specific
            – usually epididymitis
            – chlamydial
        ii) actinomyces
            – pathological features

3) *Non-infective/unknown*

    a) granulomatous orchitis
        i)   pathological features
        ii) malakoplakia

Trauma

1) *Haematoma*

2) *Torsion*

Neoplasia

1) *Germ cell tumours*

    a) seminoma
        i)   clinical features
        ii) gross pathology
        iii) microscopic appearances
        iv) (+ spermatocytic variant)
    b) embryonal carcinoma
        i)   microscopic features
    c) yolk sac tumour
        i)   microscopic features
        ii) immunohistochemistry (AFP)
    d) choriocarcinoma
        i)   microscopic features
        ii) immunohistochemistry (HCG)
    e) teratomas
        i)   mature
        ii) immature
        iii) malignant
    f) combined tumours

2) *Sex cord – stromal*

    a) Leydig cell tumours
        i)   gross features
        ii) microscopic
    b) Seroli cell tumours
        i)   microscopic
    c) granulosa cell tumours

3) _Lymphomas_

   a) primary
      i) 'mucosa associated'
      ii) B cell
      iii) large cell NHL
      iv) ? Hodgkin's disease
   b) disseminated
      i) leukaemia/lymphoma

4) _Secondary carcinoma_

(April 1984, Paper 2, Question 3)

Reference

1) Robbins, S.L., Cotran, R.S., Kumar, V. Male genital system. In: Pathologic Basis of Disease. 4th edition, p1104–1116. W.B. Saunders, Philadelphia (1989).

Discuss the cytological and histopathological aspects of the investigation of infertility in the male

A fairly straightforward question, but which might pose some problems for those candidates who have not had experience in semen analysis. The only way to really understand this technique is to become involved at some stage during training. The histopathological aspects do not only involve the use of testicular biopsy, as extragonadal causes of infertility require some consideration (e.g. pituitary disease, haemochromatosis, etc.). *(May 1973, Paper 1, Question 5)*

Reference

1) Lennox, B. The infertile testis. In: Recent Advances in Histopathology 11. P.P. Anthony, R.N.M. MacSween (eds.) p135–148. Churchill Livingstone, Edinburgh (1981).

11. Dermatopathology

Discuss the pathology and differential diagnosis of bullous diseases of the skin

A sensible approach to this group of disorders is provided in the first reference, where the distinction between vesicle and bulla is avoided by the use of the term 'blister'. Within this term there are seven groups, a mixture of anatomical and aetiological blisters; a) subepidermal b) blister following intracellular degeneration c) spongiosis   d) acantholytic e) viral f) basal cell degeneration and g) basement membrane degeneration. Several conditions fall within each group, but the main features of the most important condition should be included. Details of the role of immunofluorescent techniques in the diagnosis should be included in such an answer.   *(October 1983, Paper 2, Question 1)*

References

1) Mackie, R.M., Young, H. Use of the immunofluorescence technique in diagnostic dermatopathology. ACP Broadsheet no. 110. (April 1984).
2) Meyrick-Thomas, R.H. et al. The value of immunofluorescent techniques in the diagnosis of skin diseases. In: Recent Advances in Histopathology 12. P.P. Anthony, R.N.M. MacSween (eds.) p69–81. Churchill Livingstone, Edinburgh (1984).

Give an account of the histopathology of the skin in disorders whose cutaneous lesions are manifestations of systemic disease

Systemic diseases could include conditions as wide-ranging as infections (e.g. leprosy, tuberculosis, streptococcal sore throat, bacterial endocarditis), connective tissue disorders (e.g. SLE, rheumatoid disease), various malignancies or indicators of internal malignancy such as Cowdens, Leser-Trelat syndromes or acanthosis nigricans, and immunosuppressed states (although it could be argued that localised tumours do not constitute a systemic disease, whereas lympho-proliferative disorders could be). Other systemic diseases could be discussed such as sarcoidosis, drug eruptions, metabolic diseases (e.g. amyloidosis) as well as rare conditions like glucagonoma syndrome or acrodermatitis enteropathica for instance. There is enough potential information in the suggested categories to supply material for several essays, therefore each candidate could select these areas with which they are most familiar, while still providing a balance.
                                                                                       (November 1974, Paper 1, Question 5)

References

1) Lever, W.F., Schaumburg-Lever, G. Systemic diseases with cutaneous manifestations. In: Histopathology of the Skin. 6th edition, p190–197 (and other sections in addition). J.B. Lippincott Co, Philadelphia (1983).
2) Staughton, R.C.D. Cutaneous manifestations of malignancy. Br. J. Hosp. Med. (1978) 20: 38–47.

Discuss the interpretation of lymphocytic infiltrates in the skin

This question has been tailor-made for a candidate familiar with the article in reference 1). It should include a description of the features of malignant cutaneous lympho-proliferative conditions, including immunohistochemical features, together with the spectrum of benign infiltrates. A consideration of differentiation of benign from malignant lesions is best included after the descriptive sections. Immunohistochemical features must be mentioned but need not be expanded at the cost of an adequate discussion of benign entities. The answer should recognise that at the present time, even with immunohistochemical marking techniques, there are some cases that it will not be possible to characterise with certainty and an equivocal report will be indicated. As with all dermatopathological work, the value of clinicopathological exchange should be emphasised.

(April 1988, Paper 1, Question 5)

Reference

1) Slater, D.N. Lymphoproliferative conditions of the skin. In: Recent Advances in Histopathology 12. P.P. Anthony, R.N.M. MacSween (eds.) p83–110. Churchill Livingstone, Edinburgh (1984).

Give an account of pigmented tumours of the skin and discuss their histological diagnosis

This includes an overview of benign and malignant tumours, and would necessarily be very brief on each entity. Emphasis should be made on diagnostically difficult benign tumours (e.g. Spitz naevus, dysplastic naevus) and malignant melanoma.

(April 1976, Paper 2, Question 4)

Describe the histopathological features which correlate with prognosis in melanotic lesions of the skin

(April 1983, Paper 1, Question 3)

Discuss the difficulties in the diagnosis and assessment of prognosis of melanin-containing tumours of the epidermis and upper dermis

These answers all require concentration on malignant melanoma, but in addition lesions which cause diagnostic difficulty should be described such as shave naevus, benign epithelioid cell naevus (benign juvenile melanoma), spindle cell naevus (Reed's tumour) and dysplastic naevus. There would be a large amount of factual information to cover in the time available, and liberal use of side headings and note form would almost certainly be required for a comprehensive answer.

(April 1975, Paper 2, Question 3)

Outline a classification of malignant melanoma and discuss possible prognostic indices

Introduction

Classification
Radial and vertical growth phases – general features
General criteria of malignancy
Histologist's role in management – overview

Macroscopic examination

1) *Description and measurement*

2) *Block selection*

Lentigo maligna melanoma

1) *Radial growth phase*

2) *Epidermal atrophy*

3) *Melanocyte nests*

4) *Vertical growth phase*
   a) spindle/epithelioid cells
   b) desmoplasia
   c) neurotropism

Acral lentiginous melanoma

1) *Radial growth phase*
   a) large dendritic melanocytes
   b) small nests
   c) lichenoid lymphocytic infiltrate

2) *Vertical phase*
   a) spindle cells
   b) neurotropic

Superficial spreading melanoma

1) *Radial*
   a) epithelioid cells
   b) fine pigment
   c) nests and single cells
   d) intra-epidermal patterns

2) _Vertical_

   a) epithelioid
   b) rare desmoplasia and neutropism
   c) little inflammation

Nodular melanoma

1) _No radial phase_

   a) ? early nodular development

2) _Vertical growth phase_

   a) often nodular

Evaluation of risk

1) _Thickness range_

   a) < 0.76 mm
   b) 0.76–1.5mm
   c) > 1.5 mm

2) _Prognosis_

   a) 88% 5 year survival
   b) 61% 5 year survival
   c) 32% 5 year survival

3) _Level of invasion_

   (Clark's classification I–V – detail)
   Combined data of level and thickness – low, moderate and high risk groups.

4) _Site (BANS)_

5) _Mitotic index_

6) _Host lymphocytic response_

7) _Regional lymph node status_

                                                        (April 1979, Paper 1, Question 4)

References

1) Clark, W.H. et al. The biologic forms of malignant melanoma. Human Pathol. (1986) 17: 443–450.
2) Lever, W.F., Schaumberg-Lever, G. Melanocytic naevi and malignant melanoma. In: Histopathology of the Skin. 6th edition, p702–723. J.B. Lippincott Co, Philadelphia (1983).

Discuss the histological evaluation of malignant melanoma of the skin

(October 1985, Paper 1, Question 1)

What is the role of the histopathologist in the diagnosis and management of melanocytic lesions of the skin?

(April 1986, Paper 2, Question 5)

12. Miscellaneous

There has been a worldwide decrease in the hospital post mortem rate in recent years. Discuss the reasons for the decrease and suggest ways by which it could be reversed

Introduction

Post mortem rate ratios
Hospital and coroners' PMs
Aims of PM-Medical Audit

Reasons for decline

1) *Clinical demand*

   a) more accurate ante mortem diagnosis
   b) aesthetic objections
   c) infectious hazards
   d) fear of contradiction – legal considerations
   e) lack of prompt, relevant information
   f) lack of relevance to patient management
   g) cost effectiveness
   h) reduced demand for tissue material e.g. pituitaries

2) *Lack of pathological demand*

   a) concentration on surgical pathology
   b) alterations in teaching practice
   c) lack of clinical interest and 'prestige'
   d) infection hazards
   e) labour intensiveness
   f) demands from coroner's PMs

3) *Insufficient demand for epidemiological data*

   a) education and interaction
   b) critical assessment of data

4) *Suggestions for reversal*

   a) clinicopathological conferences
   b) improved 'aesthetics' in necropsy suite
   c) increased teaching role
   d) higher medical audit status
   e) research involvement
   f) adequate level of funding
   g) academic prestige
   h) training and refresher courses
   i) high level investigation into role of autopsy
   j) college symposia

Conclusion

1) *Personal outlook*

2) *General attitudes*

3) *Future trends*

(October 1986, Page 1, Question 5)

References

1) Robinson, M.J. The autopsy, 1983; can it be revived? Human Pathol. (1983) 14: 566–568.
2) Smith, C. The autopsy diagnosis. Human Pathol. (1986) 17: 645–647.
3) Peacock, S.J. et al. The autopsy: a useful tool or an old relic? J. Pathol. (1988) 156: 9–14.
4) Reid, W.A. Cost effectiveness of routine postmortem histology. J. Clin. Pathol. (1987) 40: 459–461.

Discuss the value of the routine hospital autopsy

(October 1988, Paper 2, Question 1)

Give a critical account of the laboratory procedures in all pathology disciplines other than routine histological studies that may be of use in an autopsy performed within four hours of death

There are clearly many procedures which can be described in this answer. The important point to remember is that a mention of many is better than an in depth comment on only a few, and will reflect a 'rounded' education. Procedures to be covered include biochemical analysis of ocular fluid (electrolytes, glucose), microbiological examination, serological examination of blood, histochemical examination of tumours, cytogenetic examination and drug screens (gastric contents, liver, urine, blood, bile). Extraction of DNA is useful in looking for genetic defects in which the gene locus can be identified, and chromosomal analysis can be performed for karyotypic disorders. Rapid removal of tissue for isolation of RNA is also useful by southern blotting or *in situ* hybridisation, especially in determining the presence of gene expression for enzymes. Fibroblastic cells may also be cultured from tissues after death to investigate gene expression disorders.   *(November 1977, Paper 2, Question 5)*

Discuss quality control in histopathological and cytological diagnosis

This is a most important area, and it is perhaps surprising it has been so neglected in the examination. There is a danger that such an essay could lend itself to an overlong and rather anecdotal discourse, so that it would be advisable to discuss the reasons for quality control in technical and clerical aspects, and suitable internal procedures, and which can be justified since these inevitably have a bearing on diagnostic reporting. The bulk of the essay is concerned with the accuracy of diagnosis, which is best assessed using external quality control schemes.

(April 1975, Paper 1, Question 1)

References

1) Underwood, J.C.E. Quality assessment and control. In: Introduction to Biopsy Interpretation and Surgical Pathology. 2nd edition, Chapter 12. Springer-Verlag, Berlin (1987).
2) Lee, F.D., Burnett, R.A. Quality assurance in histopathology. J. Pathol. (1987) 152: 247–251.
3) Cooke, R.A. Quality control in anatomic pathology: experience in Australia and New Zealand. S.C. Sommers (ed.) Pathology Annual Part 1, p221–248. W.B. Saunders, Philadelphia (1984).

In a hospital laboratory service, it is essential that there should be no errors in relating each specimen and report to the right patient. Describe how such errors may arise in a surgical histopathology service for a general hospital, and state the steps you would take to avoid them

This question is clearly aimed to those candidates with experience in a busy service laboratory, rather than the 'academic' pathologist who would be at a disadvantage. The wording clearly indicates that a very practical and simple answer is required, detailing the passage of a specimen from theatre to pathological filing and issue of the report, and could well be approached on this chronological basis, discussing each step along the way. It is important to consider responsibilities of the pathologist as head of department in the routine laboratory where the tissue is processed, cut and stained, and not merely at the dissection and reporting stages. Quality control is a rather peripheral issue to this question, but may merit some consideration.   *(April 1974, Paper 2, Question 1)*

Describe the office systems, quality controls, library facilities and continuing training required by a hospital histopathologist

Another question which is directed at the service histopathologist rather than an academic. Much of the essay would be based on a candidate's own experience within a service laboratory, concerning the specimen reception systems in laboratory and secretarial office, together with reporting and filing systems, including advantages or otherwise of computer storage and recall with pathological coding systems. Quality control is discussed in the previous essay and the library facilities and continuing training are matters of compromise between the ideal and the practicalities of a service post. Consideration of the merits of mandatory accreditation may be a suitable topic, but there is abundant scope for discussion in this question.   *(October 1980, Paper 1, Question 5)*

Reference

1) Morrow, J.S. Information systems in surgical pathology. In: Ackerman's Surgical Pathology. J. Rosai (ed.) Volume 2. 7th edition, appendix B, p1955–1978. C.V. Mosby Co, St. Louis (1989).

Discuss the role of the electron microscope in routine diagnostic morbid anatomy

(April 1969, Paper 1, Question 4)

Discuss the role of electron microscopy in diagnostic histopathology

Both of these questions are essentially similar and cover several groups of diseases in which ultrastructural features may provide a diagnostic role. At least some of these functions have been usurped by immunohistochemistry in recent years, and facilities such as scanning electron microscopy have a very limited function in diagnostic work. Transmission EM is probably of most value in the investigation of renal disease, and this may form a substantial part of the answer. Other applications include cellular pathology (e.g. detection of virus particles, or in storage disorders), and tumour pathology, where the range of applications can be very wide. Small cell tumours of childhood might provide some illustrative examples. In a comprehensive review, it would be justifiable to include a brief mention of energy dispersive X-ray analysis ('EDAX') in detection of non-organic material, and immunolocalisation at the EM level. In the future, a more critical approach to the value of electron microscopic examination may well be required, calling on the candidate to justify the use of this expensive facility.

(November 1975, Paper 2, Question 4)

Reference

1) McLay, A.L.C., Toner, P.G. Diagnostic electron microscopy. In: Recent Advances in Histopathology 11. P.P. Anthony, R.N.M. MacSween (eds.) Churchill Livingstone, Edinburgh (1981).

What methods are available to demonstrate mucosubstances (mucins) in histological material? Discuss their value in diagnosis and research. Details of technical methods are not required

This question requires a considerable amount of organisation to avoid repetition in a potentially confusing area. The first part of the answer should describe the basic composition of mucins and their distribution in tissues. A small table may suffice with different sorts of mucin (neutral, acid, sulphated and non-sulphated, etc.), the tissue/cell distribution and methods of demonstration. It is important not to forget about connective tissue mucins, and the enzymic digestion techniques used in the assessment of some mucins must also be considered (e.g.

hyaluronidase, diastase). Diagnostic uses cover the recognition of mucin in poorly differentiated adenocarcinoma, highlighting otherwise inconspicuous malignant cells (e.g. signet ring cells in gastric carcinoma biopsy), demonstration of connective tissue type mucin in malignant mesothelioma, or in benign conditions such as myxoedema and mucoid degeneration of the aorta. Research applications require more thought, but one of the major topical issues is the claim that certain metaplastic alterations of epithelia in the gut indicate pre-neoplastic potential. Other components of mucins have recently been identified, such as epithelial membrane antigen (EMA) and its use in research and diagnosis could be evaluated, along with the emergence of lectin-binding studies which bind to specific sugars in mucin side chains, and the variation in different disease states. Wide-ranging questions such as this are particularly difficult to answer in a satisfactory manner.   *(October 1986, Paper 1, Question 4)*

References

1) Cook, H.C. Carbohydrates. In: Theory and Practice of Histological Techniques. J.D. Bancroft, A. Stevens (eds.) 2nd edition, p180–216. Churchill Livingstone, Edinburgh (1982).
2) Ramesar K.C.R.F., et al. Limited value of type III intestinal metaplasia in predicting risk of gastric carcinoma. J. Clin. Pathol. (1987) 40: 1287–1290.
3) Gevers, W. Review article. Mucus and mucins. South Afr. J. Med. (1987) 72: 39–42.

Describe the techniques available to pathologists for the demonstration of immunoglobulins in tissue sections. How may these be of value in diagnostic histopathology?

The skilled eye can suspect the presence of immunoglobulins, particularly in glomeruli, in sections stained with H&E, PAS and toluidine blue. However, the question clearly requires a discussion of immunochemical methods. In 1977 only immunofluorescence was readily available, but now peroxidase and alkaline phosphatase methods are available, along with enhancement techniques such as immunogold-silver. The methodologies of the three techniques could be outlined, mentioning their strengths and drawbacks and then discussion of their applications, which presently are mainly in renal, dermatological and lymphoreticular pathology. This question is considerably easier to answer with the benefit of practical experience.   *(April 1977, Paper 1, Question 4)*

References

1) Gatter, K.C., Falini, B., Mason, D.Y. The use of monoclonal antibodies in histopathological diagnosis. In: Recent Advances in Histopathology 12. P.P. Anthony, R.N.M. MacSween (eds.) p35–67. Churchill Livingstone, Edinburgh (1984).
2) Meyrick-Thomas, R.H., Black, M.M., Bhogal, B. The value of immunofluorescence techniques in the diagnosis of skin disorders. In: Recent Advances in Histopathology 12. P.P. Anthony, R.N.M. MacSween (eds.) p69–81. Churchill Livingstone, Edinburgh (1984).

Discuss the value of special staining techniques as an aid to diagnosis in a routine histopathology laboratory.

This is a question put just when the potential of immunohistochemical staining by light microscopy was beginning to be observed, but clearly more conventional special stains would need to be discussed, a point which might have been overlooked by a candidate who had in mind the last question (April 1979, Paper 2, Question 3) which had been set in the previous examination. The following question illustrates how a different aspect of staining was included in the second paper. *(October 1979, Paper 1, Question 5)*

Describe the principles of immunohistochemical localisation of antigens in routine paraffin sections. How has this technique advanced accuracy of diagnosis in routine surgical pathology practice?
(October 1980, Paper 1, Question 3)

Discuss the value of immunofluorescence in the histopathological diagnosis and assessment of human disease

The question is directed towards the advantages of this technique in diagnosis rather than the limitations, and appropriate weight should be given to uses in renal, skin, tumour pathology and others. The assessment of human disease is a broad term but presumably relates to the applications in immunological disease or dermatopathology, for example. *(October 1979, Paper 2, Question 3)*

Discuss the role of immunofluorescent techniques in diagnostic histopathology

The answer should be broadly the same as the preceding question, but with expansion of the section on diagnosis. Nevertheless, inclusion of disease assessment could probably be justified with an appropriate introductory sentence.
(November 1976, Paper 2, Question 1)

'If all staining methods other than haematoxylin and eosin were abandoned, routine diagnostic histopathology would be quite unaffected'. Discuss this assertion

This question antedates the expansion of immunohistochemical techniques, but would naturally encompass all special stains and limited immunofluorescence and the suggested method is to assess which techniques are required in each particular system, with appropriate emphasis on their relative worth e.g. methenamine silver in renal biopsy, reticulin stain in the liver, elastic stain in cardiovascular pathology, etc. Also note that use of routine excludes research and educational usage. *(November 1969, Paper 1, Question 5)*

What are the advantages and limitations of immunocytochemistry in tumour pathology?

(April 1987, Paper 1, Question 4)

Give a general account of the uses and limitations of immunohistochemistry in histopathological diagnosis

The answer should include the uses of both fluorescent and light microscopic techniques, and contrast the limitations and advantages of each.

(April 1979, Paper 2, Question 3)

'The use of monoclonal antibodies as laboratory reagents will revolutionise diagnostic histopathology'. Give your views on this statement, mentioning the principle of the production of such reagents and giving examples of their possible uses

This question is very open-ended, and can be assessed more easily now with retrospective information. Broadly speaking the statement is true, but the crux of the matter is the relative ability of these techniques to improve diagnostic ability. The emphasis should be laid on the essential advantages of monoclonal over polyclonal antibodies. The principles of production of monoclonal antibodies should not be overstated, occupying one or two paragraphs, or preferably expressed by simple diagrams. *(April 1982, Paper 2, Question 4)*

Outline the present and possible future applications of immunohistochemistry

(October 1983, Paper 1, Question 2)

Discuss the desirable contents of a code of safe practice appropriate to a histopathology department, including the post mortem suite

(October 1981, Paper 1, Question 2)

What are the safety hazards in performing a routine necropsy and how may they be reduced?

(October 1979, Paper 1, Question 4)

Discuss health and safety in departments of histopathology. Refer particularly to the handling of fresh tissues for frozen sections and post mortems in cases of viral hepatitis and tuberculosis

(April 1980, Paper 2, Question 4)

What advice and instructions would you give to a newly recruited mortuary technician concerning hazards from infection in the post mortem suite

These questions obviously require more concentration on specific hazards in the post mortem room. The recommended approach is to discuss general aspects of dress and hygiene, post mortem room design and maintenance, technique of post mortem examination and avoidance of infective risk from trauma, aerosol, etc. and then to approach specific types of infection according to the classification outlined in the *Howie Report*. *(October 1983, Paper 1, Question 3)*

Discuss the safety measures you would require to be observed within a histopathology laboratory

These questions are clearly intended to provide an overview of the whole issue, and it is very easy to be drawn into specific issues. One example should be used from each category discussed, if at all. The use of the word 'including' means that the discussion on the post mortem suite must be maintained in proportion and not as the major aspect. *(April 1984, Page 2, Question 2)*

Reference

1) Department of Health and Social Security. Code of Practice for the Prevention of Infection in Clinical Laboratories and Post-mortem rooms. HMSO, London (1980).

Discuss the present and prospective value of quantitative techniques in histopathology

Introduction

Meaning of term 'quantitation'
General areas of application
Role of modern technology in quantitation

1) *Applicability*
   a) detection of disease showing subtle deviation from normal values
   b) improvement of objectivity in documentation
   c) comparison of therapeutic response
   d) facilitation of statistical analysis

2) _Techniques_

    a) area/volume proportion
        i) point counting
    b) surface area
        i) intercept measurement
    c) complex measurements
        i) numbers of objects/unit volume (computer assisted)
        ii) size of included features
    d) counts/unit area e.g. intestinal intraepithelial lymphocytes

Specific application

1) _Metabolic bone disease – osteomalacia and osteoporosis_

    a) measurements
        i) percentage trabecular surface osteoid
        ii) percentage trabecular volume osteoid
        iii) extent of mineralisation front
        iv) mineralisation rate (double tetracycline labelling)
        v) osteoblast/osteoclast surface concentration
    b) value
        i) borderline/early disease otherwise missed
        ii) monitoring of response to therapy

2) _Jejunal biopsy_

    a) measurements
        i) villous status
        ii) intraepithelial lymphocyte count
    b) value
        i) use in borderline villous atrophy and response to therapy
        ii) coeliac disease contains increased epithelial lymphocytes

3) _Pulmonary disease – emphysema and chronic bronchitis_

    a) measurements
        i) alveolar air spaces (emphysema)
        ii) Reid index (chronic bronchitis)
    b) value
        i) assessment of emphysema and clinicopathologic correlation

4) _Muscle biopsy – congenital myopathy and polymyositis_

    a) measurements
        i) fibre size
        ii) fibre type proportions
    b) value
        i) diagnosis of myopathy vs myositis may depend on quantitation
        ii) type of myopathy dependent in quantitation

5) *Nerve biopsy – demyelinating disease*

   a) fibres/unit area
   b) internodal lengths on teased fibres

6) *Testicular biopsy – investigation of fertility*

   a) tubule diameter
   b) spermatogenesis – Johnsen count

Prospective uses in neoplasia

1) *Tumour/stroma ratio*

2) *Cell size in hyperplasia vs. carcinoma*

3) *Nucleolar organiser regions*

4) *Mitotic indices* (e.g. in sarcomas)

(April 1981, Paper 2, Question 4)

References

1) Beck, J.S., Anderson, J.M. Quantitative methods as an aid to diagnosis in histopathology. In: Recent Advances in Histopathology 13. P.P. Anthony, R.N.M. MacSween, (eds.) p255–269. Churchill Livingstone, Edinburgh (1987).
2) Underwood, J.C.E. Introduction to Biopsy Interpretation and Surgical Pathology. p121–130. Springer-Verlag, Berlin (1987).
3) Marchevsky, A.M., Gil, J., Jeanty, H. Computerised interactive morphometry in pathology. Human Pathol. (1987) 18: 320–331.

Discuss the need for measurement in pathology

A broad question, with a danger that the candidate may be tempted to just write as examples come to mind, thus illustrating the value of an essay plan. It should be noted that this question is concerned with measurement in general and is not restricted to morphometry and stereology. One approach is to divide the answer into value of measurement in routine surgical pathology, autopsy pathology, special uses of more specialised quantitative techniques in diagnostic work and finally mention of research applications. In surgical pathology there are many situations in which macroscopic specimens require weighing, measuring for maximum dimension or assessment of volume, e.g. hyperplastic endometrial curettings. Equally, microscopic measurement can be vital e.g. determination of microinvasion in cervical squamous carcinoma, and depth of maximum invasion of melanoma. Examples in autopsy work include assessment of organ atrophy, hypertrophy, valve circumference in the heart, body measurements in neonates, etc.

More specialised quantitative techniques are required for accurate assessment of severity of pulmonary emphysema. The use of more specialised quantitative techniques is discussed in the last essay plan (April 1981, Paper 2, Question 4), where references are listed.   *(November 1975, Paper 2, Question 1)*

In recent years increasing attention has been paid to quantitative methods in morbid anatomy and histopathology for assessing the severity of disease. Describe some of these methods and their application to specific problems

This answer has a somewhat narrower scope which is a consequence of the relatively restricted range of applications at the time it was set. As can be seen from the length of the previous essay plan, which was of necessity rather overlong and yet is by no means comprehensive, the best approach may be to select a number of examples to illustrate aspects of the technique. Bone biopsies and pulmonary emphysema would probably be the most popular choices. Future questions on this theme may well restrict the scope by virtue of the wording.

(April 1972, Paper 1, Question 2)

Describe how you would measure the dimensions and area of an irregularly shaped pathological lesion in a histological section? How would you determine the proportion of an organ replaced by discrete areas of disease visible to the naked eye?

Dimensions are easily measured using a calibrated eye piece graticule, standardised by a known dimension that can be placed on the microscope stage e.g. commercially available calibrated histological slides. This process should be described from the basis of experience which all candidates should have had in measuring dimensions e.g. depth of invasion of a melanoma or micro-invasive squamous carcinoma of cervix. The assessment of surface area is more complicated but can be done by photographing the lesion at known magnification, and using a planimeter. These days it is easier to use a digitising tablet and get a computer to do the hard work!

Secondly, determination of the proportion of an organ replaced by discrete areas of disease visible to the naked eye is best achieved using the Delesse principle. This states that volume is proportional to surface area in random planes of the object, and can be readily measured by a point-counting procedure. This principle and methods of its practical application are well described in the second reference.

(October 1979, Paper 2, Question 1)

References

1) Beck, J.S., Anderson, J.M. Quantitative methods as an aid to diagnosis in histopathology. In: Recent Advances in Histopathology 13. P.P. Anthony, R.N.M. MacSween (eds.) p255–269. Churchill Livingstone, Edinburgh (1987).
2) Underwood, J.C.E. Introduction to Biopsy Interpretation and Surgical Pathology. 2nd edition, p121–130. Springer-Verlag, Berlin (1987).
3) Ellis, M.A. Metabolic bone disease. In: Recent Advances in Histopathology 11. p185–202. P.P. Anthony, R.N.M. MacSween (eds.) Churchill Livingstone, Edinburgh (1981).

Describe how you make a quantitative assessment of a) the amount of emphysema in a lung and b) the amount of osteoid in a bone biopsy

This question allows a concentration on two of the best known applications of morphometric analysis which most candidates should have had practical experience of. The necessary information is given in the previous references.

(April 1980, Paper 1, Question 3)

Describe the techniques you would use in the interpretation of a muscle biopsy. How would the results of these techniques assist in the classification of muscular disorders?

Muscle biopsy technique

1) *Procedure*

   a) site
   b) transport
   c) orientation
   d) fixation and sectioning

2) *Staining*

   a) H&E
   b) PAS
   c) reticulin

3) *Fibre typing*

   a) Gomori
   b) myosin ATPase pH 9.4
   pH 4.6
   pH 4.2
   c) NADH-TR
   d) myophosphorylase

4) *Fibre type composition*

5) *Fibre diameter*

Classification of disease

1) *Neurogenic*

   a) H&E
     i)   atrophy
   b) NADHTR
     i)   atrophy
     ii) target fibres
   c) fibre typing
     i)   type 1 and 2 atrophy
     ii) renervation

2) *Disorders of neuromuscular transmission*

   a) H&E
     i)   lymphocytes
   b) fibre type
     i)   focal type 2 atrophy

3) *Myopathies*

Polymyositis

   a) H&E
     i)   necrosis
     ii) regeneration
   b) NADHTR
     i)   'moth eaten' change
   c) fibre type
     i)   preserved

4) *Dystrophies*

   a) H&E
     i)   muscle fibre size variation
     ii) regeneration
     iii) fibrosis (reticulin)
     iv) fibre splitting

5) *Type 2 fibre atrophy*

   a) H&E
     i)   variable
     ii) myotubular degeneration
   b) NADHTR
     i)   minicore and central core disease
   c) Gomori
     i)   nemaline myopathy
     ii) mitochondrial myopathy

(April 1984, Paper 2, Question 4)

Describe the methods available for diagnostic interpretation of a skeletal muscle biopsy specimen

This question is somewhat more difficult to answer, involving greater attention to the management of the tissue and technical aspects. However, each stain or group of stains could be taken individually, and which abnormalities it may demonstrate, and so several diseases would be mentioned more than once, but this is unavoidable. There should be more emphasis on the commoner conditions rather than the obscure, rare myopathies. *(October 1984, Paper 2, Question 2)*

References

1) Weller, R.D. Muscle biopsy and the diagnosis of muscle disease. In: Recent Advances in Histopathology 12. P.P. Anthony and R.N.M. MacSween (eds.) p259–288 Churchill Livingstone, Edinburgh (1984).
2) Anderson, J.R. Muscle biopsy. Parts 1 and 2. Hospital Update (1985) 11: 199–207 and 11: 285–291.

Describe the morphological criteria and techniques which assist in the diagnosis of malignancy in serous effusions

A question clearly designed for those candidates who have had a reasonable amount of cytological training. It is quite difficult to prepare an adequate answer to this question without practical experience of the problems in these specimens, and which is difficult to glean from most texts. Several aspects could be discussed, but the major problem is the distinction of reactive mesothelial cells from adenocarcinoma and to a lesser extent mesothelioma. Other techniques could include immunocytochemistry and electron microscopy.
(April 1987, Paper 1, Question 2)

Reference

1) Butler, E.B., Stanbridge, C.M. Cytology of Body Cavity Fluids: A Colour Atlas. Chapman and Hall, London (1986).

Write a critical discussion of the role of exfoliative cytology in the prevention of cervical carcinoma

A question which is just as relevant today, as the initial hopes for cytological screening during this era were not fulfilled, partly because of organisational and technical problems. An answer should cover the factors making screening feasible (i.e. accessibility of the cervix, simplicity of the procedure), the proposed evolution of cervical cancer, complementary clinical correlation from colposcopy and biopsy and the factors which reduce sensitivity (poor technique, poor screening, etc.) and selectivity (e.g. inflammation and wart virus infection). A critical discussion should always include positive suggestions for improving the situation, which is the main purpose of setting such a question. *(April 1970, Paper 1, Question 2)*

Discuss, critically, the relative value and limitations of fine needle aspiration, percutaneous needle biopsy, and rapid frozen section of tissue removed by open biopsy, of a lump in the breast

Introduction

Role of pathologist in diagnosis and management
Clinicopathological correlations
Treatment regimes available – changes in practice

Fine needle aspiration

Advantages

1) *Patient*

   a) atraumatic
   b) rapid answer
   c) outpatient procedure at primary visit

2) *Clinician*

   a) simple, clinic procedure
   b) inexpensive
   c) rapid report
   d) planned management at primary consultation

3) *Pathologist*

   a) cost
   b) interest
   c) higher profile in patient management
   d) clinical contrast
   e) accuracy of diagnosis

Disadvantages

1) *Patient*

   a) higher rate of false negative reports
   b) repeat procedure common

2) *Clinician*

   a) false negative reports (up to 30%)
   b) ? less confidence than histological report
   c) increased formal biopsy rate

3) *Pathologist*

   a) inadequate sampling
   b) lack of familiarity with rare tumours
   c) danger of false positive reports
   d) lack of material for special staining, referrals, etc
   e) difficulties in classification e.g. lymphomas

Percutaneous needle biopsy

Advantages

1) *Patient*

   a) few false positives
   b) fewer false negatives

2) *Clinician*

   a) pre-operative tissue diagnosis
   b) planned procedure
   c) confidence in histological analysis

3) *Pathologist*

   a) familiarity with tissue diagnosis and architecture
   b) allows special staining
   c) referral for second opinions
   d) assessment of differentiation
   e) complex pathologies

Disadvantages

1) *Patient*

   a) traumatic
   b) requires second visit
   c) failed biopsy
   d) delay in receiving report

2) *Clinician*

   a) time-consuming
   b) delays in diagnosis
   c) cost

3) *Pathologist*

   a) cost
   b) failures in technique e.g. crush

Frozen section biopsy

Advantages

1) *Patient*

   a) very few false negatives
   b) very few false positives
   c) avoids separate biopsy

2) *Clinician*

   a) convenience
   b) rapid procedure

3) *Pathologist*

   a) rapid report
   b) larger tissue diagnosis
   c) macroscopic information

Disadvantages

1) *Patient*

   a) pre-operative uncertainty
   b) failure to discuss management strategies
   c) equivocal reports – delayed procedures
   d) traumatic

2) *Clinician*

   a) equivocal reports
   b) poor cost effectiveness – lack of pre-operative planning
   c) delays in report

3) *Pathologist*

   a) time-consuming
   b) cost
   c) stress

(April 1982, Paper 2, Question 1)

Reference

1) Melcher, D.H. et al. Fine needle aspiration cytology. In: Recent Advances in Histopathology 11. P.P. Anthony, R.N.M. MacSween (eds.) Churchill Livingstone, Edinburgh (1984).

Discuss the application of fine needle aspiration cytology as a diagnostic aid

The role of cytology in diagnosis and screening will certainly be taking a much greater proportion of the workload in general pathological training, and this will be reflected in the questions set for the examination. As the applications and expertise in this field expand rapidly, some familiarity with more specialised aspects will be expected, and the questions more limited in scope than this one (e.g. discuss the role in breast disease, etc), with consideration given to technique for improving cell yield. In addition, candidates may well be expected to express views on the effectiveness of various screening programmes, and how they might be improved. Several reviews on the broader aspects of fine needle aspiration cytology have been produced (see previous question).

(April 1985, Paper 2, Question 1)

Discuss the causes and effects of hypoxia in a full-term, new-born baby

The major causes of hypoxia are atelectasis neonatorum, congenital heart disease, pneumonia, and respiratory distress induced by maternal sedation, brain injury or aspiration. Respiratory distress syndrome (hyaline membrane disease) is somewhat less likely in a full-term than premature infant, but some cases occur (e.g. in diabetes). It is important to realise this in order that the answer is not dominated by a discussion of this problem. *(November 1974, Paper 2, Question 5)*

Reference

1) Robbins, S.L., Cotran, R.S., Kumar, V. Diseases of infancy and childhood. In: Pathologic Basis of Disease, 4th edition. p515–542. W.B. Saunders, Philadelphia (1989).

What are the major causes of mortality in the neonate? Describe and discuss the pathology, including pathogenesis, of one of these

The first half of the answer should comprise an overview of the causes of death as outlined in the reference. It is important to choose the subject for the second half of the answer carefully, as in all questions phrased in this manner. Thus it would be sensible to outline a well described entity which provides abundant scope for discussion of pathogenesis, such as respiratory distress syndrome, rather than an equally important but somewhat more mundane topic such as cerebral birth trauma, or pneumonia. *(April 1977, Paper 2, Question 4)*

What are the hazards and possible serious sequelae of premature birth?

(November 1972, Paper 1, Question 4)

Discuss the value of the perinatal autopsy

(October 1981, Paper 2, Question 5)

Discuss the value of the autopsy in the investigation of neonatal death

The last two of these questions relate closely to the reference below, which contains sufficient detail to enable a comprehensive answer to be compiled. The wording of the question clearly indicates that details of technique are not required, but is more an appraisal of the clinicopathological correlation and value in uncovering pathological changes not diagnosed ante mortem, or defining the exact cause of death which may be of value for genetic counselling, or in clinical management and investigation.   *(April 1985, Paper 2, Question 3)*

Reference

1) Pryse-Davis, J. The perinatal autopsy. In: Recent Advances in Histopathology 11. P.P. Anthony, R.N.M. MacSween (eds.) p65–82. Churchill Livingstone, Edinburgh (1981).

13. Short Notes Questions

Short notes questions used to be popular. Examples are:

Give short accounts of

a)   ↑ The lesions of disseminated (multiple) sclerosis
b)   ↑ The renal lesions of systemic lupus erythematosus
c)   ↑ The lesions of lichen planus

(April 1969, Paper 2, Question 5)

Write short notes on the nature and significance of any four of the following

a)   The arteriolar changes in chronic systemic hypertension
b)   The 'Philadelphia chromosome'
c)   Alcoholic hyaline
d)   'Sex chromatin' in the male
e)   Fibrinoid necrosis

(November 1971, Paper 1, Question 5)

Give a brief account of

a)   Familial amyloidosis
b)   Macroglobulinaemia
c)   Favism

(November 1972, Paper 2, Question 3)

Write short notes on

a)   Alcoholic hyalin
b)   Senile cardiac amyloid
c)   Sertoli cell tumours

(November 1973, Paper 2, Question 5)

Write brief notes on three of the following

a)   Quantitation in histology
b)   Scanning electron microscopy in pathology
c)   Histochemistry as an aid to diagnosis
d)   'Keeping up with the literature'

(May 1973, Paper 1, Question 2)

Write short notes on the following

a) Cytology of intracranial tumours
b) Clear cell adenocarcinoma of the vagina
c) Acanthosis nigricans
d) Lymphoid tumours of the rectum

(April 1974, Paper 1, Question 5)

Write short notes on

a) Medullary carcinoma of the thyroid
b) The skin lesion of pemphigus vulgaris
c) Pneumonia due to pneumocystis carinii

(November 1974, Paper 2, Question 2)

Write short notes on

a) Aschoff bodies
b) Zollinger-Ellison syndrome
c) Pleural mesothelioma

(November 1975, Paper 1, Question 2)

Describe how you would seek evidence of each of the following conditions after death

a) Air embolus
b) Immune complex disease
c) Acute alcoholic poisoning
d) Drowning

(you are not required to give the techniques of any biochemical assays)

(April 1976, Paper 1, Question 3)

Write short notes on the pathology of the following

a) Pulmonary barotrauma
b) Paraquat poisoning
c) Fibrous dysplasia of bone
d) Rabies

(April 1977, Paper 2, Question 5)

Write short notes on each of the following

   a) Pseudomembranous colitis
   b) Extrinsic allergic alveolitis
   c) The effects of paracetamol on the liver
   d) The skin in smallpox

(April 1978, Paper 1, Question 5)

Write short notes on

   a) Lymphoid infiltrations of the skin
   b) Aneurysmal bone cyst
   c) Argentaffin neoplasms

(April 1978, Paper 2, Question 2)

Write short notes on

   a) Subacute (giant cell) thyroiditis
   b) Verrucous carcinoma
   c) Takayashu's disease
   d) Synovial sarcoma

(October 1978, Paper 1, Question 3)

Write short notes on

   a) Oestrogen receptors
   b) Small cell tumours of the thyroid
   c) Psoriasis
   d) Colonic polyps

(April 1979, Paper 1, Question 5)

Write short notes on

   a) Fibrous lesions of bone
   b) Infantile respiratory distress syndrome
   c) Myocarditis

(April 1979, Paper 2, Question 2)

Write short notes on

a) Sclerosing cholangitis
b) Subepidermal bullae
c) Seminoma
d) Bone infarcts

(April 1980, Paper 1, Question 2)

Write short notes on

a) Polyarteritis nodosa
b) Scleroderma
c) Analgesic abuse
d) Renal artery stenosis

(April 1980, Paper 2, Question 1)

Write short notes on

a) Pseudolymphoma
b) Nasal angiofibroma
c) Cerebellar haemangioblastoma
d) Inflammatory fibrous polyp

(April 1981, Paper 2, Question 3)

These questions are listed as in the previous sections, but there are no outlines or references given because most of the entities mentioned are reasonably well defined, and it would be relatively easy to look them up in the texts given in Appendix 1 or from recent journal articles.

The short notes style is very similar to an essay plan, more 'fleshed out' perhaps but using recognised abbreviations and brief phrases or sentences in place of formally constructed paragraphs, so that there is a concentration of relevant facts on any subject rather than description/discussion.

No questions have been set in this format since 1981 and one reason for this may be that they merely require 'regurgitation' of facts while there is increasing emphasis these days on a candidate's ability to interpret pathological data and critically discuss disease pathogenesis, something which is difficult to achieve in notation. Moreover this type of question tends to limit the choice of subject which can be set in the remaining nine, especially if it relates to something of major topical interest which might form the basis of an essay instead. Having said all this, there is no reason to suppose that they may not be set in the future. There is, unfortunately, no way to prepare specifically for this sort of question, as any subject may be asked.

However, these questions do provide a very useful revision exercise. For each of the sections, the most effective method is to write down everything one knows on the subject and then review the answer with an appropriate article. This is a fairly painless way of accumulating information on a wide range of diseases. While this may not help in as much as these questions are unlikely to reappear in the written examination in this form, the acquired knowledge would at least be useful in many aspects of the practical examination.

The Written Examination: Practical Aspects

This is held in London, Birmingham, Glasgow and Belfast in the UK. Candidates are informed about one month in advance of the address and date for the examination which is usually held on a Tuesday. Overseas candidates may attend centres in Baghdad, Chicago, Dublin, Hong Kong, Johannesburg, Toronto and Singapore, details of which are obtained from the College as the exact location varies from year to year. In addition these applicants usually have to sit the practical examination in the UK and because of the delays in communicating results, cannot attend for the practical in that half year and have to wait six months for the next one. As the majority of candidates sit the examination in London, most of the following general points are derived from experience at that centre. The College is at present considering the possibility of arranging practical examinations overseas, and candidates should enquire about this prior to application.

There are two papers of three hours' duration each, commencing at 9.30am and 2pm. Candidates who do not live in the city should beware of leaving insufficient travelling time to the city centre, especially if staying in unfamiliar suburbs. It is far better to stay in a hotel near the centre for the evening prior to the examination and the address of suitable hotels could be obtained from the Tourist Information Service or ask any colleagues who may live there for advice. If the examination centre is not within convenient walking distance of the hotel it is best to take a taxicab there to avoid the rush hour on public transport, and avoid unnecessary further stress.

At this stage, most candidates will be aware of the instruments required for an examination, but it is worthwhile duplicating pens, etc. or carrying refills, as they always seem to cause problems during an examination. In addition, it is advisable to check that the letter from the College which has the examination number on it is in your possession, as you will need this to gain entrance to the hall, where the seats are given corresponding numbers. It is prudent to make a copy of the letter upon receipt so that there is less chance of it being mislaid.

After admission to the hall verbal instructions are given on how to fill in the front pages of the manuscript booklets, and the first task is to write in the examination number and full name. Separate slips requiring name, examination number and signature are also completed.

During the examination it is necessary to add in the sequence of the examination numbers attempted in the order in which they were answered, on the front page of the booklet, since the examination papers are divided to be sent to different examiners. In addition, each question should be commenced on a fresh right hand page, again to allow this division and put the number of the corresponding question on the top of each answer page. Rough work should be crossed out, and supplementary pages are fastened inside the booklet if needed.

If there are any particular questions about the examination arrangements or some clarification is required of the terms used in any of the questions, a senior member of the College usually attends the first 30 minutes of the examination to deal with such points, so it is best to read through all of the questions to check right at the beginning.

During the course of the examination it is essential to be very careful of the timing of the answers. It is often useful to have a digital watch or timer for this purpose which can be reset for each 40–45 minutes (but it must not have a distracting alarm). As previously outlined, the time allocated for completing the essay 'plan' (4–5 minutes) should be strictly adhered to, and it is essential to stop writing at the end of the allotted period for the question, whether finished or not. Some other questions may be finished slightly ahead of time allowing more time on the incomplete answer.

One reason for ensuring equal attention to each of the questions results from the marking system. Each question receives one quarter of the marks, 25. An overall 50% is the minimum pass-mark, and an average of 50% between the two papers is required; 46% would be regarded as an overall fail in any one paper (i.e. 46 out of a total 100), but a deficiency of marks in the range 47–49% in one paper could potentially be compensated by a corresponding surplus of marks in the other.

A very good pass would be marked as 15 out of a total of 25, and a decisive fail 10 or less, but if only a nominal paragraph on any one question is written, very few marks (5) would be awarded. Given the exponential difficulty in achieving marks over 15/25 (and indeed examiners are not encouraged to award higher marks), it is unlikely such a candidate would pass even with three excellent essays. However, it is relatively easier to score marks in the mid range (10–15) in relation to the effort expended, hence the emphasis on achieving a balanced set of essays.

Even in the event that an answer cannot be finished completely, strict observance of the time allocated to each question is recommended. An examiner is likely to be more favourable to one or two essays which are incomplete on account of the abundance of relevant information provided (rather than 'padding'), than to three complete answers and one which is rushed and half finished. They may refer to the essay plan to see how the answer would have been completed.

As an emergency measure, (and it should be regarded as an exception), an essay could be completed in short note form, to include as many key words as possible. It is still important to ensure legibility however.

Note that the essay plans should be written into the answer book, as candidates are not allowed to remove any written material from the examination hall. The plan or outline should be clearly labelled at the beginning of the question, and can be neatly crossed out with a line through it, as 'rough work', or left for consideration with the rest of your answer if it is neat enough, which is the ideal solution.

It is very important to ensure that 5–7 minutes at the end of the examination are left for completing questions and double checking the numbering, etc. Allocating exactly 43 minutes for each answer should give this leeway at the end. If more than one of the answers is unfinished it is best to return to the one which is least complete, and to which can be added useful, concentrated information.

It is important not to become over-anxious at the end as there is a grave danger of spoiling otherwise good essays by untidy scribbling, or worse still making major alterations to the main part of the essay. It is too late to significantly adjust what has already been written, and it is quite likely that a mistaken impression would be formed by a hurried 'reassessment' of an essay – critical judgement becomes very unreliable at this stage in an examination.

After completing the writing, the sequence of the questions answered should be confirmed to correspond to the order on the front of the booklet, and extra pages need to be sorted accordingly.

Candidates are notified by post of the results in approximately three weeks, although results are displayed for the nerveless at the College at 2 Carlton House Terrace, usually on a Friday afternoon. Results are never given over the telephone by the College.

The Practical Examination

Introduction

It is difficult to give advice to potential candidates on whether they should attempt to take both parts of the examination during the same half-year, or exercise the option to sit the written examination at three years, and the practical examination at five years or more. It largely depends on the breadth and quality of training received and having confidence in one's abilities, as well as constraints imposed by the demands of posts currently held. It might prove impractical to obtain the necessary study leave to allow adequate preparation for instance. It may help to take advice from colleagues who have attempted the examination recently, and from supervisors who may be more able to assess whether an individual has reached an adequate standard to have a reasonable chance of passing both. The examination can prove quite stressful, which would be prolonged over a period of two months by attempting both parts at once. Remember that after the written examination most candidates will probably not want to work for a few days, and being uncertain about the outcome of the written examination is not a very good stimulus for preparation for the practical session. This factor should be taken into account when planning a revision programme.

Assuming the written paper has been successfully completed previously or during the current session, candidates will then receive a written letter giving information about the examination centre, which is usually (but not necessarily) a university teaching hospital, about two or three weeks in advance. It is usually accompanied by some basic maps and information about the centre and who to contact. At present, the allocation appears to be completely random, and candidates could be required to travel anywhere within the UK. Most candidates will not be asked to attend a centre in which they have worked for any significant part of their training, but this is not unknown. There has been a tendency for the College to encourage non-teaching, i.e. district general hospitals, to hold the examination. Several of these centres have attracted a reputation for a difficult and punitive examination. While this is by no means true for all such centres, there appears to be a trend towards overinvestment in the practical examination as a major event. With the increasing numbers of examinations required by the new regulations, this policy may expand.

If there are any substantial objections to the centre allocated (e.g. previous differences with the head of department, or domestic difficulties), it would be best to contact the College immediately and explain the problem, (ensuring this is with the support of your head of department, who might be required to make representations). In these exceptional circumstances, alternative arrangements might be made.

After receipt of the letter, the first task is to establish how to reach the examination centre rapidly, and the departmental secretary may be able to give some guidance on this. It is important to make sure they are given sufficient details to enable them to pass on messages swiftly, as it is now usual practice to ask candidates to attend for a post mortem in advance of the main examination, and often at only one days' notice, if they are in reasonable commuting distance. Where candidates have a long way to travel, the post mortem is often performed at the time of the rest of the practical, but again, this is not always the case.

If it is necessary to stay in a hotel for the examination, arrangements should be made as soon as possible, in addition to establishing what travelling is necessary between the hotel and hospital. Some candidates have left the hotel booking until very late, travelling to London with nowhere to stay, and encountered considerable difficulty in obtaining suitable accommodation: a needless cause of stress. It is also a mistake to economise when making hotel arrangements. It is always better to stay at one which is recommended by trusted colleagues or reputable organisations, as it is not conducive to a good performance to stay in a noisy, uncomfortable environment.

Presentation

Candidates should bear in mind that they are attending an examination for a professional qualification at the level of consultant, and will be expected to look the part. It is essential to present a tidy, well dressed appearance, in order not to be 'upstaged' by fellow candidates who will also be trying their utmost to impress. Certain individuals may feel 'thick-skinned' enough to withstand this, but it is surprising how much of a 'negative' impression a scruffy candidate can make on the more conservative examiners, who may even feel somewhat insulted that the candidate does not view this as an occasion to be approached with some formality. It is a situation in which to ask a spouse or best friend for advice!

The Necropsy: Preparation to Examination Standard

It is probably true to say that most pathologists in the UK ultimately have to rely on using their own initiative in respect of necropsy training in order to perfect their technique, usually by persuading senior colleagues and their peers to help them, since there is no formal education in this skill, at least on a national level. The resulting standard achieved is a direct result of the ability of a trainee to communicate with colleagues and learn by example, fundamental qualities in a good pathologist.

Each candidate is expected to perform a competent post mortem examination using a conventional method, which would reasonably be expected to ensure the detection of most disease processes. While interpretation of the findings during the Final examination necropsy is one aspect, it is as well to note that a candidate's technical skill is also under assessment.

In the earliest stages, pathologists are usually taught a technique from senior colleagues or slightly more advanced trainees, and while learning by example is the best method initially, it is unlikely that optimal methods of dissection have been adopted in every centre and candidates who have a narrow range of experience may well become aware of deficiences only when they are pointed out by an examiner.

There are books which cover aspects of necropsy procedure, one of the best is *Post Mortem Procedures* written by Gresham and Turner (Appendix 1), which covers the layout of the necropsy suite, health and safety considerations and the role of the post mortem technician. In addition, there is a well illustrated guide to practical aspects of the dissection which would be of value for all candidates to consult prior to the examination, whatever their level of ability.

There is one specialist 3-day course designed to cover some aspects of routine and specialist necropsy procedures, and post mortem pathology, which may well be of value (Appendix 2). It might be better to attend such a course with some elementary experience, so that the recommended procedures can be established prior to the acquisition of too many bad habits. The optimal time may be soon after completing the Primary examination, but the course organiser would be able to give more detailed advice. In addition, such a course may cover the aspects of some necropsies with which some candidates have had limited experience (e.g. neonatal, paediatric and Coroner's post mortems) which they might well be confronted with as an examination case.

Even when the demands of routine work necessitate the performance of several post mortem examinations per day, it is a good policy to dissect one to a high technical standard in a relatively unhurried manner or if not take the time to examine one organ system per case according to a standard anatomical method outlined in a manual such as *Cunningham's Manual of Practical Anatomy* or an anatomical or specialised textbook which includes dissection technique (e.g. cardiac dissection as outlined in Olsen, E.G.J. *Pathology of the Heart* (Appendix 1) This requires considerable self-discipline, but the consequence of not doing so is that an individual's technique will become less than adequate, and bad habits will become ingrained and difficult to eradicate when more advanced skills are required in a particular case and in the examination. Therefore, the advice is to aspire to perfection in at least one aspect of every necropsy!

One stimulus to improvement is to become involved in the tuition of junior colleagues, and this supervision involves a considerable degree of responsibility to ensure they learn the correct methods. Questions on technique should be encouraged, and it is most important to demonstrate normal anatomical relationships as well as pathology. In order to get the maximum from this, it is often a good idea to choose one particular organ to demonstrate in detail, having revised the protocol for dissection prior to starting.

If there are no junior colleagues, demonstrations for medical students or trainee mortuary technicians are equally beneficial, in that they enable the development of an ability to comment while continuing a dissection which is an essential skill to acquire, and impressive to colleagues and examiners alike, but one which requires considerable practice.

It is essential that a consultant is responsible for supervision of the dissection and is available to give advice in the earliest stages, but at registrar level and above, they may only wish to see the major findings at the end. However, it is often possible to encourage them to actively criticise and demonstrate their expertise in dissection, especially if they have a particular specialist interest in an organ or system. Some pathologists are rather inhibited about criticising junior colleagues who have had a few years experience, afraid of this being misinterpreted as an insult. It is important to reassure them on this point, and afterwards accept any comments made with good grace. Those who put up a defensive 'shield' to avoid criticism and prefer to work in isolation severely disadvantage themselves, as there is potential for improvement in every pathologist's performance.

Communication with the clinical staff is of utmost importance, since the major reason for performing a necropsy is to assess the course of an illness, the clinical diagnosis and the effect of treatment, as the ultimate form of medical audit. It should be second nature to ensure the clinical staff attend the necropsy itself, or the presentation, and candidates would certainly be expected to request or arrange this in the examination. Always contact them prior to starting the dissection to check what might be a convenient time to hold the presentation and discussion, to fit in with their clinical commitments.

It is expected that candidates will recognise that aesthetic objections to post mortems are one of the main reasons why clinical staff may be reluctant to attend. Therefore candidates should make every effort to finish the dissection, clean up the area and arrange the organs so the findings can be demonstrated in a brisk, professional style. There is no greater deterrent to clinical colleagues than a rambling discourse from a pathologist attempting to finish a dissection, with poorly prepared organs largely obscured by blood.

As well as the clinical staff, opportunities to present post mortem demonstrations to medical students, which should be part of the teaching programme in most University hospitals, should be taken. This can be a very rewarding exercise which will quickly expose limitations in demonstration and communication, and requires an alert mind especially relating to aspects of normal anatomy, to avoid being 'upstaged' by medical students who would recently have completed an intensive preclinical course in the subject. In more formal presentations, arrangements can be made with the clinical staff to present the history prior to death and ask questions from the students on what pathological changes are to be expected. While this may be standard practice in University Departments, there is no reason why similar arrangements could not be instituted at a District General Hospital with an attachment of students.

As to more practical aspects of the necropsy, candidates should observe the recommendations of the *Howie Report* (Code of Practice for the Prevention of Infection in Clinical Laboratories and Post-mortem Rooms (Appendix 1) at all times (and may well be asked about them during the examination). Safety is a most important consideration but is surprisingly often neglected by trainee pathologists. Examiners take particular note of the steps taken in preventing injury from carelessly placed instruments, sharp bone edges, blood splashes and minimisation of aerosols.

The correct choice and use of instruments may affect the ability to dissect quite markedly. It is surprising how many trainees restrict themselves to the use of a PM40 knife and one or two pairs of scissors. However the minimum requirements are a large knife and scalpel, at least four pairs of scissors (including bowel and artery scissors), probes, bone forceps, bowel clamps and a rule. Furthermore, the correct technique for manipulating these instruments should be observed, which is again a matter for practice. In particular, producing organ slices with a single stroke of the large knife is a considerable improvement over a 'sawing' action. Use of the necropsy saw is also neglected by many pathologists, but it is not unknown for some centres to ask candidates to remove the cranial vault themselves.

The following section is intended to be a complementary rather than comprehensive guide to performing a necropsy, with comments on some often neglected aspects of the general conduct of a post mortem, together with an idea of the details of anatomy and technique which candidates might be required to know. There is an attempt to highlight those areas which are sometimes a source of particular difficulty. Some more difficult 'special' procedures are outlined and illustrated, which examinees might be expected to perform or at least be asked to explain.

Although it would clearly be impossible to follow to the letter all of the protocols outlined here in every necropsy because it would take too long, they can be adapted to suit the demands of each case as required.

The Necropsy: Procedures

One of the most important aspects of any post mortem examination is to review the clinical notes on the patient. The first task is to ensure that the permission form is in order and whether it is a hospital or Coroner's autopsy. (In the examination this would usually have been checked beforehand.) Prior to starting, the notes should be carefully read and adequate time should be given for this, but candidates should not be inhibited from asking for more if the case is particularly complicated.

During this time it is a good idea to obtain some paper and make a short summary, including age of the patient, date and time of death, and a paragraph or two on the clinical history, including relevant investigations. Trainees develop their own methods of extracting information from notes rapidly, but in a complex case, discharge and referral letters often give comprehensive, easily digestible summaries.

During or at the end of the necropsy, candidates are expected to give an accurate, brisk précis of the clinical history which is included in the written report, so it is a good idea to take advantage of this time to assemble a coherent report which can be easily transcribed. It is most important to identify the clinical diagnoses, which would indicate the site of potential pathological lesions and which would answer any specific questions raised by the clinical team.

The supervisor will conduct candidates to the post mortem changing rooms, and in most circumstances they will be shown what to wear. If unsure, specific questions can be asked about the protective clothing required, and appropriate precautions must always be taken in any necropsy in cases of serious transmissible disease. Remember that at this stage, a candidate is under the examiners' scrutiny, (either consciously or unconsciously) and it is important to convey an air of professionalism. Any opportunity the examiner may provide to discuss the clinical aspects of the case should be taken, and any special requirements which are anticipated (e.g. taking specimens for microbiology in an infective case, radiographs in neonates or traumatic fractures, special fixatives for certain tumours, etc.) should be raised and discussed, as the examiner may be kind enough to make arrangements.

The supervisor will usually make an introduction to the mortuary technician assigned to the case. It is very important to be polite and use his assistance to the greatest benefit. Many candidates are so preoccupied that their behaviour may seem offhand or even frankly rude to the mortuary staff, so it is important to make the effort to converse. It would help if the case is briefly discussed with them and the assistance which might be required outlined. Mortuary technicians are usually experienced in looking after examination candidates, and will have been briefed beforehand as to what help they can offer. However, there is nothing to lose by asking, and the response may be more favourable if a rapport has been established. Moreover, the technician is present throughout the dissection, and will closely observe the technique. Some examiners will take the opinion of the mortuary technician into account when assessing a candidate, especially if they are experienced. Thus you will not 'get away' with any bad habits while the examiners are away.

Instruments are provided, but if other types are required or preferred there is no harm in requesting if they could be made available.

However, criticism of the standard of the equipment which has been provided should be avoided at all costs. The mortuary staff will have made a special effort for the examination, and it will be unnecessary criticism and may well be taken as an insult.

Prior to commencing the dissection, the usual checks on the body should be made, and a careful external examination conducted. Visible abnormalities should be noted down at this stage for inclusion in your final report.

It is vitally important to ensure that the dissection is as tidy as possible. There is probably nothing which counts against a candidate as much as making an unpleasant mess during the dissection, especially on the floor and excessively over the working surface. Many candidates do not even take the simplest of precautions to avoid this. Expert prosectors will create remarkably little spillage of blood, but this is a skill which has to be practised. Examiners recognise that if this can be controlled, it is usually a reflection of a good pathologist. Moreover, if the appearances are obscured then there is a potential for misinterpreting the pathology, and we have already made the point that an unaesthetically presented post mortem is one of the major reasons why clinicians are reluctant to attend.

Thus it is most important that steps are taken to avoid these problems. A running water supply with a hose attachment should be provided, to wash down the body after removal of the organs, and to clean the surrounding table. The abdominal cavities should be rinsed out with water, and then a clean sponge used to allow inspection of the surfaces – a pool of blood should not be left within them. The thoracic and abdominal organs should be rinsed in cold water in a sink, transporting them in a bowl to avoid blood spillage on the table or floor. The dissection surface is kept clean by wiping down after each organ dissection with a freshly rinsed sponge. Dissection instruments should be kept to one side in a neat array when not in use (for safety reasons as much as appearances).

It is suggested that all organs are weighed as they are dissected clear, requesting the technician to note the figures down. The organs are best kept 'orientated' preferably on a large tray or board, which is used to display them for the summary presentation. In practice, it is very easy to forget which side the kidneys or adrenals have come from, and even the lungs may be very difficult to identify after dissection.

As already implied, technique in dissection will be noted by the examiner and post mortem technician. For safety reasons it is important to always cut away from one's body with scissors or a knife. The tissue should be continually inspected while being divided to avoid destroying any unexpected pathology which may be encountered. Sharp instruments should not be flourished, and care taken to minimise the risks from sharp edges of bone, especially rib ends, by covering them with cloth. Finally, aerosols and splashes should be kept to an absolute minimum by careful handling of the organs.

The following sections relate to some of the more common problems which trainees encounter but which they are expected to have mastered by the examination. It includes selected practical, technical and anatomical aspects, rather than purely pathological descriptions and it is stressed that this is not intended to be a comprehensive methodology.

Removal of Organs

The body can be opened by a conventional midline incision, or 'Y' shaped cut passing from the sternal-notch, behind the sternocleidomastoid muscles to the mastoid bone.

The skin should be reflected off the chest, including muscle, down to the level of the ribs and intercostal muscles. Removal of the sternal plate is easier if there is no muscle or soft tissue over the anterior surface of the ribs. The abdominal wall should be incised down to the peritoneum between the rectus muscles. The abdominal organs should be protected from damage by lifting the peritoneum with forceps and making an opening with scissors, the fascia being divided towards the symphysis pubis, avoiding the bowel. Ascitic fluid, if any, should be removed with a mechanical aspirator or ladles, and the quantity noted. With intra-abdominal sepsis, samples should be taken for culture. It is often best to remove the bowel at this stage and several points are often forgotten by candidates. Firstly, both ends of the small bowel should be tied off or clamped at the start of the jejunum to avoid spillage of contents. The bowel should be removed from the mesentery by holding one end at slight tension and running a PM40 knife along the junction, down to the terminal ileum. The large bowel is then dissected out in continuity. While most of the colon is easy to remove with a medium-sized pair of scissors from caecum to sigmoid colon, trainees are often not aware that the rectum, which is often left in situ, is reasonably easy to remove, and is often a site of 'missed' lesions. The rectosigmoid junction should be put on slight tension, and using scissors the peritoneal reflections are cut around the circumference of the rectum, including the rectovesical or rectouterine pouch. The incisions are extended posteromedially in the vertical plane, avoiding the ureters, and blunt dissection is used to push the soft tissues away from the wall of the rectum down to the level of the levator ani, all the time keeping a tension on the rectosigmoid colon with the other hand. When the anal sphincter can be palpated, a cut is made just above this level with a PM40, through the anal canal. The bladder (with prostate in the male) can be removed intact with a similar combination of peritoneal incision, blunt dissection and incision across the upper urethra. Significant pathology can be missed if bladder and rectum are left inside the body and it is far more impressive when correctly removed and dissected.

The intact intestines should be placed immediately after removal into a bowl or in a sink, and after opening longitudinally the contents washed away with cold running water, to allow inspection of the mucosal surface. The colon is best opened along the anterior taenia coli. Make sure the intestinal contents are not allowed to contaminate the working surfaces or dissection table, either by seepage when left in an untidy pile or by careless spillage during opening.

Removal of the remaining organs is rather dependent on an individual's preferred approach but it is as well to have attempted both the Letulle and Virchow techniques before making a final choice (see Gresham and Turner, Appendix 1). Many pathologists use Virchow's method, taking out the liver and biliary system followed by the remaining intraperitoneal and retroperitoneal organs prior to opening the thorax. Using this approach, it is important to dissect carefully around the gastro-oesophageal junction to avoid penetrating the diaphragm. Care should be taken to remove the ureters as intact as possible. In the event of potential disease in the genitourinary system, remove the bladder, ureters and kidney intact. This should be possible if a careful approach has been taken during the rectal dissection.

Opening the chest can be fairly straightforward, but elementary mistakes are usually a consequence of rushing. A brief check for pneumothorax is advisable, (and is a commonly asked question in examinations), usually by opening 'under water' in a pouch formed by the reflected skin and the lateral chest wall. After the incision of intercostal muscles over the 9–11 rib spaces anteriorly, a careful inspection for pleural adhesions needs to be made before removing the ribs, to avoid cutting into the surface of the lungs if they are adherent, in which case they may be severely distorted. The line of the separation is best just medial to the costochondral junction up to the first rib. This might be easiest with a knife (unless there is heavy calcification, in which case bone forceps should be used). Clean incisions through the cartilage avoid the danger of jagged rib edges which are often left after cutting the bone. Care needs to be taken when removing the sternum, which should be carefully lifted and dissected off the underlying lungs, pericardium and anterior mediastinum. If the lungs and pleura are adherent it is usually possible to use blunt dissection to find a plane between pleura and chest wall, pushing the lung away from the chest wall if this plane is not completely separated (laterally and posteriorly as well). Removal of the lungs causes severe tearing and distortion of the parenchyma, providing artefacts and masking the pathology.

The thoracic pluck is best removed 'en bloc', starting from the tongue. Using the 'Y' incision, the skin of the neck is reflected up over the face, and then a cut made around the inner border of the mandible to include the submandibular salivary glands, and vertically to include the posterior border of the sternomastoid muscle down to the level of the cervical vertebrae, dividing the muscle at the level of the mastoid bone. By this method, the internal and external carotid arteries are included in the dissection, and the detection of parathyroid glands is considerably easier (see page 281). When removing the thoracic pluck a releasing incision along the inner border of the first rib needs to be made, posteriorly extending downwards through the parietal pleura parallel to the aorta. It is important to remove the diaphragms intact, by cutting the muscle flush with the thoracic wall.

In removing thoracic organs with or without the abdominal contents, it is not an excuse to exhibit 'brute' force by 'tearing' the tissues away using traction on the tongue and neck contents. Not only will this disrupt delicate anatomical relations, it inevitably leads to unnecessary aerosols and blood splashing. Instead a knife or scissors should be used to release fascia and soft tissues (wherever possible under direct vision), holding the tissues under slight tension to facilitate this.

The abdominal organs can be removed attached to the thoracic block if required, according to the method of Letulle (Gresham and Turner, Appendix 1) but care should be taken to dissect around the lateral and posterior aspects of the kidneys, extending the vertical incisions down to the level of the thoracic vertebrae behind the psoas muscles. The latter can either be transected lateral to the ureters, followed by medial extension of the incision across the lower edge of the pelvic brim, or if the ureters and bladder are to remain intact the incision is brought anteriorly, dissecting out the anterior and inferior aspects of the bladder, which is then reflected upwards, and with gentle traction on the base of bladder, the ureters can be teased away from the connective tissue with a scalpel up to the level of the pelvic brim. The organs can then be removed en bloc as above, with a releasing incision through the psoas muscle and fascia over the anterior sacral promontory.

Immediately on removal, the organ block(s) must be transferred to a sink to be rinsed in cold water, ensuring they are placed into a bowl during this transfer to avoid the spillage of blood over the body dissection area and floor which would inevitably occur otherwise, again creating a very bad impression.

At this stage, the outside and inside of the body should be cleaned using sponges. Then the iliofemoral vessels should be dissected out, especially where there is a history suggesting deep vein thrombosis or pulmonary thrombo-embolism. In all cases the femoral vein should be opened, which involves cutting across the inguinal ligament, at least to the origin of the great saphenous vein. At this stage, in males the testes should be everted into the inguinal canal and removed together with the spermatic cord. It is common for candidates to forget this part of the dissection. The external genitalia should always be examined in addition.

Having sponged out the thoracic and abdominal cavities, the peritoneal surfaces should be closely inspected and the spine assessed for gross abnormalities. A strip of bone should be removed from the anterior vertebral bodies, after which the cut surface needs to be washed and sponged to assess for collapse of vertebral bodies, or metastases in malignant disease. Some bone should be taken for fixation at this point (otherwise, this is frequently forgotten). At some centres it is routine practice to dissect around each rib to check for fractures. This may or may not be part of each individual's usual approach, but it is prudent to establish whether this is routinely done at that centre, and the post mortem technician would be aware of this. Others prefer a close examination of the inner aspect of the ribs to look for haemorrhage (which invariably accompanies significant fractures) combined with palpation and subsequent dissection if fractures are suspected.

The breasts are often overlooked. It is recommended that several neat, parallel vertical incisions from the chest wall aspect are made, and which do not breach the skin. One of these should be level with the nipple, and at least two equidistantly spaced either side, following which the cut surfaces should be palpated as well as inspected. At this stage it is convenient to check for axillary lymphadenopathy.

Systematic Dissection

Cardiovascular System

Heart

The dissection technique outlined by Olsen (*Pathology of the Heart* Appendix 1) is well illustrated and sufficiently comprehensive for nearly all situations. The heart is such an important organ to examine and yet is paradoxically very badly dissected by many candidates, usually due to bad habits which have developed to save time. Some of the more practical points related to the dissection are highlighted below.

a) Removal of the Heart

The protocol laid down in the above reference should be closely followed. It is very easy to leave parts of the atria behind when cutting the pulmonary veins and venae cavae, which can be lessened by putting slight tension in the heart prior to cutting these structures with scissors. Examiners often check for this by asking to be shown the location of the sinoatrial node. The pulmonary trunk should be incised before removal of the heart (and preferably while still in the body) to check for massive pulmonary thromboembolism. The pericardium should also be included in any demonstration and commented upon in the report.

b) External Examination

The epicardial surface should be inspected very closely, with the heart orientated as if in the body (after recognition of the acute right border and oblique left border). As well as gaining an idea of the heart size, evidence of early infarction may be apparent, where the more flaccid myocardium is depressed, and may show some very fine epicardial vascular congestion. These changes can be obscured on sectioning.

c) Coronary Arteries

All candidates should be familiar with the normal anatomy (and variations) as ignorance about the location of the main branches will count heavily against them. It may be quite difficult to find the arteries after dissection of the heart, but useful landmarks are the tips of the auricular appendages and the great vessels. The right coronary artery emerges between the right auricle and pulmonary trunk, the left between the aorta and left auricle. It is an essential skill to identify these structures swiftly, and with some 'panache', for demonstration of vessels to clinicians and examiners alike. In the event that the vessels are still difficult to identify on external examination, a look inside the sinuses of Valsalva from the top will identify the orifices, (which should be demonstrated in any case). There is nothing more irritating or depressing than a mumbling pathologist trying to find the coronary arteries and failing to act with any degree of confidence.

The arteries may be sectioned longitudinally with artery scissors, or by transverse sectioning. In the latter technique, regular cuts at 0.5 cm intervals should be made (closer in the more proximal segments), and care taken that they are transverse to the direction of the vessels. Heavily calcified arteries could be removed for decalcification and subsequent sectioning in appropriate cases, as there is a risk to attempted section of such vessels with a knife, but in the examination advice could be sought from the supervisor on this point.

d) Valves

An attempt should be made to inspect all of the valves before they are divided, to look for distortion or vegetations. As a general rule the incision is made through the centre of valve cusps, or through the commissures of the mitral and tricuspid valves. The valve diameters are measured (and candidates are expected to know the normal values). Vegetations should be carefully searched for, as they can easily be overlooked. It should be remembered that papillary muscles and chordae tendinae are also part of the valve structure and often receive scant attention.

e) Atria

The usual structures are identified and a check made for small atrioseptal defects, (apart from 'probe' potency of the foramen ovale). In atrial fibrillation the auricular appendages may be thrombosed, and need to be fully opened. The annulus of the mitral valve should be inspected after division of mitral valve and ventricular wall. It can be calcified and predispose to incompetence of the valve.

f) Myocardium

It is difficult to advise whether the ventricles should be removed from the remainder of the heart when there is a pathological abnormality present. In general, in macroscopically normal hearts, they are best removed and weighed separately. When there is an abnormality, it is often better to keep the atria and ventricles intact for demonstration purposes, after opening the heart as for the standard protocol (it is often advantageous to make a transverse slice first of all about 1 cm above the apex to inspect the chambers and examine the myocardium). With valvular disease, the ventricles should be relatively intact, the chambers being opened according to the direction of blood flow. In myocardial disease, the ventricles are opened and the myocardium sliced transversely at 0.5–1 cm intervals, keeping the epicardium intact so it can be 'reconstituted' as a structure for demonstration – this is virtually impossible if the slices are completely severed. In doing this the coronary arteries should be disturbed as little as possible, otherwise further cuts are made in them and can ruin your neat dissection when the outer surface of the heart is demonstrated. The myocardium should also be washed after sectioning, as subtle changes such as fatty heart, papillary muscle disease or early myocardial infarction are very easily obscured by even a small amount of blood.

Conducting System

No candidate would really be expected to perform a detailed study of the conducting system, but they may be asked to give an outline of how it might be approached. It is relatively easy to find the major structures with a little practice which could be pointed out if asked. The sinoatrial node is located at the junction of the superior vena cava and a line extending from the superior border of the right auricular appendage. The atrioventricular node can be located at the intersection of a line passing through the papillary muscle of the conus with one passing horizontally through the opening of the coronary sinus. This point is variable when the myocardium is flabby, so a block of muscle needs to be removed from the general area and divided into two or three small blocks. With practice, it is possible to see both nodes macroscopically. Candidates should have some knowledge of the general course of the bundle of His, the right branch passing into the intraventricular septum, and the left travelling above the membranous portion of the intraventricular septum before passing inferiorly.

Anatomical Structures

Candidates may be expected to demonstrate the following if asked, so it is useful to have the ability to point them out rapidly and clearly, explaining the orientation and outlining any anatomical variations which may occur.

1) Orifices of right and left pulmonary veins and venae cavae
2) Auricular appendages
3) Left coronary artery, main named branches, orifice in sinus of Valsalva
4) Right coronary artery, branches and orifice
5) Posterior descending coronary artery (the main branch leading to this is called 'dominant')
6) Range of total (defatted) heart weight, weights of right ventricle, left ventricle and septum, and ratio LV+S : RV; relationship between LV&S and RV; relationship between hypertrophy and weight
7) Valve circumference and diameters
8) Right atrium – foramen ovale, crista terminale, coronary sinus opening
9) Left atrium – fossa ovalis
10) Right ventricle – myocardial thickness, papillary muscle of conus, crista supraventricularis
11) Left ventricle – myocardial thickness, membranous part of interventricular septum
12) Sinoatrial node, atroventricular node, bundles of His (approximate location)
13) Location of ductus arteriosus

Common General Questions in Examination

If there is a pathological abnormality in the heart, candidates would be asked to demonstrate it and discuss aspects of the diagnosis. More general points that may be asked by an examiner include:

a)   Anatomical Features

Most important is the weight of the heart and ventricles. If asked, it is best not to give one weight, or even an approximate range, but preface the answer with 'In a male/female of this height and build (which should have already been established from the clinical notes), I would expect the heart weight to range between X and Y grams'. After this the case in question should be compared to the expected result and assessed accordingly. If there is hypertrophy affecting the left and/or right ventricle, weight ratios should again be quoted in support of the assessment. Examiners will expect a fluent discourse from a candidate, so the explanation should continue until interrupted. However, the aim is to include as many facts per sentence as possible, avoiding the temptation to ramble. It is common for examiners to go on to ask the causes of ventricular hypertrophy, isolated and combined, which should also elicit a rapid, full answer.

b)   Further Macroscopic Techniques

Some procedures may be performed on the gross specimen to demonstrate specific pathology, such as the nitro-blue tetrazolium (NBT) test for myocardial infarction. Candidates should be aware how to perform this test, (although it is unlikely they will be asked to perform it), and of its limitations. Amyloid can be demonstrated with Lugol's iodine/dilute sulphuric acid, and may be very useful since cardiac amyloid is very common in the aged. It is important to know how to take bacteriological samples in cases of suspected infective endocarditis, prior to opening the heart.

Aorta and Arteries

If the patient had severe arteriosclerosis producing major ischaemic effects on other organs besides the heart, it may be useful to keep the aorta and major branches as an intact dissection, which can be accomplished relatively easily, especially in the Letulle method.

The subclavian, common carotid arteries, internal and external carotids should always be opened (or at least the first 1–2 cm where much of the major pathology lies), and the major branches of the abdominal aorta. The distal iliofemoral arteries are best demonstrated in the body. In cases of ischaemic renal disease or hypertension, remove the abdominal aorta with both kidneys (cutting across the inferior vena cava), to open them as an intact dissection – remember to look for accessory renal arteries. With intestinal ischaemia or embolism, identify the superior mesenteric artery and cut down it with the aid of a probe. This will be facilitated if you have left the mesentery intact when removing the bowel. You are usually only expected to dissect down the first two or three branches however.

Abdominal aortic aneurysms are best opened from the posterior aspect. A transverse cut may help to demonstrate the structure of the wall. It is best to check the extension of any thrombus down the iliac vessels and for potency before attempts are made to open them. It is very difficult to demonstrate any residual lumen in a calcified, atherosclerotic iliac artery once it has been opened unless great care is taken.

Dissecting aneurysms require particular care, and in suspected cases the removal of organs needs handling with care. Transverse sections of the aorta may help to demonstrate the pathology, and careful inspection may be required to identify internal breaches.

Anatomical Structures

It is necessary to be familiar with the following arteries and their variation.

1) Subclavian and carotid arteries (including branches of the external carotid arteries)
2) Vertebral artery origin (see 'Special Procedures', page 283)
3) Coeliac axis and major branches
4) Superior mesenteric artery
5) Renal arteries
6) Inferior mesenteric artery (may be a very inconspicuous branch in some cases)
7) Iliofemoral vessels

More distal parts of the arteries are often covered under specific organ systems e.g. internal carotid and vertebrobasilar arteries in CNS, hepatic and splenic arteries in alimentary system, etc).

Common Questions

1) Anatomical relations
2) Clinico-pathological consequences of atherosclerosis

Venous System

It is most important to check the iliofemoral veins in all post mortems by opening them at least to the origin of the great saphenous vein. In cases of significant pulmonary thromboembolism, thrombus will be found up to this point in almost all cases even if some has detached. In addition, a careful search for leg oedema should be combined with measurement of the leg circumference around calves and ankles.

The inferior vena cava should be opened from the posterior aspect, but the renal artery should not be sacrificed if there is any significant pathology to demonstrate. The orifice of the hepatic vein should be inspected for thrombosis or tumour when the liver is diseased.

When the thoracic duct is to be examined (see 'Special Procedures'), it is better to leave the venae cavae in situ to act as landmarks.

Alimentary System

Mouth and Oesophagus

The mouth is often neglected, but should always be quickly inspected for obvious dental abnormalities and mucosal disease such as thrush. The submandibular salivary glands and tongue are dissected when examining the thoracic pluck, but are often neglected. The parotid gland must be examined with great care because of the risk of damaging the face, and is best left alone unless there is a gross lesion. The tonsils should be inspected in cases of lymphoreticular disease.

The oesophagus can be removed after locating the parathyroid glands, by dividing it 1 cm below the larynx, holding the upper border with forceps, and freeing the fascial attachments to trachea, oesophagus and diaphragm with scissors. It is very easy to remove it in continuity with the stomach if required, by dividing the diaphragmatic attachments, when the organs have been removed by the Letulle technique. This is desirable when there is suspected gastro-oesophageal disease such as hiatus hernia, carcinoma or varices. Hiatus hernia can only be convincingly demonstrated with an intact diaphragm, and division of the crus will make it very difficult.

The oesophagus is opened from the posterior aspect after mobilisation of the stomach, but the demonstration of varices requires particular care as they become collapsed and inconspicuous on conventional dissection. The unopened oeso-phagus, freed from its attachments, is tied at the upper end with string, and mobilised along with the stomach (see below). The latter is opened midway along the greater curve, to within 10 cm of the cardia. After removal of gastric contents, a long Spencer-Wells forceps can be inserted through the cardia to grasp the mucosa at the upper end. Withdrawing the forceps evaginates the oesophagus and the dilated veins are well demonstrated.

Stomach

It is necessary to clamp or tie off gently (avoiding crushing) the gastro-oesophageal junction and duodenum prior to removing the stomach. The stomach is best opened along the greater curvature, putting the contents into a clean bowl (extending it to open the oesophagus if required). In forensic cases the gastric contents may need to be kept for analysis. Candidates who allow gastric contents to spill over the organs or over the dissecting table will create an unfavourable impression.

After removing the stomach, with or without the oesophagus, the mucosal surface should be gently washed in clean water. Even when the mucosa appears 'autolysed', significant abnormalities such as chronic ulcers and neoplasms are usually discovered because of their fibrous tissue base. The first part of the duodenum should be closely inspected as it is a frequent mistake to miss chronic ulceration at this site.

Small and Large Intestines

The removal and inspection of the intestines were covered earlier. It is important to wash the surface well and inspect the bowel thoroughly – it is often a neglected part of a necropsy. The duodenum should be opened along the lateral border, and examined with the pancreas and common bile duct. Opened small bowel can be arranged fairly compactly on a board (if required), as a series of folds resembling a ploughed field.

Liver and Biliary System

The liver is often removed from the surrounding tissues with scant attention paid to the surrounding structures. Before this stage the biliary system should be dissected, starting by opening the lateral border of the duodenum, exposing the Ampulla of Vater. Patency of the common bile duct can be demonstrated by gentle compression of the gall bladder.

The unopened gall bladder is mobilised from the liver attachments, and the cystic duct identified with judicious incisions with a small scalpel in the surrounding connective tissues. It can then be opened with small scissors, and followed into the common bile duct which is opened with artery scissors up to right and left hepatic ducts, and downwards, into the duodenum via the ampulla. If there is no ductal disease, the gall bladder, still containing its bile, can be freed by dividing the cystic duct; bile should not be allowed to contaminate the dissection, but is discharged into a small container, and the gall bladder opened along its length.

The portal vein should be opened in all cases, and a comprehensive dissection of the branches included in any case of portal venous hypertension, where it is better to leave the splenic and gastric veins intact with the pancreas, stomach and oesophagus for demonstration purposes.

The liver is often poorly sectioned with apparently random strokes, by many candidates. In cases where no liver pathology is suspected, or where there may be focal disease (such as metastases), the organ should be placed on its inferior surface, and vertical antero-posterior incisions made from the superior border almost to the level of the inferior capsular surface (to enable the slices to remain in relationship to each other). As in all solid organs, a large knife is used to make a single clean stroke, rather than a sawing action which produces an unsatisfactory, ragged cut surface.

Another elegant but little known method can be used in cases of biliary or venous disorders. The liver is rested on its superior capsular surface and probes placed into the right and left main hepatic ducts to serve as guides for bisection of the organ in the plane, thus giving a good view of the biliary tree. Section of the lobe demonstrates the hepatic venous system. Slices can be either side of these cuts as before to inspect the remaining parenchyma.

Pancreas

This seems to present problems for many candidates, and is often very badly dissected. Palpation of the firm gland parenchyma around the borders will allow for swift removal of the softer retroperitoneal fat with a pair of medium scissors. The head of the organ should be excised from the duodenal loop except when there is ampullary or biliary disease, and then the isolated organ is sectioned transversely at 1 cm intervals, leaving the anterior capsular surface intact. In rare cases with suspected pancreatic duct disease, a single transverse slice at the junction of head and body will reveal the main duct, which can be opened through to the duodenum with the aid of a probe. A well-dissected pancreas enhances the final presentation and will impress examiners.

Anatomical Relations

1) Arterial supply to stomach, liver and pancreas
2) Arterial supply to small and large bowel
3) Portal venous system
4) Surface anatomy of the liver
5) Distinction between anatomical and functional liver lobes
6) Intra and extrahepatic bile ducts
7) Structure of the porta hepatis
8) Normal liver and pancreas weight ranges
9) Length of normal small bowel and colon

Common Questions

1) Structural effects of portal hypertension
2) Causes of biliary obstruction
3) Cholelithiasis – frequency and pathogenesis
4) Mesenteric ischaemia – venous and arterial
5) Classification of cirrhosis
6) Recognition of true cirrhosis vs. hepatic fibrosis
7) Aspects of gastrointestinal neoplasia
8) Malabsorption syndrome – causes and effects

Respiratory System

It is best to decide whether you wish to inflate one or both of the lungs with formalin prior to starting the dissection, so that the post mortem technician can make preparations. However, it is quite a time-consuming procedure in an examination situation, and with recent guidelines restricting the use of formalin to a suitably ventilated area, it is not always practicable. However, candidates should be familiar with the technique of formalin liquid and vapour inflation (Dunnill, M.S. *Pulmonary Pathology* Chapter 6, Emphysema p81–82. Churchill Livingstone, Edinburgh, 1982). If in doubt it is best to ask if facilities are available. It is a desirable procedure in a number of cases where primary pulmonary disease is a major factor in the patient's demise, in particular in a case of pneumoconiosis or emphysema. The usual compromise is to inflate one lung for later examination (which a candidate may well be asked to perform subsequently!) and to dissect the other at the time. It is important to be aware of potential artefacts produced by lung inflation (usually by too high an inflating pressure), and enough main bronchus needs to be left to enable it to be tied off.

Dissection Procedure

a) Chest Wall

Since the rib cage and parietal pleurae also form part of the respiratory system, they should have been inspected for rib fractures, pleural plaques, metastatic deposits, etc. earlier, when the organs were first removed.

b) Larynx and Major Airways

The larynx is usually opened from behind in the midline, cracking the thyroid cartilage. In cases where patients have died suddenly in hospital or those which give rise to suspicion of inhalation of food, it is important to visualise the larynx before removing the organs, as material is often dislodged during manipulation. The material in the airways should be examined closely (e.g. mucopus, viscid mucus, food), and note whether there are associated mucosal inflammatory changes.

c) Lungs

It is important to keep both lungs orientated both during and after the dissection. It can be surprisingly difficult to identify right and left lungs, especially if they are diseased, and is an embarassing mistake to make in front of an examiner or clinician. Lungs should be displayed in the antero-posterior direction, and the surface topographic features identified.

The pleural surface of the hemidiaphragm should be included in the assessment, and attempts made to correlate any pathology (e.g. adhesions, plaques, etc.) with corresponding abnormalities on the visceral pleura. In cases of rib fracture, a close inspection should be made for damage to the underlying lung.

Before starting to dissect the lungs, they are weighed and then placed in cold water to assess the density. While a poor discriminator of inflation during life, a disproportionate heaviness in one lobe might indicate some localised consolidation.

It is important to strike a balance when searching for pulmonary thromboembolism. Some candidates seem to forget to do it entirely, while others follow the pulmonary arterial vasculature almost to the periphery. A compromise is to open to the 4th or 5th branch of each artery which should locate significant pulmonary thromboemboli. Smaller ones are better detected on the cut surface of the lung (see below).

Similarly, the airways are opened to the level of the segmental bronchi. There is little point in going further however, unless grossly diseased.

Sectioning of the lung always seems to cause problems for pathologists in training. Many compress the lung with a sponge, and try to bisect the lungs by sawing their way through the parenchyma with a large knife. This invariably produces a flabby, poorly orientated mess, which is impossible to demonstrate adequately.

It is better to take a slightly more refined approach, taking each lobe in turn and making a single lateral to medial incision from the parietal surface towards the hilus, holding the lung firmly on a flat surface without heavy compression. It should be possible to make more than one cut, especially in the lower lobes, one in the anterior half and one in the posterior. The right middle lobe is best displayed by a horizontal incision.

The cut surfaces require close inspection, with sponging or washing where necessary, and the lungs palpated (without squeezing), which is equally effective in locating abnormalities, but is often neglected. Bronchopneumonia and small thromboemboli are often palpable rather than visible. Parenchymal disease is often missed, especially the more subtle forms of emphysema or fibrosis. Examining the lungs under water may improve the architecture, but squeezing the parenchyma should be avoided as it draws water in. When demonstrating the lungs, an explanatory statement to the examiner to the effect that pathology is best seen in inflated lungs should be made and that immediate dissection is a compromise.

Specimens should be taken for bacteriological or virological examination in suspected infections, but this should ideally be performed before removal of the lungs from the body to lessen the risk of contamination.

Anatomical Relationships

1) Pulmonary lobes
2) Segmental bronchial nomenclature
3) Pulmonary lobular architecture
4) Vasculature (pulmonary and bronchial arterial, venous)

1) Weight of normal lungs
2) Pulmonary thromboembolism. Frequency and predisposing features
3) Methods of pulmonary inflation
4) Classification of emphysema
5) Macroscopic appearance of carcinomas
6) Spread of bronchial carcinoma
7) Appearances of pulmonary tuberculosis
8) Function and requirements of Pneumoconiosis Medical Panel.

Urinary System

Kidneys

The renal dissection should be tailored to the abnormalities anticipated from the clinical history or inspection in situ. In hypertension or renal arterial disease the aorta and renal arteries should be kept intact with both kidneys. When there is lower urinary tract disease, keep both kidneys, ureters and bladder (+/- prostate) as an intact dissection as described on page 257.

When there is no obvious renal disease, it may suffice to 'enucleate' each kidney from the perirenal fat, (after dissection of the adrenal glands), with the renal vein and artery transected (which should also have already been opened and inspected). The ureter is divided at the pelvic brim or bladder wall. One disadvantage of using the Letulle method is that the bladder is usually left behind in the body (and often forgotten by candidates).

The kidney itself should be examined by removing the renal capsule, by making a nick and separating the plane between cortex and capsule with a finger. The kidney is often then bisected without inspecting the subcapsular surface closely, and it is advantageous to make the cut through any lesions on the convex border (e.g. scars, abscesses, haemorrhages) angled towards the hilus. The aim should be to bisect the kidney with a single cut, so that the surface is smooth. The two halves can 'hinge' on the renal pelvis, which should remain intact medially. Close inspection should be made of the parenchyma for other lesions, and transverse or vertical incisions made as required, but in a systematic fashion so that the kidney can be reconstituted.

The ureters should be opened longitudinally, preferably following them into the bladder. The latter is best opened from the urethra up the anterior wall to display the trigone. The prostate requires examination by making two or three transverse cuts – this is often neglected.

Anatomical Relationships

1) Weight of kidneys
2) Thickness of cortex
3) Topography of cut surface
4) Number of calyces
5) Diameter of ureters

Common Questions

1) Causes of subcapsular scarring
2) Effects of renal artery stenosis
3) Effects of hypertension
4) Pyelonephritis vs. glomerulonephritis – macroscopic appearances

Female Reproductive System

The ovaries and uterus are inspected in situ, and can be removed separately from both rectum and bladder. It is easier once the rectum is removed, to cut across the upper vagina, and using scissors to remove the broad ligaments flush with the pelvic wall, avoiding the ureters. The organs may then be displayed in the anatomical orientation, with incisions in both ovaries, Fallopian tubes, and the uterus and cervix opened either with multiple transverse incisions or a single vertical incision on the anterior wall, exposing the endometrium. If pathological lesions are present these should be dissected as for a specimen received in a routine surgical dissection.

Central Nervous System

Removal of the brain is often performed by post mortem technicians during most of the routine post mortems performed by a trainee, and examiners are well aware of this. Removal of spinal cord is described under 'Special Procedures' (p 282). However, the examinee may well be asked to remove the brain, under the scrutiny of the examiner, and if this procedure has not been practised it is relatively easy to damage and disrupt the delicate tissue. It is not unknown for candidates to be asked to remove the cranial vault in addition. On the other hand, in a routine case, the supervisor will let it be known if the post mortem technician may remove the skull and brain. In cases of suspected meningitis or abscess, CSF should be taken from the fourth or third ventricles area by syringe puncture for microbiological studies.

In cases where intracranial pathology is suspected, the brain should be removed by the candidate. During this the brain needs to be well supported (ask for assistance). The first task is to reflect the meninges to inspect the subdural space. The vault is inspected for signs of extradural haematoma, and other conditions such as Paget's disease or hyperostosis frontalis interna, etc. In removing the brain, special care must be taken to cut the delicate cranial nerves at their foramina, rather than letting them tear if the brain is allowed to fall backwards under its own weight. If the spinal cord is not to be removed, a deep cut with a scalpel is made well into the foramen magnum to transect the upper spinal cord, and care taken to include the vertebrobasilar arteries which are often left behind.

Detailed dissection of the brain is described in Gresham and Turner (Appendix 1) and you should follow the general guidelines for a routine dissection. The first thing to establish is whether it is the usual practice at that centre to dissect the brain at the time, or to suspend it in fixative for later examination (which will therefore not be by the examinee!). An opportunity to point out that this is always preferable with suspected intracerebral pathology should be taken.

The carotid sinus, pituitary fossa and meninges need to be inspected and commented upon. The eyes should not be removed except with express permission or suspected intra-ocular pathology. The pituitary gland should always be removed at this stage, by incising the diaphragm of the sella, displacing the posterior clinoid process.

The outer surface of the brain should be closely inspected. In suspected cerebrovascular disease, all of the vessels on the base of the brain should be identified and displayed, including the vertebral artery, but also the internal carotid artery within the carotid sinus should be inspected by removing the lateral bony wall of the sinus. It is unlikely that a candidate would be asked to expose the vertebral arteries, but the origins should be inspected along with the intracranial segment.

Sectioning of the brain will not be covered in detail here, but in a soft, unfixed brain, compression should be avoided, using a single stroke to make each slice. The cut surface should be wiped with the knife blade held at an angle, to remove blood before inspection of the white matter and if there is vascular disease the major vessels should not be divided before they have been demonstrated to the examiner. The medulla and cerebellum should be removed and dissected separately usually with horizontal slices.

After sectioning, the slices are best displayed in a neat, orderly array, preferably on a board. This may be difficult at times with unfixed brain, but is still no excuse for presenting a rather jumbled mound of brain slices which have received only a perfunctory inspection.

Candidates would not normally be expected to remove the spinal cord for a routine post mortem, but if there was a specific clinical indication to do so (e.g. muscle wasting, paralysis, sensory deficit, motor neurone disease, etc.) which was directly connected with the cause of death, it should be performed without prompting. On occasion, candidates have been asked to remove the spinal cord as a special procedure (see page 282), but only usually with an otherwise straight-forward examination (e.g. probable myocardial infarction, etc.)

Anatomical Relationships

1) Weight range of brain
2) Cranial nerves – origin and identification in skull
3) Cerebral arterial supply
4) Vertebral and carotid arterial supply
5) Surface anatomy of the brain
6) Main anatomical regions of brain
7) Major deep nuclei in midbrain and thalamus
8) Ventricular system
9) Hippocampus
10) Internal capsule
11) Pineal gland (candidates should ensure they are able to locate this structure, which is often left behind in the cranial fossae if the brain is not carefully removed).

1) Morphological sequelae of coning phenomenon
2) Appearances in senile dementia
3) Types of cerebral haemorrhage
4) Cerebral infarction. Sites and appearances
5) Demyelinating diseases

Endocrine System

The pituitary gland is commonly neglected, but should always be carefully removed and bisected, usually transversely. It is important to be familiar with the normal macroscopic appearance.

The parathyroid gland dissection is described more fully in 'Special Procedures' (page 281), and should ideally be performed at the start of the dissection of the thoracic pluck prior to removing the oesophagus.

The thyroid gland should be carefully removed from around the trachea, and from surrounding muscles, in one piece. Both lobes and the isthmus should be vertically sectioned, leaving the capsule intact on the anterior surface of the gland to allow it to be orientated afterwards.

Both adrenal glands should be dissected out prior to removing the kidneys, as afterwards they may be difficult to find, and are often damaged. They are best located by palpation, and separated from the surrounding fat using small dissecting scissors, so that the gland is not disrupted. Glands removed cleanly from the fat are impressive to examiners, and are another sign of the expert prosector. After removal, several parallel cuts made into the gland allow inspection, but one border should be left intact to allow reconstruction.

Although not strictly endocrine, it is as well to be familiar with the location of the carotid bodies and other paraganglia, which is sometimes raised in discussion.

Anatomical Relationships

1) Normal gland weights – especially adrenal glands and differences between autopsy and operative gland weights.
2) Vascular supply of pituitary gland
3) Surface anatomy of adrenal glands
4) Aberrant locations of thyroid/parathyroid glands

Common subjects for discussion

1) Atrophy of thyroid gland – recognition and effects
2) Adrenal cortical hyperplasia in hypertension
3) Significance and frequency of adrenal cortical nodules
4) Effects of hypo/hyper function of glands
5) Methods of assessing ante mortem gland function from necropsy material (blood, vitreous humour analysis, etc.)
6) Parathyroid and adrenal gland weights

Lymphoreticular System

This is often disregarded as a system unless there is a specific disease such as leukaemia or lymphoma, and frequently no specific comment made in the final report. It is necessary to examine certain node groups as a matter of routine, including axillary, cervical, mediastinal, para-aortic, mesenteric and inguinal, keeping them to one side, or in a small dish, in a specific order, as the dissection proceeds. Otherwise it becomes all too easy to forget and overlook more subtle forms of nodal pathology. Such attention to detail will always create a favourable impression with the examiner.

The spleen is fairly straightforward to dissect. (The splenic artery and vein should be examined before removing the pancreas.) The capsular surface is inspected carefully, and the parenchyma is examined either by a single horizontal cut from the anterior border, or as a series of vertical transverse cuts along the length of the organ on the inferior surface, leaving the superior capsule intact. The choice of approach is largely dictated by the consistency of the spleen, and when 'autolysed' a single horizontal cut may be all that is possible. The cut surface needs to be carefully washed in order to examine and display the parenchyma, otherwise some features may be obscured by blood.

The thoracic duct dissection is described in detail under 'Special Procedures' (page 283).

Anatomical Relationships

1) Drainage areas of the major nodal groups
2) Normal splenic weight range
3) Anatomy of thoracic duct

Common Questions

1) Causes of splenomegaly
2) Causes of local and generalised lymphadenopathy
3) Spleen in portal hypertension
4) Location of accessory spleens
5) Spleen in Hodgkin's disease/NHL

Musculoskeletal system

Much of this should be covered by the external examination of the body. All deformities should be carefully noted, and the corresponding joints examined. Lesser degrees of rheumatoid disease may be easily overlooked and the hands require particularly careful assessment. A check should be made for alignment of the legs, especially for true leg shortening, as a fractured neck of femur is easily missed otherwise.

The rib cage should be examined as previously described. The cranial vault is inspected when the brain is removed, and it is worthwhile measuring the thickness of the skull if there is any suspicion of Paget's disease. The spine must be assessed for deformity, and a careful examination of the atlanto-axial joint and other cervical vertebrae should be made in Coroner's cases, especially where there has been trauma. In the thoracic and lumbar spine, collapsed vertebrae are easily overlooked. This may be facilitated by removing a strip of bone from the vertebral column. Blood and bone dust should be removed from the cut surface, preferably with a sponge, as the finer detail is usually obscured otherwise.

In cases of bone disease diagnosed ante mortem, the clinical history and radiological studies may well dictate the bones and joints to be examined, and this should have emerged during assessment of the clinical notes. It is often useful to make a note of any bones requiring particular examination, writing a reminder on the board in the post mortem room, as it is something that is easily forgotten, since it is customary to perform detailed examination near the end of the dissection.

Removal of the femur is described under 'Special Procedures'. However, it is regarded as an essential part of the procedure in some centres, a point which should be established with the post mortem technician, who must also have the materials available for reconstruction. Dissection of the temporal bone (middle ear) is also described under 'Special Procedures' (page 281).

It is worthwhile examining any joint that has had an operative procedure performed on it, especially in the case of prosthetic replacements such as an artificial hip. The orthopaedic surgeons may well find it of value to have a careful assessment of the state of the prosthesis, and its integration with the surrounding tissues.

The muscles are rarely examined in detail at post mortem, but any wasting should be carefully noted, and the cause for this established if possible, in conjunction with examination of the nervous system.

Presentation of the Post Mortem

Candidates may find that they are unable to make a formal presentation of the findings at the end of the examination, but should always prepare just the same. It is a mistake to attempt to 'sort out' the organs at the end of the dissection, as the examiner may return at any time to inspect the findings, and may wish to make several visits. Therefore each organ should be laid out on a separate board or dish as it is finished, ensuring it is washed and dried to avoid too much seepage of blood. It is often useful to rest the tissues on paper towelling, which can be later removed.

It is important to keep in control of the presentation, and anticipate the questions that are likely to be asked. In certain cases, a skilful presenter will be able to suggest an interpretation, prompting the examiner to discuss the differential diagnosis. In this situation, the best candidates have prepared good reasons for supporting their interpretation in the light of the clinical information, and indicate that they considered alternatives, discussing the reasons for their decisions. This requires careful advance 'planning' during the course of the dissection.

The manner of the presentation is most important. It is best to commence with a concise clinical history (if it has not been discussed with the examiner previously). After this, attention should be turned to the major pathology, stating initially the opinion as to the cause of death as it would be phrased for death certification. The evidence to support this should be presented in a logical order. In pulmonary thromboembolism for example, the starting point is the pulmonary arteries and on to the lung parenchyma, moving then to the inferior vena cava and leg veins. After this the factors considered to have predisposed to this pathology are discussed (e.g. recumbency due to fractured neck of femur), which are in effect underlying causes of death, rather than the acute event. In appropriate cases it is useful to comment on the clinical course and effects of therapy on the disease. If the clinical staff responsible for the patient attend they should be engaged in the discussion, and the presentation aimed as much to them as the examiner. They may provide some observations which will aid in the interpretation of the case, and the examiner will always be impressed by a pathologist who clearly demonstrates an ability to establish a rapport with clinical colleagues.

After discussion on the cause of death and major associated pathology, then other findings should be considered, starting with the most important, leaving the trivial abnormalities until last. If a long time has been spent on the major pathology these findings may not be required by the examiner. Many candidates approach the presentation in the opposite way, starting with minor, irrelevant or peripheral abnormalities, as if to impress the examiner with the thoroughness of their dissection. Unfortunately this has the opposite effect, merely providing distractions and using up valuable time which could be better spent on the main pathology, and runs the risk of irritating the examiner, who may interrupt and take the initiative away. Trainees should enquire from senior pathologists about their presentation style, and whether they achieve the right balance and emphasis.

As well as verbal presentation, every effort should be made to be specific when illustrating the pathological changes. Rather than vaguely pointing things out, a probe or similar blunt instrument should be used but not a knife. The organ or tissue must be displayed to the best advantage, orientating it towards the examiner and held steadily. The skill of communicating while manipulating the tissues should be developed by constant practice in order to maximise the information which is to be conveyed in a most succinct manner. Avoid giving lists of negative findings.

After the presentation, candidates are given time to finish the examination. Tissues are taken for histological examination and it is important to take special care over this, as examination of these may comprise part of the examination subsequently. It is always best to take uniform blocks during training, and if possible regular slices no greater than 5 mm in depth which will fit into a standard cassette. These will fix well, unlike larger, poorly orientated lumps of tissue. It is up to personal preference whether tissue is taken for histology as each organ dissection is finished, or at the end of the necropsy. The advantage of the former method is that it is possible to 'picture' where the blocks have been taken from when the sections are examined, and candidates are less likely to forget to include tissues from any site, a distinct risk if things are rather rushed at the end of the necropsy. Extra pots can be labelled separately for particular lesions or sites, in order to make the subsequent histological assessment easier. A record of the blocks taken should be kept and put in the post mortem report. It is common for examiners to enquire what tissues are required for histological examination and what constitutes an adequate or optimal number to examine.

When satisfied that the dissection is complete, the area should be tidied and all instruments located for safety reasons. Then a note of the organ weights and other abnormalities identified on external examination written on the post mortem room board, should be made.

Writing the Report

In many centres candidates are asked to write up the report on blank A4 paper, as this will constitute part of the submitted examination data. Therefore they must be able to set out a report in this fashion, which may be a problem if they are used to standardised sheets with pre-typed headings and sections. Conversely, in some centres they may be given these sheets to complete for the report which, while this will avert any errors of omission, may be in a different format to a form which a candidate is used to so needs to be read through carefully prior to starting.

The following is an example post mortem report which is considered perfectly adequate for examination purposes. It is not intended to be a counsel of excellence. The same principles as for essay writing should be followed in the actual written report on examination with attention paid to legibility, subheadings, etc. It is always better to submit a neat handwritten report (some centres may allow you to send the completed report the next day, especially if the dissection was in the afternoon, but it should not be typewritten). In general, it is best to complete the report at the centre the same day, otherwise there is a temptation to embellish and modify findings after discussion with colleagues.

POST MORTEM EXAMINATION

Hospital:
Name of Patient:
Date of Birth: 13.6.20   Age: 69
Nationality: British   Ward: X   Consultant: Dr ....
Date of latest admission: 13 July 1989 13.40 hours
Date and time of death: 23 July 1989 04.10 hours
Date and time of necropsy: 24 July 1989 0900 hours
Weight of patient: 74.5 Kg   Height: 5'9"
Coroner's report submitted: No
Prosector: Dr ....

Cause of death

I   a) massive pulmonary thromboembolism
        due to
     b) thrombosis of the iliofemoral veins
        due to
     c) recumbency following acute myocardial infarction
II   Ischaemic heart disease and essential hypertension
     Maturity onset diabetes mellitus

Summary of pathological findings

1) Thrombus in main pulmonary arteries
2) Bilateral thrombosis iliofemoral veins and major branches of legs
3) Acute myocardial infarction (10–14 days)
4) Myocardial scarring and left ventricular hypertrophy
5) Coronary artery atheroma with thrombotic occlusion of the left anterior
   descending branch
6) Systematic atherosclerosis
7) Bilateral renal cortical scarring
8) Nodular hyperplasia of adrenal cortex
9) Small oesophageal nodule (? leiomyoma)
10) Splenic mesothelial cyst
11) Seborrhoeic keratoses chest wall
12) Previous appendicectomy

Clinical history

The patient had been treated for mild hypertension for 7 years, and maturity
onset diabetes was diagnosed 2 years later (controlled by diet). His only health
problem prior to this was an appendicectomy in 1955. Three years ago he was
admitted to this hospital for suspected anterior myocardial infarction, and had
been followed up since that time in the outpatient clinic, during which he was
requiring increasing levels of therapy to control his hypertension. He had also
noted increasing angina of effort in the past year.
   On 13 July 1989 he was admitted via the accident and emergency
department with a 4-hour history of breathlessness and severe anginal pain

resistant to sublingual glyceryl trinitrate. Acute myocardial infarction was confirmed by ECG examination. Over the next few hours he developed signs of acute left ventricular failure, managed by diuretic therapy.

The patient made slow progress over the next 6 days, but was generally weak with poor mobilisation. On 19 July, 7 days after admission, he was noted to have swelling of the right lower leg, and ultrasound examination confirmed the suspicion of deep venous thrombosis. Anticoagulant therapy had been commenced 2 days previously, and mobilisation was encouraged. Despite this he developed thrombosis in the left leg.

At 03.35 hours on 23 July he suffered a cardiac arrest. Resuscitation attempts, including injection of streptokinase via a central venous line and intracardiac injection of calcium and adrenaline, were unsuccessful, and the patient was declared dead at 04.10 hours.

External examination

The body is of a mildly obese, elderly white male. Recent needle puncture wounds are noted in the right and left antecubital fossae, left neck and subclavian region, and over the fifth and sixth intercostal spaces on the anterior chest wall. A 7 cm appendicectomy scar is present. There is marked pitting oedema of both lower limbs (mid calf circumference 22 cm right, 21 cm left), with pitting oedema over the sacrum. A few seborrhoeic keratoses are noted over the anterior chest wall.

INTERNAL EXAMINATION

Cardiovascular System

a) Veins

Thrombus occludes both femoral veins, to the origin of the giant saphenous vein on the left, and the origin of the internal iliac vein on the right. A fragment of thrombus 2.0 cm by 1.5 cm is found in the inferior vena cava. The superior vena cava, subclavian and jugular veins are normal.

b) Heart

The pericardium has an area of fine fibrous adhesions over the anterior surface of the heart, and there is a small amount of fibrinous exudate mainly over the lateral and posterior wall of the left ventricle, with 80 ml of yellow, slightly turbid pericardial fluid.

The heart weighs 510 g. The orifices of the venae cavae and pulmonary veins are normal. The atria are normal, and the auricular appendages are free from thrombus.

The tricuspid valve is normal (circumference 12.5 cm). The right ventricle is of normal size (defatted weight 60 g) and the pulmonary valve is normal (circumference 7.5 cm). The pulmonary arteries contain pieces of cylindrical thrombus (see Respiratory System). The left ventricle and septum are diffusely hypertrophied (combined weight 215 g), and there is a transmural fibrotic scar 1.5 x 1.0 cm in the anterior wall consistent with an old healed infarct. The myocardium over the anterolateral border is softened over a 3 cm diameter area, and is pale, with a distinct hyperaemic margin. Areas of yellow/grey mottled appearance are seen on the cut surface, and there is a small amount of adherent thrombus on the endocardial surface. The appearances are consistent with acute myocardial infarction of 10–14 days duration.

The mitral valve shows slight mucoid nodularity of the leaflets but is otherwise normal (circumference 11.0 cm). The aortic valve is normal (circumference 7.0 cm).

The right coronary artery shows two foci of severe (75%) atherosclerotic narrowing, 2 cm and 3.5 cm from its origin. The left coronary artery shows marked narrowing of the main branch and the anterior descending branch is occluded over a 1.0 cm length by recent thrombus. There is severe narrowing over the first 3 cm of the circumflex branch, but no occlusion is present. The posterior descending artery is formed from the right coronary artery and is patent. The coronary ostia are patent.

c) Arteries

Atherosclerotic plaques are present in the aortic arch and in the common carotid arteries near the bifurcation, the left having surface thrombus. Increasingly severe complicated atherosclerosis is encountered in the distal thoracic and abdominal segments of the aorta, the latter showing confluent ulcerated plaques with heavy calcification of the wall. There is severe atherosclerosis of the iliac and femoral arteries. The renal arterial orifices are surrounded by atherosclerosis but are not occluded.

Respiratory System

a) Airways

The larynx, trachea and major bronchi appear normal.

b) Vascular Supply

The pulmonary trunk and both the right and left main arteries are occluded by fragmented and coiled cores of thrombus.

c) Parenchyma

The lungs are mildly oedematous (right 530 g, left 470 g). A few emphysematous bullae are noted in both upper lobe apices, but there is no gross emphysema elsewhere. There is some fibrotic scarring at the left apex in addition, possibly a result of old healed tuberculosis. The parenchyma elsewhere is slightly congested. Some of the medium-sized branches of the pulmonary arteries contain thrombus visible on the cut surface. There is no evidence of infarction or bronchopneumonia.

d) Pleural Cavities

The left and right pleural cavities each contain 100 ml of serous fluid.

Alimentary System

a) Alimentary Tract

The mouth is edentulous. The tongue oral cavity and pharynx are normal. There is a 0.9 cm, light grey, ovoid, firm nodule in the wall of the lower third of the oesophagus, probably a leiomyoma. The gastric mucosa is partly autolysed but appears normal. The duodenum, jejunum and ileum all appear normal. The large intestine is normal apart from occasional diverticula in the sigmoid colon. The anus appears normal.

b) Liver and Biliary System

The liver is of normal weight (1470 g), but has a mildly congested appearance on cut surface. The hepatic and portal veins are normal. The gall bladder is distended with bile but no calculi are found. The common bile duct is normal, and bile could be expressed from the ampulla prior to dissection.

c) Pancreas

Normal appearance (weight 145 g).

Genitourinary System

a) Kidneys

Both kidneys are generally atrophic (right 120 g, left 115 g), with adherent capsules and a finely granular subcapsular surface, with focal small scars up to 0.5 cm across. The cortical width is reduced averaging 0.4 cm, but the corticomedullary distinction is maintained. The medulla and renal pyramids are normal. The renal pelvis and calyces are normal. Both renal arteries show atherosclerosis, but this is considerably less than in the adjacent aorta and no occlusion is demonstrated. The renal veins are normal.

Both ureters are of normal size. The bladder appears normal. The prostate is nodular but not significantly hypertrophied. The penis and testes are normal.

Central Nervous System

The meninges are normal. The brain is of normal size (weight 1390 g). There is mild atheroma of the internal carotid and vertebrobasilar arteries and atheromatous plaques are visible on the arteries of the circle of Willis. No occlusion is demonstrated. The cut surface of the brain parenchyma is normal to inspection. The cerebellum, mid-brain and brainstem are all normal. There is no visible abnormality of the cranial nerves within the skull. The eyes appear normal. The middle ears were not examined. The spinal cord was not removed.

Endocrine System

a) Pituitary Gland

Normal appearances.

b) Thyroid Gland

Normal appearances Weight 28 g.

c) Parathyroid

Three glands were identified and all appeared normal.

d) Adrenal Glands

Both adrenal glands were enlarged (left 11 g, right 10 g). This was due to nodular hyperplasia of the cortex, with the fine nodules ranging from 1 - 4 mm across. The medulla appeared normal.

Lymphoreticular System

There was no significant lymphadenopathy. The splenic artery was rather tortuous and calcified but no occlusion was demonstrated. The spleen was of normal size (weight 190 g), with normal appearances on cut surface.

Musculoskeletal System

The skull and vertebrae appear normal. The left 6th and 7th ribs are fractured anteriorly near the costochondral junction, but the lack of associated haemorrhage indicates this was almost certainly a result of resuscitation attempts. The consistency of the bones generally appeared normal.

Comments

The post mortem findings are in keeping with those expected from the clinical history. The renal and cardiovascular abnormalities present are consistent with long standing hypertension, complicated by atherosclerosis and ischaemic heart disease. Diabetes mellitus may well have accelerated the development of atherosclerosis. Nodular hyperplasia of the adrenal glands is considered to be a frequent finding in long-standing hypertension, but its exact functional significance is obscure.

The patient died from pulmonary thromboembolism due to venous thrombosis of the legs. The latter was predisposed to by the patient's poor mobility, myocardial infarction with an element of left ventricular failure and severe atherosclerosis of the lower aorta and major arteries of the legs. Blocks taken for histological examination:

1) Heart x 4
2) Coronary artery x 2
3) Lung x 6
4) Brain x 2
5) Kidneys x 4
6) Liver x 1
7) Pancreas x 3
8) Spleen x 1
9) Pituitary x 1
10) Thyroid x 1
11) Adrenal x 2
12) Lymph node x 1   Signature..

This is a conveniently straightforward case, but which is designed to illustrate the general layout of a report. The 'Comments' section is a particularly useful device to interpret the pathological findings, emphasising the most important and providing clinicopathological interpretation usually appreciated by clinical colleagues who can otherwise be somewhat unsure of the possible sequence of events and the relevance of certain abnormalities to the overall picture. It is best to limit this section to one or two fairly succinct paragraphs.

It is even more important to provide this information for the Coroner in complex cases. However, if in the examination you are asked to perform a

Coroner's necropsy then a senior member of staff or your examiner will usually take an interest and assume responsibility for completing the official report and notifying the Coroner's office of the findings. You should conduct the necropsy as for a detailed hospital case, and not as an exercise to determine the immediate cause of death.

Special Techniques

1) Parathyroid gland dissection
2) Middle ear dissection
3) Removal of brain and spinal cord
4) Removal of femur
5) Identification of thoracic duct
6) Vertebral artery dissection

Parathyroid Glands

It is a favourite examination task to be asked to identify one or more parathyroid glands. Some candidates often find this difficult and possibly because they attempt to find them too late in the dissection, when many of the crucial landmarks have been distorted. It is not unreasonable, however, to expect pathologists to identify the glands in every post mortem.

The suggested method starts with examination of the neck viscera after removal from the body. It is facilitated if the carotid arteries are removed as previously suggested (page 258). From the posterior aspect, the oesophagus and both carotid arteries are identified. Then gentle dissection between the two using vertical strokes with a scalpel will eventually reveal the lateral margin of the thyroid gland and trachea. The fine fascial tissues between the posterior border of the thyroid gland and the lateral border of the oesophagus are teased away using a scalpel which is facilitated by putting the tissues under slight tension. The posterior and medial aspect of the thyroid lobes are then revealed, and the parathyroid glands should become visible, attached to the thyroid gland capsule. The upper glands are found midway down the posterior border, the lower pair at the inferior margin or just underneath the thyroid lobe, although these can be very variable. Examined under a strong light, they are quite distinct from lymph nodes or nodular thyroid, with which they may be confused on superficial inspection. The parathyroid glands have a distinctive tan coloration, with a very delicate vascular network under the capsular surface. At least two glands should be identified. However, with practice it is possible to identify all four glands as a routine very swiftly.

Middle Ear Dissection

It could be argued that the proper way to examine the middle ear is to remove the temporal bone intact, decalcify it and section it in a large microtome, but few pathologists have the expertise or patience to accomplish this. However, alternatives such as cracking off the roof of the temporal bone with bone forceps or chisel are equally unsatisfactory, often destroying much of the detail. The following method is relatively quick, but does require practice to get the optimal alignment of the saw cuts.

The first task is to remove the dura mater over the petrous temporal bone with forceps and a scalpel (or as much as possible). A 'T' blade is put into the necropsy saw, and the first antero-posterior cut is made vertically 1 cm in from the squamous portion of the temporal bone, and passes into the external auditory meatus. This cut should be 2 cm deep. The second antero-posterior cut is 1 cm in from the edge of the sella turcica, again 2 cm deep. Cut three runs in between these two, parallel to and 1.5 cm anterior to the superior border of the petrous temporal bone.

The fourth cut is the most difficult. This should be made parallel to the edge of the petrous temporal bone, 3–4 mm below the superior border. It will require assistance to support the head and hold it forwards to effect this. It is important not to cut in too deeply, 3–4 mm at most. Then a bone chisel with a 'T' bar is inserted, and with a rocking motion the plate of bone between the cuts is levered off. It may need a few sharp taps with a hammer to loosen it. The bone plate usually comes off intact but occasionally loose fragments are left. However, the structure of the middle ear is clearly revealed, after bone dust is gently washed away. With practice, the procedure can be accomplished in 2–3 minutes.

Removal of Spinal Cord

Candidates are unlikely to be asked to remove the spinal cord unless there is a specific indication in the history, of if the necropsy is otherwise very simple (e.g. myocardial infarction with no other pathology present), to provide some more stringent assessment of the capability of the candidate. However it is not uncommon for the candidate to be asked to remove the cranial vault, since it is recognised that this task is frequently neglected by delegating it to the mortuary technician. The following method includes the removal of brain and spinal cord intact. The cord is best removed from the posterior aspect, as it is very hard to remove the anterior spinal bodies to gain access, although it is perhaps less time-consuming for the technical staff.

A longitudinal incision is made over the whole length of the spine, and the erector spinae reflected over the medial aspects of the ribs, so that the 'field' is clear. It is most important to scrape away the muscles over the vertebral arches so that a clean cut can be made with the saw. This may take 10 minutes to perform, but it is reasonable to ask the mortuary technician to assist.

Having done this, transverse processes are transected using a circular or T-shaped blade on the necropsy saw, angling the cut at about 30° to the vertical, 2.5 cm from the midline. It is best to start on the mid-thoracic vertebrae where the arches are thinnest. It is important not to penetrate too deeply or the cord may be damaged. If the penetration of the spinal canal cannot be felt (there should be a sudden 'give' when cutting the arch), the cut is either too lateral or the blade is held in too vertical a plane.

These cuts are continued either side, leaving a gap of at least 3 cm between the two. When completed the cervical vertebral region is transected between C2–3 or C3–4, severing the interspinous and posterior ligaments (but not the cord), the vertebral arches can be peeled back by holding them with large Spencer-wells forceps, progressively dividing ligaments with a scalpel.

If the saw cuts have been made at the correct angle, the dura mater will still be intact, but it requires some practice to get this exactly right.

The arches are removed down to the level of the sacrum. Then the dura mater is gripped in the lumbar region border with toothed forceps, gently elevated and nerve roots progressively divided near their exit from the canal with a sharp scalpel, up to the level of the cervical spine. Keep the dura on slight tension while doing this, and avoid any flexion or kinking.

If the brain has already been removed, the whole cord from the C1–2 level downwards should be excised from the canal still within the dura. If not, the spinal cord is usually transected at this level and removed separately. In particular cases, both are to be removed in continuity. To do this an incision needs to be made in the dura around the foramen magnum from inside the skull, to release the dura mater. The brain is mobilised in the conventional fashion, but it is still quite a difficult exercise to cut the dura around the foramen magnum with the brain in place, to enable the cord to be delivered via the foramen. This is quite time-consuming, and hence not really appropriate for examination purposes, but may be of value when there is suspected pathology in the medulla/upper cervical cord.

Removal of Femur

This procedure is not very complicated technically, but requires some thought to minimise the effort involved, and to avoid the possible hazards in deep dissection. One method is well illustrated by Gresham and Turner (Appendix 1).

A lateral longitudinal incision is recommended, from the iliac crest to below the knee. It is easiest to incise deeply and remove all the muscles and ligaments around the knee, cutting into the joint to mobilise the lower end of the femur. The femur is manipulated to allow muscles up to the hip joint to be dissected off. Assistance may be needed to hold the femur out laterally to gain access.

Having freed the muscle attachments lower down the bone enables it to be manipulated to remove the gluteal hamstring muscle insertions, and the joint capsule around the acetabulum is incised. If there is a fracture of the femoral neck, great care is required as the bone splinters are a considerable hazard.

After removal, the femur is immobilised with a clamp and longitudinally sectioned with a tenon saw, bisecting the head and neck. The cut surface is washed as bone dust obscures much of the detail.

Thoracic Duct

This structure is largely ignored by most pathologists but it is useful to be able to find it if required, perhaps for demonstration to medical students. Candidates have been asked to demonstrate it on occasion, particularly in malignant necropsies.

The duct is a thin-walled, pale cord which can be observed on the posterior aspect of the thoracic viscera, at its lower end (cisterna chyli) by the right side of the aorta and right crus of the diaphragm, ascending between the right side of the aorta and main azygous vein, where it lies adjacent to the left side of the aorta.

Vertebral Arteries

While it should be a matter of routine to inspect the origins of the vertebral arteries as they enter the cervical vertebral transverse process, and the intracranial segments proximal to the vertebrobasilar artery after removal of the brain, the intracervical segments of the vessels are more of a problem. It is certainly not an easy process to remove and inspect these but there may be a specific clinical indication to do so, and the candidate may be asked to perform it in an otherwise straightforward necropsy, or at least asked how it could be performed.

One elegant methodology is described in detail in the reference below and is very useful in that the cervical spine does not have to be removed. The instruments required are two particular types of scalpel and a pair of curved, wire-cutting scissors. It is unlikely that a candidate would be faulted for not being capable of performing this dissection but, as already pointed out, it is expected they would be able to point out the origin of the vessels.

Reference

Bromilow, A., Burns, J. J. Clin. Pathol. (1985) 38: 1400–1402.

Paediatric and Neonatal Necropsies

Although most of the technique of post mortem examination of foetuses, neonates and children is similar to that in adults, there are a few critical differences, which candidates are often unfamiliar with because they have had access to far fewer paediatric than adult necropsies. Examination candidates should appreciate that they may well be required to conduct such an examination. Failure to do so has resulted in several candidates being surprised when faced with such a task, with consequent very poor performances. The frequency with which candidates are required to undertake neonatal and paediatric necropsies may well rise in the future, as the numbers of suitable adult necropsies decline, which is often the case at many of the examination centres. Nor will the argument be accepted that the request to perform a neonatal/paediatric necropsy is unfair, as it is as much a function of a consultant pathologist as a routine adult case.

Each candidate should take the necessary steps to obtain experience in these examinations during the course of their training, and preferably not just before the practical examination. Specialist paediatric pathologists, or consultant pathologists with an interest in this field, could be approached with a view to arranging some supervision in these necropsies, which could be made on an informal basis or as a formal part of a training rotation, with the approval of the departmental chief. (The ACP might be able to arrange a secondment in certain cases).

The necropsy itself differs in many respects from the adult, and it is worthwhile reiterating the major alterations in emphasis and technique which may provide problems for trainees. Examiners usually recognise that examination candidates have particular difficulty in performing such necropsies, because for the majority an opportunity to perform them is restricted to some degree, and will thus make some allowances. This does not extend to awarding a pass standard for hopelessly incompetent performances, even with the advantage of a 'sympathy vote'.

In the external examination, it is extremely important to accurately weigh the body and make certain measurements, especially foot length, head circumference, crown-rump and crown-heel lengths. The last three are prone to inaccuracies, especially as a result of intrauterine death, where widening of the sutures and joint laxity may occur. Weights and measurements should be assessed against appropriate gestation or age-related normal values in tabular form, which should be available in the mortuary. (It is not expected that candidates should learn such values). It might be prudent to take copies of such tables to the examination centre, however, just in case.

Radiographic examination of the body should be suggested in all cases of suspected congenital abnormalities, sudden infant death syndrome, growth disorders or deformities, among others. Arrangements would probably have been made in advance by the mortuary technical staff to perform this in the hospital radiology department but a well-equipped mortuary usually has a self-contained x-ray unit such as a Faxitron for this purpose. Having requested radiographs, it would be as well to have some knowledge of bone development and appearance of the major ossification centres, and be aware of a reference source for more detailed appraisal.

If there are clinical reasons to suspect congenital abnormality or if dysmorphic features are apparent then medical photography should be requested. This again is something to be discussed with the supervisor or mortuary technician who will advise of the usual procedure in that department.

In addition to the pathological assessment of the body, the position and appearance of any drains, catheters or vascular lines should be noted, and preparation made for taking bacteriological samples from these during the dissection.

In neonates and infants an inverted Y incision is usually adopted to allow reflection of the bladder and umbilical vessels. In the older child a conventional Y incision is usually made. In cases from intensive treatment units or where ventilation has been given, testing for pneumothorax should be made. Use of a small manometer attached to a hypodermic needle may be useful in this assessment.

One of the major problems with the assessment of a paediatric post mortem is a familiarity with the relative size of organs, and this is difficult to assess from theoretical knowledge rather than practical experience. Tables are available of organ weights compared to the gestational age and should be consulted.

The conventional removal of organs is well described in the reference at the end of this section, but there are three main blocks: neck structures, thoracic and upper abdominal viscera, and intestines, urogenital tract and related vessels. The liver should always be removed in continuity with the thoracic viscera in cases of congenital heart disease. In intrauterine death, congenital heart disease is a major unsuspected discovery and this is therefore the recommended technique in this situation.

From a practical point of view, organs must be dissected resting on a sponge to maintain them in a static position, essential for accurate and safe sectioning. The detailed examination of organs is comprehensively described and illustrated in the given reference texts, and are generally modifications of the adult dissection.

Examination of the cranial contents is always a problem for the inexperienced. It is tempting to incise along suture lines once the scalp is reflected, but this destroys the venous sinuses and dural folds, structures which are much more important in neonatal and infant pathology than in adults. Bony 'flaps' should be made and folded back to expose the brain, but the latter's removal is often a problem to candidates because of its delicate, easily disrupted tissue. Assistance from the post mortem technician in supporting the brain is invaluable. Some authorities have advocated removing the foetal brain under water to provide this support, but this can be awkward and is a matter for personal preference.

Reference

1. Berry, C.L. Examination of the Foetus and Neonate. In: Paediatric Pathology, p1–39. Springer-Verlag, Berlin (1989).

Surgical Pathology Slides

These are the most important part of the examination and a poor performance in this section is unlikely to be retrieved by anything other than exceptional performances in the others, and usually not even then. Candidates are expected to demonstrate a sound and thorough approach to examining histological material. However, no one is expecting perfect answers to all of the slides, as this would be highly unusual in the examination situation. It is therefore very difficult to convey any consensus opinion on the standards required, so the following discussion attempts to provide some guidelines on the way to approach the answers, which may reflect the attitude of a competent histopathologist.

In most centres, candidates are asked to examine about 20 slides, ranging from 18 to 26. It is always better to use a familiar type of microscope, preferably the one used in routine daily work. It can be very difficult to adapt to one provided by the examination centre, and leaves a candidate at some disadvantage. If this is unavoidable, it would be reasonable to ask if the instrument could be made available to enable some familiarisation with it prior to the examination itself.

The examination is conducted in a quiet room, usually with one supervisor present. Candidates are instructed about the nature of the examination and in general terms what is required. A typewritten sheet with brief clinical histories relating to each of the slides is distributed.

The first thing to do is work out how many slides there are, and what is the average time allowed to answer each of them. This calculation is most important. With 20 slides, there are about 8.5 minutes for each one, allowing 10 minutes at the end of the period. It is absolutely vital to be aware of how long it takes to examine a section of the appropriate degree of difficulty, and write a report on it, during revision preparations. Misjudgement of the time available is one of the major reasons for candidates running into problems with this part of the examination. It is therefore of great importance to be very strict with the timekeeping. This really requires a small clock or watch, if possible with a timer (but not an alarm!), and sufficient self-discipline to adhere to the allocated time for each section. It is usually possible to return to some of the cases at the end of the period.

Recommended Approach to Examination of Sections

It is difficult to dictate to pathologists who are considering applying for the Final examination on how to examine a tissue section, which is after all the main skill which they have developed. However, it is surprising how often deficient technique is responsible for misinterpretation, as all pathologists have to admit (if they are honest). It is a useful exercise to ask senior colleagues to admit to misdiagnoses they have made, and describe the factors that led to these problems.

More than that, however, are the unconscious lapses in technique which the examination may well uncover. These are either a result of inadequate training and supervision, or a mistaken belief that a diagnosis is usually reached by examining sections under high power magnification.

Assessment of the Clinical Information

This was mentioned in the introduction but its importance cannot be over-emphasised. All of the information provided must be taken into account, as it is there for a purpose. Although exceptions can occur, it is unlikely that a section of something which is inconsistent with the usual age and sex incidence of a particular entity will be introduced, unless it is a very distinctive lesion. Conversely, great consideration should be given before suggesting a diagnosis which would be distinctly unusual in that setting (e.g. a liposarcoma in a 5 year old child, Gaucher's disease in a bone marrow biopsy of a 70 year old woman).

The site, size and duration of the lesion, plus any other clinical information, must be taken into account. The amount given in the examination is variable, but is usually no more than one or two sentences, or even just a few words. It is vital that each lesion is assessed in the light of this information and the answer directed accordingly. The differential diagnosis of any particular problem may also vary considerably, and candidates will be marked down if they are incapable of adapting to this in order to make a rational assessment. In cases where the clinical information is particularly scanty or vague, then it usually means either that the diagnosis would be very straightforward if the exact location is given, or that the lesion is difficult to define and only a differential diagnosis is required (with indications as to how to resolve the problem). The former situation is much more common.

The macroscopic description of a lesion may also be given. If so, there is usually a very good reason, probably that this may help in the differential diagnosis between two similar lesions.

On the other hand, having read and digested the clinical information, it is important not to form an opinion on a preconceived notion of the likely diagnosis prior to examining the slide, as then the risk of 'seeing what you wish to to see' occurs. Some people find it better to look at the section 'blind' to form an impression and then read the clinical information. Whatever the individual preference, it must be stressed that the clinical information is taken into account before forming a final opinion.

Naked Eye Examination

It is remarkable how often some experienced pathologists, as well as trainees, fail to look at the slide with the naked eye or even low magnification, merely examining it under medium to high power to make the diagnosis. While this may be effective with a number of cases, dangers lie in missing focal lesions or architectural clues.

The recommended approach is to examine sections against a sheet of blank white paper in a good light. Holding it up to the window is not really adequate as features may be obscured. (An old x-ray viewing box or transparency viewing box is ideal but not really practicable for examination purposes.)

The first thing to assess is the distribution of the material on the section. (Candidates in the habit of circumscribing the limits of the area to be examined with a felt pen, should ensure that a washable one is used and the slide wiped clean afterwards.) A mental note of the number of tissue fragments is made to ensure all of them are examined under the microscope. It is a favourite manoeuvre of examiners to include cases where only one of a number of biopsy fragments includes the diagnostic features.

Secondly, the architecture of the section is assessed. It is important to try to identify any normal tissue landmarks, especially at the margins. If there is an obvious lesion present, the circumscription or otherwise is noted, together with variations in staining, and any patterns which may be visible. A magnifying glass or loupe may help reveal these features. There may be a single focus or multifocal lesions. A wealth of information can be gleaned from examining sections in this way, and its real value can only be appreciated by constantly examining sections. Sadly this appears to be neglected by many trainees (who have possibly followed the example set by senior colleagues) and is responsible for many errors.

The section should then be examined under the microscope in the usual fashion, but again the low magnifications often reveal more information. Good diagnostic pathologists will make great use of all of the magnification powers available. Oil immersion is often valuable for looking at subcellular features which are difficult to resolve with the higher power lenses. Confirming or excluding the presence of cross-striations in primitive sarcomas is one example. However, it can be somewhat time-consuming to do this and should only be used in selected cases.

As with naked eye examination, discipline is required to inspect all of the material with a low power magnification, which following practice becomes a habit with good histopathologists. Inexperienced ones often wish to use the high power lens at first sight of a potentially diagnostic field, and this is sometimes the reason for misinterpretation.

Writing the Report

It might seem obvious, but the main function of the report is to convey a diagnosis or interpretation to the examiners in the shortest and most unequivocal manner possible. About a paragraph of writing is adequate for most of the cases, using concise descriptive language as for a report to be issued to a clinician. The format will vary from case to case and according to personal preference, but it is often a good idea to write a few words or one sentence giving the major diagnosis (or diagnoses) at the beginning, followed by a few lines to a paragraph describing the major features, other conditions considered in the differential diagnosis (and the evidence against them), and a sentence outlining which special stains or other procedures (e.g. electron microscopy) might be performed to support the diagnosis. An alternative format is to place the diagnosis at the end. The most important point is not to 'lose' the main diagnosis in amongst the description, as examiners recognise this is an important cause of misunderstanding in the interpretation of reports.

Another general point is that ambiguity must be avoided at all times. In some of the cases, there may well be uncertainty about the diagnosis, in which event a clear differential diagnosis should be stated, followed by an outline of the procedures necessary to resolve this problem. There is a great temptation to word the report in order to disguise the inability to reach a definitive diagnosis, the most crass examples being to avoid stating whether a particular tumour is benign or malignant and leaving it as a 'neoplasm' hoping this will be a good 'each way' bet. There are numerous other examples which all candidates will be only too aware of, as of course are the examiners.

Types of Cases Used in the Examination

It is not unusual for senior colleagues and contemporaries to declare that a particular section or case is of 'MRC Path standard'. Usually this means that it is particularly hard and that they have reached a diagnosis after much deliberation and consultation of the literature! In reality such cases actually form a minority in the examination, and are more likely to be a device for keeping an up and coming trainee in their place. Most centres aim to achieve a balance of material from reasonably straightforward to impossible, and naturally this is highly variable. In general terms, about half of the cases could well be encountered fairly often during routine practice and have a fairly distinctive histological appearance (examples are given at the end of this section). It is very reassuring to identify these cases, but the relative proportions do vary widely among centres (so it is not a cause for undue concern if an individual finds relatively few in their particular examination!) Candidates would be expected to identify most or all of these, giving a reasonable description and a confident diagnosis, or a limited differential diagnosis. As far as can be ascertained, no centres have 'automatic fail' slides, but any candidate making more than one or perhaps two serious errors in this lower category will be marked down very heavily, (unless some mitigation of the mistake can be made in the *viva voce* – see later).

Around one third or more will be more difficult problems. These fall into several groups (anecdotal examples given for illustrative purposes).

1) Good examples of rare diseases e.g. epithelioid sarcoma

2) A reasonably common lesion in an unusual location e.g. non Hodgkin's lymphoma in the uterus

3) Rare entities which may simulate commoner diseases e.g. progressive multifocal leucoencephalopathy resembling astrocytoma

4) Common diseases with an uncommon or potentially misleading histological appearance e.g. lymphadenitis due to EB virus, healing fracture simulating osteosarcoma

5) Subtle changes in tissues (the history is often a major help in such cases) e.g. amyloidosis in the gut or heart

6) Sections containing a small area having the diagnostic features, which gives some idea of the ability of a candidate to comprehensively examine sections e.g. focus of CLIS in otherwise benign breast disease

7) Dual pathology. Either two related entities e.g. villous atrophy with small intestinal lymphoma, hepatocellular carcinoma in cirrhosis, or two unrelated diseases which are identifiable in a single tissue section (often a local lesion and a systemic disease) e.g. adrenal myelolipoma with metastatic carcinoma in residual adrenal parenchyma.

Many candidates worry unduly about the incidence of groups 5) and 6) in examinations, suspecting every slide may hold a potential trap. While it may be a useful discipline to make a check for other pathology in every section, it is most important not to become too obsessed with this. If the right approach to examining sections has been adopted, the main diagnosis will usually be identified. In the case of 'coincidental' dual pathology, both conditions should be readily identifiable in a properly examined section; candidates would not be expected to make a 'spectacular' diagnosis if there were only a small group of cells at the periphery of the tissue for example.

Some of the sections, usually (but not always) less than a quarter, will be particularly difficult. There are several aims to putting such examples into an examination. It is not always expected that a definitive diagnosis should be made but rather that a reasonable differential can be proffered. The examiners take note of a candidate's method of approaching such problems and follow the method of reasoning. If they can see that the assessment is sound, and suggested further investigations would probably lead to a correct diagnosis, then this is all that is expected. These cases should not cause too much despair if they cannot be sorted out immediately. It is far better to move to the next case and return at a later stage, when the problem may even have resolved itself by subconscious processes! The problems seem to arise when candidates panic, and write disjointed, ill-thought-out answers which either suggest rare, unlikely diagnoses (which if they bear no resemblance to the lesion in question, further compound the error) or, worse, come to a certain diagnosis because the candidate thinks it is an appropriate lesion to be in an examination and interprets the appearances in order to make them fit this diagnosis. This is one of the major pitfalls of any diagnostic histopathologist and is a habit into which any pathologist must gain some insight. This is considered further in the next section.

Preparation for the Surgical Histopathology

General Principles

Candidates have different ideas on how to prepare, but there appears to be a prevalent belief that wading through masses of sections from various sources in the few weeks leading up to the examination will somehow enhance their diagnostic ability, resulting from the rather restricted attitude that to have seen a certain entity will ensure its future recognition. It is unlikely to yield significant improvements in proportion to the effort expended. It is necessary to adopt other tactics to enable the information to be usefully retained, otherwise it is merely an exercise in 'wallpaper matching'. The following sections suggest methods of improving the retention of information during revision exercises, and for enhancing *interpretation* as opposed to merely *recognition*.

Instead of examining random collections of slides, examples should be arranged in systematically organised groups. The advantage of this is that comparisons can be made between different pathological changes within the same tissue, which are a potential source of confusion. It is a great deal easier to identify the more subtle differences when concentrating on a particular tissue, and can recall the appearances of other conditions which have been examined in conjunction. When many slides are examined on a random basis, it is far more difficult to retain the mental 'image' of the section when it is a condition with which you are not familiar.

One reason for this phenomenon may be the selective nature of recall necessary to make a differential diagnosis, where the major differences are the crucial elements, while insignificant or common features require less active interpretation. When other completely different sections are interposed between two conditions which may be confused, it is more difficult to get a perspective on the most and least important differences between them. Collaborative exercises involving active interpretation rather than passive recognition are the key to committing the information to long-term memory.

It is always advisable to further reinforce the effective yield from any revision session by writing a report as for the examination, and it will help to organise the interpretation of the condition. It is a mistake to make a particular diagnosis and assume that the report will be easy to write. If a conscious effort is made to justify the reasons for reaching a particular conclusion in descriptive terms, and how it may be confirmed further, the interpretative element of the answer will not be lost. Recognition alone is not sufficient. The ability to compile reports in concise, accurate and relevant detail is a skill to be acquired as much as examining the section, and unfortunately requires constant practice. (It is probably unnecessary to write longhand reports in the later stages of revision; note-form will suffice and will actual highlight the key words in each sentence of a report, and indicate the overall structure.)

It should be obvious that maximum benefit would be gained by examining sections with the help of clinical information only, prior to being given or looking up the correct diagnosis, otherwise opinion will be biased and will not accurately reflect the level of ability. It may be necessary to take steps to remove the diagnoses from vision or preferably from easy reach during the session. After or during each microscopic session, it is absolutely essential to read up on the conditions examined, using either comprehensive textbooks (e.g. *Ackerman's Surgical Pathology*) or specialist books. This is another reason for examining one system at a time, to avoid searching for different subjects in a multitude of books at each session, which is time-consuming and generally discouraging.

The relevant section of each text can be quickly scanned in cases where the diagnosis is certain, and the key words in the report serve as a guide. Those items found to be incorrect or were omitted from the written report can be revised, which is a very efficient way of revealing deficiencies and for remember-ing them. If the reports are used as a basis for a revision session following the microscopy, perhaps later in the evening, it may also provide an opportunity to read up on related subjects.

It is perhaps even more vital to write reports for sections where the diagnosis is not straightforward and only a differential diagnosis can be made, or where further investigations are required. These are the sorts of cases which provide practical difficulties in the examination, and are most revealing about a candidate's ability to deal with a particular problem. Writing down the interpretation of a slide as a report during revision can reveal whether incorrect emphasis is given or assumptions made when the subject is reviewed with the aid of a textbook. It is important to be honest about one's own capacity and the only way to do this is to have it written down. Otherwise a degree of self-deception will inevitably be acquired, as no one likes to admit they are wrong!

If there are a large number of slides to be examined which are relatively straightforward, or the time of the examination is very near, then in order to save time it might be helpful to mentally compose a report rather than note it down. However, it is most important to know exactly what would be written word for word as a report. If circumstances permit, it may be an advantage to dictate the report aloud. The danger lies in reverting to only having a vague idea about what to say, and it would still be better to avoid this as far as possible.

Adopting a different theme every few days will help to maintain interest in the material, which is most important to gain maximum benefit. On the other hand, there can be too much of a good thing, as attempts to examine large numbers of cases only result in a superficial coverage of each subject. This is often the case with senior colleagues' personal slide collections, compiled from randomly selected 'interesting cases'. While these certainly have a role to play (see later), they are often the staple diet of the examination 'crammer' and one which is often too rich for examination purposes. Very often, these are not filed on a systematic basis, and it would be inadvisable to disrupt the order unless the owner is in full agreement. However, it is an idea to work through the key to select out cases pertaining to the system currently under review. If such collections are the only or major source of revision material, it is most important to take this extra effort. While it may be initially discouraging to learn from boastful colleagues that they have examined in excess of 100 slides in a day, it is important to remain confident that a more circumspect inspection of even a quarter or less of that total coupled with a written report and brief reading will be far more productive in the long run, with more detailed information being retained and understood, whereas it would have largely evaporated from the mind of the former. If confidence in the approach is still lacking, it is suggested that some simple trials are conducted (well in advance of the examination) to test this hypothesis!

As already explained, personal collections can form the bulk of many candidates' revision, but the following sections deal with the use of alternative sources of material which could form the basis of a more structured and comprehensive approach. Of these, there is no doubt that routine surgical reporting is the best method of achieving proficiency, and every effort should be made to gain experience at this, even at the expense of formal revision sessions.

Material Sources and their Utilisation for Surgical Pathology Revision

The key to a good revision programme is to arrange the material source in an organised fashion, at least in the early stages, which involves some effort and not a little ingenuity at times. We suggest that the following sources be tapped.

Routine Surgical Files

All hospitals have interesting and unusual pathological material in the files, but there can be a problem in extracting it. The best way is to plan in advance, making notes on selected cases or keeping a special file. Unfortunately, trainees are often not in one department for long enough to establish anything substantial in the way of numbers. There may be a departmental filing system in operation for such cases.

Running through coded files to identify potentially interesting cases is often unsatisfactory and disheartening. This is because the material is often of poor quality, perhaps a small biopsy or not a typical example. Also, there may be many sections to examine, which is time consuming. The sections may be misfiled or frequently 'missing', a not uncommon experience with interesting cases. The expenditure of effort is therefore quite large for a relatively small return, and the place for examination of routine files is considered more in conjunction with routine surgical reporting.

Post Mortem Files

Surprisingly, these often yield substantial amounts of pathology, which while not strictly surgical pathology, may well be useful material to review. It is relatively easy to leaf through post mortem reports, and select some which might yield material. The advantage of post mortem sections are that they are often large and relatively well orientated, although the preservation may not be optimal. Post mortem files are more likely to be intact, and are useful because it enables material to be extracted and grouped into systems. This is inadvisable with routine surgical files because material may be removed which has some relevance to the current specimens.

Teaching Collections

Some departments have teaching collections specifically compiled for trainees. However, the quality can be variable and the material may not have been updated for some years.

Course Material

Slides given out during a teaching course or symposium are an invaluable source of revision material, as they are usually accompanied by an explanatory text. It is often unclear which courses will provide sections to take away, but it is useful to make enquiries of the organisers, or better still speak to previous applicants. Courses designed specifically to meet the needs of trainees, covering a wide range of subjects, are the most useful in this respect (see Appendix 2), as well as other courses organised in some of the major teaching centres, in Britain, Australia, USA or elsewhere.

Symposia or courses on more specialised fields of pathology are also organised regularly, and may well provide a slide set, sometimes for an additional fee. It is usually worth investing in one, and if finance is a problem it may be possible to purchase a set with departmental funds to include as part of the teaching collection, or the cost spread amongst several colleagues.

There are more compelling reasons for attending the courses other than the acquisition of a teaching set however, which should not be a primary reasons for deciding whether or not to attend. After all, the most important factor is to have the opportunity to examine the material and be involved in a discussion and review, so that the appearances would be sufficiently explained to enable a recognition of the entity again, even in a slightly different form. Again, the best way of doing this is to look at the sections with the clinical data, write a report, and then see how the answer tallies with the correct diagnosis.

It is important to decide at what stage to attend such courses. All regional teaching sessions should be attended throughout training. Comprehensive courses are best attended around two years prior to the examination, so that there is time to absorb and read around the course material, and perhaps identify any areas of particular weakness that the course may uncover. In this event, arrangements can be made to attend some more specialised teaching sessions or symposia to redress this.

Some trainees prefer to attend some of the advanced histopathology sessions just prior to the practical examination. While this may provide some advantage in that the entities examined will be fresher in the memory, there may be little time to correct any deficiencies. It may be better to go to such courses six or seven months prior to the examination for this reason. On the other hand, certain individuals find that they are better motivated close to the examination.

It is important to take full advantage of these courses, in particular to discuss various problems with the supervisors. Many trainees appear inhibited, a problem which appears to increase the nearer the examination is. However, course students who fully participate in discussion during microscopy revisions and reviews undoubtedly gain a great deal more, and it is important to make a determined effort to ask questions, in order to gain maximum benefit.

While it is advisable to attend as many courses as possible in the year before the examination, it is also just as important to be selective. Some courses may be too narrow, being concerned with a subject more suited to post-MRCPath specialisation, and it is best to take advice from your Head of Department or even the course organisers to find out if you would benefit merely in terms of examination revision. Further comments on this aspect are made in Appendix 2.

Personal Slide Collections

All pathologists should compile a personal slide collection, as this will be useful in future teaching of junior colleagues, presentations and in revision, where they are able to pool resources with others in a similar position (see later). One of the major failings of many pathologists is to forget to catalogue the slides with an adequate clinical history. It is virtually impossible to do this just before the slides are needed, if they are in a large disorganised pile when the relevant information has been forgotten or is incomplete. Therefore each slide should be filed, preferably in a purpose-made slide box, as soon as it is obtained. Over the course of a few years several hundred examples will accumulate, and will be an invaluable collection if properly documented. (One way of keeping the history and diagnosis intact is to write it on the back of the slide with a permanent fibre pen marker.)

Slide Clubs

It is most important for every pathologist to join a slide club. This may be difficult as a junior registrar because the post may be relatively transient, but is easier at a senior registrar level. The purpose is to exchange slides of interesting cases and have regular meetings to present and discuss the diagnoses. If properly organised, it can be a great source of material, but there are many other advantages to such a club. As well as the academic exchange, insight will be gained into the problems colleagues are facing, as well as information about courses and teaching opportunities.

In order to investigate this possibility, colleagues should be contacted at various hospitals to enquire if they are members of a slide club, whether it is possible to join. Otherwise it is necessary to initiate a group *de novo*. Optimal numbers vary, but 10–12 contributors are probably about right, from different hospitals to maximise the input of material. The benefits of a slide club far outweigh the effort expended in organising and maintaining it.

Having obtained material from a personal slide collection, including that of the slide club, it is useful not only for revision, but in order to pool resources with other colleagues taking the examination, in the later stages of revision. The cases can be used for practice examinations, and reciprocation made with personal material. In order to do this, it is necessary to simulate examination conditions, being in a quiet room, and remaining undisturbed for three hours – this can be difficult to arrange but is most essential.

These exercises should be commenced three or four months prior to the examination, increasing the frequency to one or two per week in the final month. The number that can be performed is limited by the availability of material and this in turn is dependent on the number of colleagues it is possible to exchange slides with. This is why slide club contacts and organising revision with colleagues is so important, maximising the exposure to this kind of revision. Even a few such tests are of great value for organising timing and fluency of the report writing.

As well as contemporaries, senior colleagues may be willing to set mock examinations. They may be more keen to do this than lend their valuable slide collections, since they are only on loan during the test session, and are hence less likely to be lost or damaged. Moreover, they would have a better idea of the examination standards required, and are able to criticise the technique of answering.

These sessions are very important, as it is all too easy to wade through a great number of slides during private revision, but be deceived into believing that this could be repeated under examination conditions.

Current Literature

Although it is not usually possible to have the opportunity of examining directly sections of recently described entities, (unless encountered at certain symposia) it is useful to keep a continued awareness of recent advances by reviewing the major pathology journals up to the examination. Again, it is important to be selective, and read only about lesions which appear to be of recurrent interest and argument, or concern major or common lesions, or which attract editorials and comments. Only a small proportion of published material is liable to achieve any substantial or lasting influence. However, it is not unusual for 'topical' pathology to appear in the examination, and while candidates would be unlikely to fail for not being aware of it, an opportunity to impress may be lost.

Much of the current literature is concerned with the application of monoclonal antibody technology in restricted fields of pathology, and while this is an exciting area of research, it is vitally important not to draw too many conclusions relating to their application in diagnostic pathology. There are innumerable instances where an initially promising reagent has not proved to be of truly restricted specificity which enables any reliance to be placed on the results. The range of antibodies used for diagnostic purposes is relatively small and has been verified in several laboratories over a period of time. The pathologist who displays a rather naive over-enthusiasm to utilise the newly described antibodies might give the impression that such results may heavily influence the diagnostic criteria for a particular lesion, without taking proper account of the morphological details. Therefore while it is all very well to be aware of the latest reports, the assessment should be tempered with the appropriate degree of scepticism, especially in the presence of more experienced and conservative examiners. Review articles by respected pathologists experienced in the field of immunohistochemical techniques in diagnostic surgical pathology are a better source of information, and often give much more insight into the limitations.

Routine Surgical Reporting

This is by far the best method of improving technique, and it is a great advantage to arrange a work rota which will include at least two months' reporting in the six months prior to the examination. This may be difficult in a heavily staffed University Department, but it may be possible to arrange a locum position in a district general hospital with other senior registrars or consultants, if possible in a department previously attended to avoid the need to become familiar with the environment.

Since the examination aims to assess whether candidates are competent to undertake the responsibilities of a consultant pathologist, routine experience is very valuable and helps to develop the attitudes and qualities which the examiners are looking for, whether the candidate is aware of them or not. It may be a mistake to avoid routine duties as much as possible to concentrate on other forms of revision, especially as it may not be viewed too favourably by one's peers.

In addition to undertaking or assisting with reporting, at other times attempts should be made to review interesting cases which have passed through the Department each day. To do this effectively requires the cooperation of the reporting team who may be able to select cases. Each case should be evaluated with the clinical information only, and appropriate further investigations chosen. If possible these cases should be followed up (with the permission of the reporting team), including the results of various special stains where indicated.

Specialised Pathology

If any particular areas of weakness can be identified in terms of specialised material not available during training, attempts to remedy this by arranging to visit pathology departments within the region or as secondments may help. In some cases, such as neuropathology, this may be the sole concern of a particular unit, in which case the concentrated experience would be invaluable.

Particular needs should be discussed with the head of the department, who may be able to arrange this or else personally contact the consultant in charge of the particular unit.

While it would be unduly optimistic to expect individual attention, there may be teaching sets available; many specialist pathologists welcome the opportunity to teach using routine material. However, arrangements should not be left too late, so that it does not become an attempt to 'cram' all the information into a couple of days, without displaying any real enthusiasm for the subject. This is not only discourteous, but is often a waste of effort.

Cytology

Cytopathology is assuming greater importance in diagnostic pathology and this is being reflected in the emphasis given to proficiency in this discipline in the examination. Part of the reason is the increasing number of specimens from fine needle aspiration as advances in guided needle biopsy techniques enable access to virtually all sites in the body, resulting in a very varied workload. As confidence in the technique among clinicians rises, it may, in some instances, supplant the need for surgical biopsy. Other reasons are that cytological preparations are also obtained in increasing numbers to complement endoscopic biopsies (e.g. in the respiratory and alimentary tracts), and are now routine practice in most centres.

Although diagnosis is still largely morphological, certainly in gynaecological cytology, conventional histochemical and immunocytochemical methods can be applied to cytological preparation to refine the diagnosis, and in many cases prompt and optimal fixation techniques may allow a greater flexibility than with surgical biopsy.

Thus the number and variety of cytological cases included in the examination have increased markedly in the last decade, and greater importance is laid on the ability to interpret cytological preparation than has hitherto been the case.

Most centres now allocate a separate session for cytology in the examination timetable, lasting anything from 30–90 minutes, though the recommended duration is one and a half hours. There is a minimum of six cases, and candidates may be asked to examine up to 10 or 12, about a third to a half of which are usually gynaecological.

This means that the time spent on each slide could be from 5–7 minutes, to include a standard (fortunately brief!) report, but which is still less time than a professional screener would take to review a case. Examiners appreciate this, and almost invariably the cases are selected as 'classical' examples, or perhaps have a focal but very obvious abnormality designed to assess the screening ability of a candidate.

General Principles in Examination Preparation

Even more than in surgical pathology, 'hands on' experience in cytology is the only route to proficiency. Expert guidance from a consultant cytologist(s) is essential in assessing progress, and of far more value than any textbook. While several excellent monographs and atlases are available, it is probable that photographs are less useful than in surgical pathology, perhaps because it is impossible to reflect the more subtle features of particular cells in a single field, without relating them to the whole content of the preparation, something which can only be achieved by direct examination.

'Wallpaper matching' can be a risky business in cytology, and one of the most important principles is to identify the normal population(s) of cells in any cytological preparation before starting to look for abnormalities. Not only will this give you some idea of the size of normal cells, the scale of which can be easily forgotten when examining abnormal cells only, but will provide a subconscious wealth of experience with which to compare an abnormal cell population.

Teaching collections have a role in the recognition of straightforward entities, but many trainees find it difficult to develop the skill necessary to interpret less well defined conditions such as severe inflammatory change versus dyskaryosis in a cervical smear. The sound knowledge of normal cell populations and their variations, and modifications in disease states, can only really be acquired by examination of routine material. The clinical relevance of current cases, which have to be correctly examined, may provide the motivation which is absent in archive material, and which otherwise could not sustain an interest for very long.

One other practical point is that some laboratories prefer air-dried to alcohol-fixed preparations, and some centres may provide only one or the other in the examination. Most laboratories prepare both types, and it is important to gain experience using each of them as they are to some extent complementary.

At least two months of full-time cytological training is necessary in order to reach a reasonable standard for the average candidate, but to be capable of providing a good clinical service, this period would be considerably longer. Early in their training many pathologists appear reluctant to become involved in cytology, and posts still exist which do not involve cytology rotation. It is important to gain this experience, so if this is the case representations should be made to the Departmental Head to obtain an attachment to a busy laboratory. Moreover the sponsor for the examination must also certify an applicant has completed three months training in cytology as a condition of sitting the Examination.

In order to maintain a level of competence in cytology, it would be an idea to examine about ten mixed cases a week, which should not be too time-consuming. It may be of value to examine them without a preliminary opinion, and it would be ideal if the consultant cytologist could be persuaded to select some cases, and review written reports with the aid of a discussion microscope, demonstrating any mistakes. It is most important not to imagine that it is possible to retain a static level of ability in cytology without practice, as it is perhaps easier to lose perspective in this discipline than in any other in pathology.

In addition, the biopsy specimens which are taken concurrently or subsequently following the cytological report should be followed up, with actual examination of the histology rather than just reading the report. Not only does this act as a quality control but it enables an appreciation of the differences in cell morphology by these different techniques.

Having stated that texts in cytology are of limited value, nevertheless it is important to have access to some books to reinforce the interpretation of certain conditions. *Diagnostic Cytology* (Koss, L.) is a large, two volume book, which although admirably comprehensive, is virtually impossible to digest prior to the examination. It is of great use as a 'bench book' for reference to certain diagnostic problems. There are copious illustrations, and it is useful just to examine these rather than read the full text, which is an undemanding exercise which can be accomplished relatively swiftly, helping to fill in some gaps in experience. Similarly some cytology atlases (Cardozo, L) are useful (although the one quoted only contains air-dried preparation). Review articles on fine needle aspiration biopsy abound, but the following is suggested as initial reading (Lever, J., Melcher, D.H., Lineham, J.J., Smith, R.S. Fine Needle Aspiration Cytology. In: Recent Advances in Histopathology 11. P.P. Anthony and R.N.M. MacSween (eds.) Churchill Livingstone, Edinburgh 1981).

Approach to Cytology Specimens

In the examination, each case will have appended a brief clinical history, which should be read carefully. Each interpretation must be placed in its clinical context, as in the surgical histopathology. Even with information as brief as 'cervical smear', the age of the patient must be taken into account. For example, in a 70 year old female it is unlikely to be an example of mild dyskaryosis. Similarly, if other information is given in a case, such as 'vaginal discharge', it is almost certain there is something present to account for this, but of course there may be a combined pathology, (e.g. dyskaryosis plus infection). In non-gynaecological specimens the histories are often more relevant. For instance, a cellular breast aspirate from a 65 year old is highly unlikely to be from a fibroadenoma.

Although not as important as in surgical pathology, the slide should be looked at with the naked eye, before placing it under the microscope, to assess the distribution of material, which may indicate the most rewarding areas. The number of the slide should be double-checked at this stage.

In cytological practice, most of the slides have been pre-screened, but candidates are expected to have developed sufficient skills to identify abnormalities themselves, and so no preliminary opinion is provided in the examination. Any dots that may remain on the slides may have been put there by a previous candidate or screener and are potentially misleading, so while these should of course be examined, it is not to be assumed that these indicate the major abnormality on the slide. Furthermore, it is all too easy to become reliant upon having a screening opinion in routine cytological practice. During preparation, it is important to continually practise reaching an independent opinion rather than being directed to abnormalities by a screener. This is the basis of good screening technique, which might not be developed otherwise, and it is worthwhile to consider this separately.

Screening Technique

This skill seems to receive insufficient attention in many centres so that candidates often appear undisciplined in screening, randomly scanning the slide. It is a major factor in poor cytological acumen.

The x10 objective should be used since the magnification given by x4 is not sufficient for recognising most abnormalities. (It is often a good idea to remove the x4 objective from the microscope during training for cytology!) The slide is placed on the stage and moved to one corner, and the examination proceeds in a vertical or horizontal direction in order to scan all the area under the coverslip. To obtain a 'feel' for the movement required from one scanning line to the next, the stage should be moved so that a cell at the right or left of the field crosses to the opposite side. With a x10 objective, this distance is about 2 mm.

If this is difficult, it is a useful exercise to take a plain glass slide and make a careful grid with several horizontal or vertical lines one x10 field apart, using a ruler and fine permanent fibre tip marker pen. This can be used to follow the edges of the lines to gain some idea of the necessary discipline and fine control of the microscope. Later a grid could be superimposed on an old or duplicate cytology slide to give some perspective to cell size and distribution. This exercise needs repeating at regular intervals until an ability to scan accurately develops and becomes 'second nature'. A random, undisciplined scanning pattern is the cause of many errors in cytological interpretation.

Cytological Reports

These are usually brief and do not require much descriptive detail. It is usually best to start with a firm, unequivocal diagnostic assessment in notation style if necessary. Some qualification is usually given to refine any diagnosis and put it in a clinically useful form, as for example in an ascitic fluid specimen in suspected ovarian carcinoma 'Malignant cells present consistent with an origin in an ovarian adenocarcinoma'. No further descriptive detail is required. In gynaecological smears, it should be stated whether malignant cells are present or not. If dyskaryosis is seen, an assessment should be made of the grade of CIN in which the cells may have originated e.g. 'Dyskaryotic cells present consistent with an origin in CIN II. Colposcopy and biopsy advised'. The significance and further management of the case are also unequivocally stated. All reports are based on similar principles. Even when the diagnosis is not established, there should be a clear statement of the abnormalities present and of the steps which would be necessary to identify the underlying pathology. In such cases, it might be reasonable to compile a report such as in a surgical case: 'A few glandular cells present showing nuclear enlargement and atypia in an inflammatory smear. Endocervical biopsy advised'. Equivocation should be restricted as far as possible to the few cases where it is genuinely not possible to make a diagnosis. Using such devices to avoid coming to a conclusion in most instances will certainly detract from a candidate's overall assessment, in cases where a firm diagnosis could reasonably have been expected. Again, it comes down to experience, and it is probably more difficult to recognise the cases which require caution to be exercised than others which permit an unequivocal opinion.

If there are no identifiable malignant cells, this must be stated in the first sentence, and then an outline given of whatever other diagnosis is made in concise terms, e.g. 'No malignant cells seen. An inflammatory smear pattern with a trichomonas infection. Repeat after treatment'.

Non-gynaecological specimens may occasionally require slightly more in the way of description, but in general little more than two or three sentences are required. The sequence should run 1) abnormality, 2) origin and 3) underlying pathology.

Standards in Cytology

A list of the conditions which most often appear in the examination, with which candidates would be expected to be familiar, is given at the end of this chapter, but it is worthwhile making explanatory comments on some of these, acknowledging that it is not attempting to be a comprehensive account.

The choice of examination material is somewhat restricted compared to everyday practice as the cells need to be well preserved and present in such a form or sufficient numbers to enable unequivocal interpretation. Furthermore, it is highly unlikely a 'normal' specimen would be included in the examination. If this is the assessment it is almost certainly mistaken and it is best to review the case at the end rather than attempt to guess. Further ideas may come to mind while concentrating on the other cases. If a case is left then it is important to ensure enough time is left to try again.

Of the gynaecological specimens, it is usual to be given at least one or two cervical smears, including examples of dyskaryosis which should be graded. Adenocarcinomas of endocervical or endometrial origin crop up relatively often but are suprisingly easy to overlook sometimes. In this respect candidates should ensure they are fully familiar with the range of appearances in post-natal and atrophic smears which can look very alarming to the inexperienced, due to the immaturity of their cell populations, with relatively large nuclei.

Infections may be easily overlooked, especially *Trichonomas* and *Candida*. Active herpetic infection is fairly characteristic but again may be mistaken for dyskaryotic cells. Endometrial brush specimens are sometimes taken for assessment of carcinoma, but in general the same criteria for adenocarcinoma apply here as elsewhere, except that squamoid cells are common features as seen in histological sections. Ovarian cyst fluids are usually very straightforward, but it is important to be familiar with granulosa cells from a follicular cyst, which can look quite alarming, sometimes with mitotic figures.

Non-gynaecological cases are very varied. Sputum examination is included in most examinations since it comprises such a large proportion of routine workload. Candidates are expected to be able to distinguish between keratinising and non-keratinising squamous cell carcinoma, adenocarcinoma, large cell undifferentiated carcinoma and small cell carcinoma. The latter can be particularly difficult to identify and requires some degree of expertise. Some clusters of reactive bronchial epithelial cells can show a worrying appearance, but one of the best guides is to see if any particular cluster contains ciliated cells at the periphery. If these are present, they should never be called malignant!

Benign conditions in sputum are relatively limited but it is useful to identify asbestos fibres which can be surprisingly variable in morphology, and be aware of the appearance of various fungal organisms such as aspergillus.

Endoscopic brushings from the upper gastrointestinal tract are generally taken to distinguish between benign and malignant ulcerative lesions. Squamous carcinoma of the oesophagus is relatively straightforward but reactive changes in glandular cells can produce considerable pleomorphism. In malignant ulcers, there is often a large number of fungal organisms, whose presence should prompt a thorough search for malignant cells.

Fine needle aspirates can be from many sources as already pointed out. A lot of the interpretation is purely common sense, applying principles which anyone with a good working knowledge of surgical histopathology would easily understand. The breast is an important site in which to have a very sound working knowledge, and misdiagnosis of these aspirates would be viewed with concern. Within the benign breast diseases, it is most important to recognise fibroadenoma with its cellular clusters and 'naked' nuclei, apocrine cells which are pleomorphic with a large nucleolus, reactive breast epithelial changes in duct ectasia, and lactational changes in which the cells are very active-looking and vacuolated. Malignant cells are often accompanied by cell debris and are often easier to assess under oil immersion. Not all carcinomas are ductal in type but unless the features are particularly striking candidates would probably not be expected to subtype any breast carcinoma.

Other sites of fine needle aspiration are many and varied and general principles are applied in diagnosis in most sites. However, the thyroid gland is a particularly common and favoured site, mainly because of the superficial location and the relative difficulty of obtaining a diagnostic surgical biopsy, so it is as well to have a working knowledge of the appearances. Hashimoto's thyroiditis is an important benign condition favoured in examinations because it can be easily confused with malignancy.

Serous fluid specimens are also frequently set. The distinction between reactive mesothelial cells and malignancy is an everyday problem in cytological practice and one which examination candidates are expected to resolve. Malignant mesothelioma can be a difficult diagnosis to make but, as a general rule, if there is difficulty in making a decision in the examination situation (as opposed to real life), then it is best to err on the conservative side. One point worth making is that not all laboratories cytospin their fluids because there can be loss of cytological detail, cell crowding and some nuclear aberrations due to this technique. Therefore it is worthwhile to become familiar with these changes, so if the local laboratory does not do it as a routine, they could be requested to perform it in surplus fluid specimens.

Urinary cytology can be a minefield for the inexperienced as reactive changes in urothelial cells can closely mimic malignancy. Post instrumentation, in urinary tract infection or calculus disease, and even odd cells from the seminal vesicle or prostate can lead to a potential misdiagnosis of malignancy. Transitional cell carcinoma is generally obvious when poorly differentiated, but the diagnosis of grade I transitional cell carcinoma is really for the experts. One benign condition, but which is sufficiently distinctive to be included in the more difficult slides for the examination, is polyomavirus infection in the immunosuppressed.

Cerebrospinal fluid specimens are generally for the diagnosis of a primary brain tumour invading the meninges (e.g. medulloblastoma, which can look very like lymphoma), leukaemic/lymphomatous infiltration or infection. There can be a marked excess of lymphoid cells in conditions such as tuberculosis but the important thing to note is that these cells are not morphologically atypical. Oil immersion examination is particularly useful in CSF cytology.

Imprints are of somewhat less use in diagnostic cytology as the main diagnosis will be based on histological examination in the majority of circumstances, but may be a better source of material for immunostaining. More importantly, they can provide experience of a wider range of appearances which can later be applied to fine needle aspiration cytology and thus it is not merely an academic exercise. This is particularly applied to lymph node pathology where the distinction between reactive changes and lymphoma can be difficult to assess. Candidates might be expected to recognise Reed-Sternberg cells in Hodgkin's disease or granulomatous lymphadenitis on an impression or aspirate so it is wise to obtain some familiarity with these conditions.

Smears of central nervous system tumours have been set in the examination. While some are fairly easily recognisable the fact that such specimens are not universally available is acknowledged by examiners, and these are probably only included as an exercise for the more advanced candidate. However, a wild diagnosis of malignancy when most of the cells are bland would indicate that the candidate is unable to apply the general principles of cytological assessment. It is far better to be circumspect, make a limited report and admit one's deficiencies in these rarefied cases rather than guess.

Common Cytological Specimens in Examinations

Gynaecological

1) Dyskaryosis
2) Inflammatory changes
3) Infection – wart virus (HPV), candida, herpes simplex, trichomonas, ? chlamydia
4) Endocervical cells – inflammatory and neoplastic
5) Post-natal and post-menopausal smears
6) Endometrial cells – normal and neoplastic
7) Radiation changes
8) Ovarian cyst aspirates

Non-gynaecological

Sputum

1) Inflammatory changes and asthma
2) Asbestos bodies
3) Fungi (e.g. aspergillus)
4) Malignancy

Endoscopic Samples (brushings, washings, suckings)

1) Inflammatory changes
2) Squamous cell and adenocarcinomas
3) Specific infections (e.g. herpetic oesophagitis, fungal pneumonia)

Serous Fluids

1) Reactive mesothelial cells
2) Adenocarcinoma and mesothelioma
3) Lymphoma/leukaemia

Urine

1) Reactive changes (post instrumentation, calculus disease, urinary infection)
2) Malignancy (transitional cell carcinoma, prostatic carcinoma, renal carcinoma)
3) Specific infections (e.g. polyomavirus)

Fine Needle Aspiration

1) Breast (fibroadenoma, duct ectasia, lactation, apocrine cyst, papilloma, ductal and lobular carcinoma, medullary carcinoma with lymphoid infiltration)
2) Thyroid (colloid nodule; papillary, follicular and medullary carcinomas)
3) Liver (normal hepatocytes, secondary carcinoma and carcinoid tumour, hepatocellular carcinoma)
4) Pancreas, testis, lung (commoner malignant tumours)
5) Lymph nodes (large cell NHL, Hodgkin's disease, granulomatous lymphadenitis)

Cerebrospinal Fluid

1) Meningitis – pyogenic and viral/tuberculosis
2) Lymphoma/leukaemia
3) ? primary CNS tumour

Imprint

1) Lymph nodes
2) ?CNS tumour

Surgical Dissection and Macroscopic Examination

One or two of the examiners usually conduct this part of the examination, the main aim of which is to assess how a candidate would deal with specimens received in a routine surgical laboratory, and for discussion of practical aspects of macroscopic inspection, block selection, laboratory safety and procedures for ensuring correct block labelling, etc.

In many centres, the specimens are selected from the routine material awaiting dissection and require examination, description and block taking for processing. In others the specimen may already have been dealt with, and a candidate would just be expected to identify and describe tissue, illustrating which areas should be sampled.

There are usually one or two larger specimens (such as a pneumonectomy, colectomy or nephrectomy for example), and several smaller ones (e.g. thyroid gland, breast lump or skin tumour). The specimens should be examined as for a routine surgical 'cut up', including checks on the labelling of the specimen, request form (and cassettes if blocks are to be taken). The clinical information should also be taken into account.

During the inspection and dissection, the examiners will be looking for the practical skill and awareness of the candidate as much or more than any theoretical knowledge. It is therefore important to ensure the working surface is kept clean, instruments are cleaned after each use, and selected blocks placed in order away from the main specimen, measures which are necessary to minimise 'carry-over'. The tissues should be washed with a spray or hose attachment after each phase of the dissection and comments made as appropriate.

A description should be given to the examiner or dictated to an assistant as for a routine specimen, and not over-elaborated merely because it is the examination. Only relevant information should be included, as well as measurements and weight. Similarly, blocks should be selected according to standard protocols, and only a reasonable number taken from standard sites and visible lesions.

It is important to pay attention to safety at the conclusion of the session, by tidying the area, removing scalpel blades and cleaning the work surface.

Preparation for Surgical Dissection

Surprisingly there are few sources which give advice on dissection of surgical specimens, apart from the appendix in *Ackerman's Surgical Pathology* (Appendix 1), which gives the most comprehensive recommendations. These guidelines are very useful and candidates might be advised to review them prior to the examination. Specialised texts sometimes give further information on the correct dissection of some organs, and the Association of Clinical Pathologists have Broadsheets, advising on the dissection of particular specimens (e.g. No 116, July 1987 – Examination of Breast Specimens). However, most trainees are expected to learn by practical experience at the SHO or junior registrar level from more qualified colleagues. The adequacy rather depends on the level and care of supervision in this respect, which can be very variable. There is no guarantee that the methods adopted for each specimen are detailed enough to satisfy an expert within that particular field. Therefore it is important to take each type of specimen individually and critically assess the method of dissection, seeking advice from senior colleagues, especially if they have a specialist interest.

Many common surgical specimens show a surprising variation in the selection of blocks and thoroughness of the dissection. Examples include mastectomy or colectomy specimens for carcinoma, as a review of archive reports and sections in many Departments would reveal. The optimal methods of dissection, which really need to be viewed as a skill rather than a chore (as is the case in many busy Departments) require constant motivation which is not always easy to achieve. Many trainees do not seem to be aware that their diagnostic acumen in surgical histopathology is limited by the effort expended on the macroscopic specimen, with a critical and careful selection of blocks. Unfortunately, many trainees are not encouraged to gain this insight, possibly because the necessary tuition is extremely time-consuming for supervisors. It is largely up to the person concerned to engender the necessary attention, and persistence usually pays off.

Special Stains

This is often a separate section from the surgical pathology, but is very variable in format and may not be included in some centres. In other cases, candidates may be provided with additional stains on request to supplement the surgical histopathology section. One danger here lies in requesting too many, since it does not impress examiners to request a plethora of unnecessary stains, which not only would not be made available, but indicates a pathologist who adopts a 'blunderbuss' approach, rather than intelligent discrimination.

If this is a separate session, the slides are provided in a format similar to the conventional surgical pathology, with brief clinical histories. H&E stained sections may or may not be provided. Candidates are normally expected to comment on the presumptive diagnosis, and the architectural or cytological features which are being demonstrated.

In some centres, several short questions may be asked on each stain, and the citation of other instances where the stain may be of value in diagnostic pathology is frequently required of candidates. Alternatively an H&E section may be provided with a variety of stains, all of which should be relevant to the diagnosis or which at least exclude some aspect of the differential diagnosis. The choice of stains given will almost certainly aid in reaching the correct diagnosis but it is the pattern of staining that is important. There is a great tendency to make apparently contradictory staining patterns fit the diagnosis, by 'seeing what one wants to see'. This must be avoided at all costs as anomalous results can occur and there are certain diseases which simulate others on conventional stains but have different staining characteristics (e.g. systemic kappa light chain deposition disease vs. amyloidosis in the kidney). It is therefore important to keep an open mind until all of the material has been examined, and then review the findings in total.

Selection of Material

There are a wide range of stains available to choose from, but in many centres there is a tendency to try to concentrate on more established histochemical techniques which are often neglected by trainees who have recently become more obsessed with immunostaining. Among the former, stains for various mucins are frequently included, as they can reveal a good deal of valuable diagnostic information, and be confusing to the pathologist who only has a superficial knowledge of these techniques. For example, Alcian Blue will stain acid mucopolysaccharides at pH 2.5, sulphated acid mucopolysaccharides at pH 1.0, connective tissue mucin at pH 2.5 is removed by hyaluronidase digestion, etc. It makes little sense to list all the various conditions which may be illuminated by the use of special staining techniques, as this should come from application of them during training, with a knowledge of recent advances in the literature. It is also helpful to read some of the textbooks on histochemical and immunochemical techniques and applications (Bancroft, J.D., Stevens, A. *Theory and Practice of Histological Techniques*, 2nd edition, Churchill Livingstone, Edinburgh, 1982).

Necropsy Histology

This section is again variable, depending on the examination centre and may be replaced by a clinicopathological conference. If included, it may take the form of examination of the sections from the candidate's post mortem or a mixture of post mortem sections from a variety of cases.

A candidate is unlikely to be asked to examine the sections from their own case if performing the necropsy during or just before the major part of the examination (although rapid processing of one or two selected blocks may be possible on occasion). However, if the examination was one or two weeks beforehand, they may well be given for evaluation and reporting.

This is where careful selection of the material for histology during the necropsy can pay dividends. It is difficult to make generalisations on how many blocks need to be taken from each necropsy since at the commencement of training each pathologist should take a large number to obtain an idea of normal histological appearances and of artefacts due to autolysis. By the time of the final examination, a pathologist has usually acquired sufficient skill to recognise when a more restricted number of blocks is required, usually as a routine from major organs, the minimum being one or two from heart, lungs, brain, liver, spleen and endocrine glands, when these are ostensibly normal, and obviously from any macroscopic abnormality.

It is a useful habit to take blocks from standard sites as a routine so that the recognition of any subtle abnormality is not obscured by difficulties in interpretation of architecture (especially in the kidney or brain, for example). Selecting too many blocks will not create a good impression with the examiners and will not facilitate concentration on the more important aspects during subsequent histological evaluation, especially during an examination.

If there is a suspected diffuse abnormality in an organ, it is useful to have a policy of selecting several blocks from defined sites which are recognisable by their outline on naked eye examination of the section (perhaps by including adjacent distinctive structures) or by cutting the tissue to a distinctive shape. This avoids wasting any time during histological examination. To ensure that the trimmed tissue which is processed will represent the area of interest, it is very important to select the area, a block of which would fit within a standard processing container and which is about 0.5 cm in thickness (if it is thinner the tissue may become distorted during fixation; it can easily be thinned later). Placing such neatly prepared tissue into the container will dictate the appearance and orientation of the subsequent section. It also enables a prompt fixation. On the other hand, a somewhat randomly selected, large lump of tissue, which pathologists often take at autopsy, results in poor fixation and in less well chosen blocks. By such selection, the number of blocks put through for processing is also known. The reports can be formulated according to the scheme of block selection, e.g. in cardiac cases; sinoatrial node, atrial wall, left and right ventricles, conducting system, valvular pathology, etc. or in the CNS, meninges, cerebral cortex, hippocampus, internal capsule and basal ganglia, medulla, cerebellum, upper spinal cord, etc. Clearly, the emphasis will depend on the pathology, both in the examination and in routine practice. Where further histological examination may be of value, larger samples of tissue can be stored in a separate container.

If there is a particularly difficult problem, there is no reason why tissues cannot be labelled in individual pots. This is suggested as an exception rather than a routine, and will not be viewed too favourably by the examination centre because of the extra work this involves, unless there is good justification. In cases of pathological abnormality, a well orientated junction with normal tissue should be included in cases of focal abnormality (e.g. in tumours or infection), or tissue selected where the changes are likely to be maximal in cases of more diffuse disease (e.g. hippocampus in Alzheimer's disease, lower lobe of lung in asbestosis, etc.). The histology must also be viewed in the light of other results from bacterial or viral culture, blood levels of hormones, etc. Naked eye examination of post mortem sections is just as important as in the surgical cases, and is otherwise evaluated in the same methodical fashion.

Post mortem reports should be as concise as possible, since many of the conclusions will already have been drawn from macroscopic examination. The report should be related to the visible abnormalities and the correlation comment-ed on, being very brief if merely confirmatory. If the result is contradictory, a more detailed appraisal is called for, the length varying according to the importance of the abnormality. In other words, the temptation to make too much of a minor insignificant change with little clinical relevance should be avoided. The examiners will be looking for the ability to interpret the post mortem findings for the benefit of the clinical staff in terms of their diagnosis and management, which may be obscured by over-indulgence in pathological minutiae.

The report should start with the organs showing the major pathological abnormalities, and leaving incidental findings and normal tissues until last. A concluding paragraph may be helpful along the lines of that given at the end of the initial report, indicating where further procedures such as EM or special stains, may be of value. This final paragraph should put the major histological abnormalities into context related to the clinical progress, mode of death and findings at necropsy.

In the event that slides are not available from the examination necropsy, material from other cases may be provided. Apart from gaining a wide experience of tissue changes encountered in necropsy material during training, there is little in the way of specific revision which can be performed. These cases overlap to a large degree with a following section on clinicopathological conferences, which contains further observations on the way to approach this material.

Mounted Museum Specimens ('Pots')

These are often used during the course of *viva voce* examinations, during the clinicopathological conferences or to complement the post mortem histology slides so that some correlation of macroscopic and microscopic appearances can be made.

The technique for examination of mounted specimens can often be poorly displayed by examination candidates and severely disadvantage them during the course of a *viva voce*, and it is useful to consider the basic approach.

Firstly, the container should be placed upright on the table surface and rotated as required. It should never be shaken or inverted. The specimen should be examined from the front, sides and back and, if examiners are present, placed in such a position that the specimen is clearly visible to both candidate and examiners, and so the relevant features pointed out. The time taken to complete this initial examination should be kept to a reasonable minimum and the initial comments on the nature of the tissues or organ displayed should be made during this time to avoid a prolonged silence, which might precipitate unwanted questions or prompting by the examiners.

After determining the anatomical site of the specimen, comment should be made on the way in which it is displayed or dissected, as bisected solid organ, opened viscus or blood vessel for example. Note should be taken whether any tissue has been removed during this process, e.g. in cardiac dissections, where portions of the ventricular wall or valve leaflets are sometimes removed.

As a routine, the size, configuration, colour, architecture and anatomical relationships are all assessed for any specimen, with any deviation from the expected normal appearances commented on, as will be the case with most diffuse pathological abnormalities, and which may be rather subtle (e.g. amyloidosis). Methods of enhancing such changes on tissues can be commented on at this stage (e.g. Lugol's iodine/dilute sulphuric acid in amyloidosis, NBT in myocardial infarction) and may even have been performed in the mounted specimen.

If a focal lesion or lesions are present, they will usually be at the focal point of the specimen, which in most cases is central. It is best to concentrate on this area for the detailed description, gradually including the effects of any lesion which may be produced on the surrounding tissue (e.g. indurated lungs in mitral stenosis, hydrocephalus in ventricular obstruction), or possible predisposing factors to any lesions (such as thrombotic occlusion of an artery in cases of possible infarction). The potential existence of these secondary changes can often be inferred from an understanding of the pathogenesis of any particular lesions and searching carefully for this underlying cause.

After the appraisal of the specimen, which should occupy two or three concise sentences, a likely diagnosis to account for the appearances should be suggested. In appropriate cases, a differential diagnosis should be presented (in descending order of likelihood) together with brief reasons for not regarding them as the primary diagnosis. The aim is to produce a logical, fluent appraisal of each specimen, where the candidate dictates the direction of the discussion, rather than making rather tentative suggestions requiring frequent prompting by the examiner. However, the reaction of the examiners to any suggestion should be carefully assessed, and the approach taken modified accordingly until a satisfactory response is obtained.

As well as the primary disease process present, there are sometimes subtle changes of an associated but entirely distinct condition (e.g. scarring due to asbestosis in a case of lung carcinoma, or hepatocellular carcinoma in cirrhosis) so that it is as well to bear this in mind as these are often favoured specimens for mounting. Occasionally specimens with two entirely unrelated pathologies are included, but are fortunately uncommon.

The ability to describe a 'pot' in a fluent fashion is a matter of practice, which to be effective should not merely entail a silent inspection of museum specimens, but demands active demonstration. The best method is to demonstrate to or interrogate medical students with such specimens, usually during tutorial sessions. Alternatively, arrangements could be made with a colleague to provide each other with half a dozen or so specimens, each being assessed on a 'mock' examination basis, with criticism centred on the style of assessment as much as the diagnosis.

Case Discussion or Clinico Pathological Correlations

This is a frequently used format for the introduction of post mortem material and hence is more likely to be a part of the examination in centres where the necropsy is not done a week or so in advance. It enables a more 'standardised' level of material and allows for the introduction of various other items such as special stains, electron micrographs, microbiological and biochemical investigations, etc. as appropriate. There is no way to prepare for these cases, as the exercise is designed to assess practical and interpretative skills acquired during training.

However, there are ways of approaching these sessions which are helpful in making a good presentation.

The clinical history given in these cases is often quite lengthy and must be read carefully since if often contains many valuable clues to the primary disease process present, and to the anticipated pathological changes.

The candidate will usually be asked to examine a set of slides, possibly in conjunction with macroscopic photographs or other material as indicated above. The point to remember is that the cases are usually selected because they illustrate either the effects of and progression of a systemic disease throughout the body (e.g. systemic lupus erythematosus, rheumatoid disease in a coal miner), or are concerned with a primary disease and its complications (e.g. carcinoid syndrome and heart disease, or parenchymal disease of the lung and pulmonary hypertension). There may well be iatrogenic changes in addition, and this being the Final Examination, the pathology may be slightly atypical as there may be unrelated disease processes present.

The most important task is to identify the 'theme' or primary disease process present and evaluate whether the remaining organs fit in with any predicted patterns. Having said this, the temptation to make the features fit the anticipated change must be avoided. The case may have been so constructed to lure candidates into this trap, so it is vital to keep an open mind until certain. It is helpful to imagine whether it could be demonstrated as a convincing example of the pathology (an idea which could be adopted in other parts of the examination).

The answers, which may be written or verbal, should be concise and to the point. In oral sessions, after answering the direct question, a reason for the conclusion should be given with a short qualifying sentence or two. In some instances, the sequence of events present has been identified, the next question can be anticipated, in which case the next step in the predicted disease process can be suggested, or what information might be required to confirm any suggested diagnosis. The examiners may supply the material, e.g. EM plates, and ask for comments. It is important to avoid interrupting examiners however and always let them finish asking the question since they may give some guidance to the required answer, consciously or otherwise.

'Viva technique' may be of great value in these sessions and is a factor many candidates fail to take into account. It is important to look at the examiners both when they are asking questions and when giving replies. The response to the answers or comments given is very valuable in assessing how accurate it is, and whether it is the required information. Guarded questions from the examiner (e.g. 'why would you think that?') often indicate a candidate has failed to justify their statements or have deviated from the expected line of the discussion. Overlong attempts to justify any conclusion are a mistake if it is clear from the responses that the arguments have failed to convince the examiner. It is far better to concede the issue and move to another subject than argue over a point which may be of little consequence, risking antagonising the examiner.

Case conferences usually last 40 minutes to an hour. There are often two or even three cases, one a longer, more complicated case, the other rather shorter, which usually illustrates one or two specific diagnostic features or includes the use of special techniques. In some cases, candidates may be expected to examine fixed organs, which should be demonstrated as outlined in the necropsy or macroscopic dissection sections.

Electron Micrographs

It is possible that ultrastructural pictures would be included in case conferences, or perhaps during the viva voce examination. At some stage in training candidates should have had access to EM facilities, and it is as well to develop at least a rudimentary knowlege of various cellular features. The following list contains many of these, together with an appropriate cell type in which it is found, and suggested references where such a feature is well illustrated. Many of these may be found in reference 2, a fairly comprehensive book which should be available in most EM departments. However, *Diagnostic Ultrastructural Pathology*, by the same author (reference 4), is an excellent, well-illustrated book containing 50 ultrastructural interpretation exercises, (hence the unpaginated references) and it is ideal preparation for an examination candidate.

One word of caution is that it is vital to take account of the magnification in ultrastructural pathology, especially when looking at subcellular particles: these sometimes appear very different or inconspicuous at lower magnification.

Feature	*Cell type or location*	*Reference*
Glycogen	e.g. renal tubular cell	1) p912 2) p181–183
Lipid	e.g. liposarcoma	2) p370–373
Mucin	e.g. adenocarcinoma	2) p88–91
Lipofuscin	e.g. hepatocyte	1) p25
Dense bodies	e.g. leiomyoma	3) p253
Intermediate filaments	e.g. keratinocytes	2) p350–357
Mallory body	e.g. hepatocellular carcinoma	2) p353
Short microvilli	glandular cells	4) question 4
Long microvilli	mesothelial cells	2) p101
True desmosomes	epithelial cells	2) p65–84
Desmosome-like structures	e.g. synovium, Schwannoma	2) p80
Lamellated bodies	alveolar cell carcinoma	2) p418–419
Muscle striations	e.g. rhabdomyosarcoma	3) p369 2) p190–193
Melanosomes	melanocytes and melanoma	2) p106–121 4) Question 13
Birbeck granules	Langerhans cells	2) p427–429 4) Question 17
Luse bodies	Schwannoma	2) p212
Crystalloid bodies	alveolar soft part sarcoma	2) p395–398
Renin crystal	juxtaglomerular cell	5) p796
Reinke crystalloids	Leydig cells	2) p286
Weibel-Palade bodies	endothelial cells	4) p413
Lysosomes	granular cell myoblastoma	2) p166
Megamitochondria	hepatocytes or oxyphil adenoma	1) p29 2) p159
Sphingolipid (Tay-Sachs)	ganglion cell	6) p247
Gaucher body	macrophage	4) Question 8
Zebra body	neurone	7) p107 4) Question 4
Adrenoleucodystrophy	adrenal cortical cell	1) p1438

Neurosecretory granules	diffuse endocrine cells	2) p123–147
Alpha, beta, delta granules	endocrine pancreas	1) p993 4) Question 7
Plasma cell		2) p257–263
Myeloma	plasma cell	6) p251
Dutcher body	Waldenstrom's macro-globulinaemia	5) p1287
Sezary cell	blood/lymph node	7) p290
Podocytes	glomerulus	1) p1013
Membranous GN	Glomerular basement membrane (GBM)	1) p1035
Mesangiocapillary GN	GBM (I and II)	1) p1040 4) Question 37
Amyloid	mesangiioma	1) p217 4) Question 42
Hereditary nephritis	GBM	1) p1026 4) Question 44
Minimal change GN	podocytes	6) p243
Lupus nephritis	GBM	6) p251
Virus-like particles (SLE)	mesangium	5) p755 4) Question 47
Virus particles	e.g. herpes virus, CMB	4) Question 25 6) p246
Bacilliform bodies (Whipple's disease)	macrophages	6) p249

References

1) Robbins, S.L., Cotran, R.S., Kumar, V. Pathologic Basis of Disease, 4th edition. W.B. Saunders, Philadelphia (1989).
2) Ghadially, E.N. Diagnostic Electron Microscopy of Tumours, 2nd edition. Butterworths, London (1985).
3) Enzinger, F.W., Weiss, S.W. Soft Tissue Tumors. 2nd edition. C.V. Mosby Co, St Louis (1988).
4) Ghadially, F.N. Diagnostic Ultrastructural Pathology – a self evaluation manual. Butterworths, London (1984).
5) Rosai, J. Ackerman's Surgical Pathology, 7th edition. C.V. Mosby Co, St Louis (1989).
6) McLay, A.L.C., Toner, P.G. Diagnostic electron microscopy. In: Recent Advances in Histopathology 11. Anthony, P.P., MacSween, R.N.M. (eds.) Churchill Livingstone, Edinburgh (1981).
7) Anthony, P.P., Woolf, N. (eds.) Recent Advances in Histopathology 10. Churchill Livingstone, Edinburgh (1981).

Cryostat Sections

It is advisable to make your own arrangements with the laboratory staff to cut spare sections of selected cases, or else contact the Head of the Department to institute a more formal policy to provide material for a teaching set.

Alternatively, it may be possible to arrange for frozen sections received in the department to be collected within the laboratory after return for filing, and reviewed on a weekly or monthly basis depending on numbers received, perhaps in conjunction with a surgical meeting or on an informal basis with colleagues. In addition, the paraffin sections should be obtained for comparison at the same time, to get some idea of the differences in morphology that may be produced in cryostat sections.

On this point, one of the major problems in interpreting cryostat sections is the failure to appreciate that the cell and nuclear size is considerably greater than in conventionally processed tissue, and minor differences may be greatly exaggerated, which may give a misleading impression of nuclear pleomorphism. Furthermore, the sections are much thicker, which makes any lesion appear more cellular than in paraffin section. Another factor is that cellular and cytoplasmic fine detail may be largely obscured, such as the nuclear membrane and chromatin pattern, nucleolus and cytoplasmic staining properties. These differences are well illustrated in examples such as sclerosing adenosis of the breast, or reactive lymph nodes, both of which can look very alarming on frozen section but are easily assessed on paraffin sections.

Some of the other difficulties encountered in frozen section diagnosis are in part due to poor technique. In routine practice, there is always the macroscopic inspection of the tissue and selection of material which provides valuable inform-ation, but this is admittedly lacking in the examination. However, many trainees fail to adopt the principles of examining a section outlined on page 288, and try to make a diagnosis using medium and high power objectives. On cryostat sections, as already explained, most of the detail at these magnifications is lost. Therefore it is considerably more important to be able to make a diagnosis on the basis of naked eye followed by low and medium power microscopic examination, reserving the high power to confirm details such as mitotic figures.

Using the previously cited tissues as examples, compare cases of sclerosing adenosis and invasive ductal carcinoma or reactive lymph nodes and lymphoma, first with the naked eye/hand lens and then under high power objectives. The amount of information gleaned from the former should be much greater in nearly all circumstances, and it will demonstrate how pattern and architectural considerations are of greater value than cytological detail. This is not to say that frozen sections should not be examined under high magnification, but that the information it reveals must be placed in the context of the previous impressions gained. If there is some contradiction in the two, the case, including clinical information, must be critically reviewed, avoiding the temptation to make a rushed decision.

The examination format is usually intended to provide an assessment of a candidate's approach to frozen section diagnosis within the setting of a routine surgical pathology laboratory, so that most (but not all) of the cases are relatively straightforward. The usual number of slides is between six and eight and very brief clinical information is given, apart from the patient's age.

The time allocated to each section is usually 4–5 minutes, and overall duration of this part of the examination is 30–45 minutes. It is possible that other candidates be in the room but more often each assessment is performed on an individual basis. The examiner may interrupt and ask questions during this time, unlike the surgical pathology section. Indeed, some candidates are asked to look at the sections in a double headed microscope with the examiner, resembling a *viva voce* examination. If this happens to you, you just have to grin and bear it, or take the positive view that this is an ideal opportunity to explain the reasoning behind the diagnosis, and impress the examiner with a careful technique. In addition, the alert candidate will act on the verbal and non-verbal clues as to the accuracy of any particular answer, and adjust their tack accordingly.

The form of the answers expected is somewhat different to those of the surgical histopathology. Less description is required, as a surgeon merely wishes to have a diagnosis on which to base a decision on the operative management. This is also the form in which the report is expected in the examination and long descriptions will definitely detract from the answer. The majority of cases are concerned with tumours, and the first sentence should clearly include the words benign or malignant, with an exact classification where possible.

Equivocal diagnoses, or avoidance of a decision (e.g. 'await paraffin sections') where a decision ought to be made, are usually marked down heavily in the examination, as it indicates a weakness and lack of experience in the candidate. Equally well, there are situations where a distinction between benign and malignant should not be made on frozen section. For instance, while a large nodular malignant melanoma is usually not a problem, deciding whether a small melanotic skin lesion in a young person is a malignant melanoma or Spitz naevus is often impossible on cryostat sections. Similarly, small, well-differentiated papillary lesions of the breast are difficult to assess, as are some endocrine tumours, which may even be impossible to categorise as benign or malignant even after multiple paraffin sections (e.g. phaeochromocytoma). There may be one or two cases which fit into this category, but it would be manifestly unfair to have the whole section composed of such examples, (although this is often the pre-examination 'dread' of a candidate). It should be appreciated that they serve to indicate a degree of maturity in a candidate who recognises his limitations and will not take risks in overdiagnosis.

Benign and non-neoplastic lesions of all types may be included in the cases, and one of the purposes is to ensure trainees do not become conditioned into thinking that frozen section equals tumour. It is an attitude which may lead to a misdiagnosis when an unexpected inflammatory, hamartomatous or degenerative lesion is encountered which simulates a tumour.

Therefore the material selected for the examination may obviously be from a very wide range of pathologies (and is often dependent on local surgical practice including occasional 'idiosyncratic' or rare cases encountered), resulting in a particular composition in each centre. The list given at the end of this chapter includes a selection of entities which are either known to have been included in the examination in some centres, or which a candidate may be expected to have seen during training or recognise de novo on frozen section. It clearly cannot be a comprehensive list, but it may be useful to work through any archive material of cryostat sections to examine such entities, or make some special effort to perform a cryostat section should fresh material become available. One way of doing this is to review the operating lists for the following day when on a surgical pathology rota and make arrangements with the surgical team.

Although it is a rather superficial generalisation, there are three broad categories of case submitted for the cryostat sections in the examination:

A) Lesions which the candidates may commonly encounter in clinical practice, or are particularly distinctive, and in which the surgical management is dependent on a correct, unequivocal diagnosis. Misdiagnosis in this category would be regarded as a serious error.

B) Lesions which are encountered reasonably often but which might be confused with other entities, or in which a diagnosis may not materially alter the management. Misdiagnosis of malignancy in a benign condition (and vice versa) may be viewed as a serious mistake in some of these, but the inability to make a firm diagnosis would not result in failure, and some equivocation or differential diagnosis might even be expected.

C) Rare but distinctive lesions, or commoner lesions in an unusual site, the diagnosis of which (or failure to diagnose) would not be a matter of failure in an examination. Nevertheless, a correct appraisal would obviously be impressive.

Clearly, each type of lesion in the examination would vary in the degree of difficulty depending on the material available and some might fall into more than one category (e.g. chronic pancreatitis can be very difficult to diagnose on biopsy and yet is of considerable importance in surgical management decisions). In such cases, category A/B or B/C is given and there are several such examples quoted.

It is worthwhile to make specific points relating to some of the entities mentioned in the following, but it should be appreciated these are selective. There can be no adequate substitute for practical experience in first hand (supervised) cryostat section diagnosis.

Breast Lesions

(A)	Invasive carcinoma NOS
(A)	Intraductal carcinoma
(B)	Lobular carcinoma in situ
(A/B)	Medullary carcinoma with lymphoid infiltration
(A)	Mucoid carcinoma
(B/C)	Ductal papilloma
(C)	Papillary carcinoma
(A)	Fibrocystic disease with epitheliosis
(A)	Sclerosing adenosis
(A)	Duct ectasia/lobular mastitis
(A)	Fat necrosis
(A)	Lactating breast/lactational adenoma
(B)	Phyllodes tumour

It is extremely common for breast carcinomas to be included in the examination for obvious reasons. Diagnosis of malignancy is the prime objective but some cases are sufficiently typical to allow distinction between lobular and ductal carcinoma, but it is by no means imperative to make this decision. In situ ductal carcinoma can be difficult to recognise, but in in the examination a fairly obvious example such as comedocarcinoma would be included. Lobular carcinoma in situ is more of a problem, and since it may not materially alter the immediate surgical management paraffin section assessment may be preferable. The less common sorts of breast cancer should be sufficiently distinctive to be fairly easily recognisable.

Of the benign conditions, epitheliosis and sclerosing adenosis can look alarming with high power objectives on cryostat section, and the architecture is all important. One of the classic 'traps' for an unwary pathologist is the lactational adenoma, which can look very aggressive even in paraffin sections but in which the history will be helpful. Similarly, all pathologists should be familiar with the cellular changes of lactation in the normal breast. The other conditions mentioned are straightforward matters of recognition.

Respiratory System

(C)	Nasal glioma
(C)	Rhinoscleroma
(C)	Foetal rhabdomyoma of larynx
(C)	Sclerosing haemangioma
(B)	Rheumatoid nodule
(A/B)	Oat cell carcinoma of lung
(A)	Squamous carcinoma
(A)	Adenocarcinoma
(A)	Large cell carcinoma
(A)	Carcinoid tumour
(A/B)	Secondary deposits (including chondrosarcoma (B), choriocarcinoma (A/B), leiomyosarcoma (A/B), renal cell carcinoma (A/B))
(A/B)	Epithelioid malignant mesothelioma
(B)	Spindle cell or mixed malignant mesothelioma

Rare lesions in the upper respiratory tract and nose at the top of this list have been included at some centres but these are presumably to provide some scope for the more advanced candidate. The importance of distinguishing between various main types of bronchial carcinoma has been mentioned previously but the most important distinction is oat cell from non-oat cell varieties. The more distinctive types of secondary deposits are included as a measure of awareness since these may occasionally pose a problem in practice and can easily be misdiagnosed. Mesotheliomas are rarely biopsied but it has been known. The distinction from adenocarcinoma or spindle cell carcinoma is often impossible on cryostat sections.

Lymphoreticular System

(A)	Granulomatous lymphadenitis – sarcoidosis (B), toxoplasmosis (B), tuberculosis (B)
(C)	Silicone lymphadenopathy
(A)	Reactive follicular hyperplasia
(A/B)	Castleman's disease – hyaline vascular
(B)	Castleman's disease – plasma cell
(A/B)	Secondary carcinoma and melanoma
(A)	Non-Hodgkin's lymphoma (follicular/diffuse)
(B)	Hodgkin's disease
(C)	Splenic kala-azar
(B)	Splenunculus (laparotomy)

It is important to be familiar with the range of appearances in lymph nodes on cryostat sections and architectural changes are of far more value than cytological features. A diagnosis of lymphoma can usually be made but subtyping is often difficult, and large cell lymphomas may look like undifferentiated carcinoma or melanoma. Splenic frozen sections are rarely performed and are often rather difficult diagnoses, as in the quoted examples. Splenunculi are a not uncommon clinical request, especially if enlarged by processes such as CML. They may be misdiagnosed as lymph nodes or lymphoma by the unwary.

Endocrine Glands

- (A)   Follicular adenoma/colloid nodule of thyroid
- (A/B) Follicular carcinoma of thyroid gland
- (A)   Papillary carcinoma of thyroid gland
- (B)   Medullary carcinoma of thyroid gland
- (A)   Grave's disease
- (A/B) Hashimoto's disease
- (C)   Riedel's thyroiditis
- (A/B) Dyshormogenetic goitre
- (A)   Parathyroid adenoma/hyperplasia
- (B)   Phaeochromocytoma of adrenal
- (B)   Adrenal cortical adenoma/carcinoma
- (B/C) Paraganglioma (e.g. carotid body)

Benign thyroid nodules are very common and in most cases pose little problem. Follicular carcinoma should only be diagnosed on frozen section in the presence of clear vascular invasion or other compelling evidence. The nuclear pleomorphism of benign thyroid tumours can be grossly exaggerated on cryostat section and very misleading. 'Orphan-Annie' nuclei in papillary carcinoma are also much less obvious but for examination purposes other helpful features such as psammoma bodies will usually be present. Medullary carcinomas can look very odd in cryostat sections and the distinctive amyloid seen in paraffin section is often pale and inconspicuous. It is often worthwhile to automatically ask 'could this be medullary carcinoma?' in thyroid lumps, before considering the more common possibilities.

Hashimoto's disease can be problematic as the oxyphilic cells are often large and pleomorphic. Dyshormonogenetic goitre is a rare but recognised 'trap' but a consideration of the patient's age and the lack of normal tissue are strong indicators of this possibility.

An enlarged parathyroid gland is frequently included as the surgical management of hyperparathyroidism is strongly influenced by the pathology and it provides a convenient subject for discussion between examiner and candidate on the practical aspects.

Alimentary System

- (A)   Pleomorphic salivary adenoma
- (A)   Adenoid cystic carcinoma
- (A)   Low grade mucoepidermoid tumour
- (B)   High grade mucoepidermoid tumour

(B)   Granular cell myoblastoma of tongue
(A)   Smooth muscle tumour ('bizarre leiomyoma') of gut
(B)   Inflammatory fibroid polyp
(B)   Gastric lymphoma – low grade
(A)   Gastric lymphoma – high grade
(A)   Pancreatic carcinoma – poorly differentiated
(A/B)   Pancreatic carcinoma – well differentiated
(A)   Chronic pancreatitis
(B)   Islet cell tumour
(A/B)   Adenoma or adenocarcinoma of ampulla/lower CBD
(A)   Bile duct adenoma of liver
(C)   Linguatula (tongue worm) cysts
(A)   Von Meyenberg complex (bile duct hamartoma)
(A)   Hepatocellular carcinoma – typical
(B)   Hepatocellular carcinoma – variants
(A)   Secondary carcinoma or leukaemic infiltration in liver
(C)   Epithelioid haemangioendothelioma
(B)   Secondary malignant melanoma in gut or liver
(A)   Rectal biopsy for ? Hirschprung's disease
(A)   Peritoneal endometriosis/endosalpingiosis

Despite the length of this list, cryostat sections are relatively infrequently requested presumably reflecting the use of endoscopic and needle biopsy. Salivary gland tumours are usually fairly characteristic and it would not be expected for candidates to recognise the rare variants. Adenoid cystic carcinomas can be particularly difficult on frozen section. The distinction of chronic pancreati-tis from scirrhous pancreatic carcinoma is a clinical and pathological problem, and is one situation where higher power examination of the cytological features can be of value in a particularly fibrotic biopsy. At least in the examination situation, a distinction should be possible. One feature of pancreatic carcinomas is that they tend to fragment, so it is important to check for material lying adjacent to the main biopsy tissue on the section.

Bile duct adenomas are sometimes biopsied at laparotomy because of their resemblance to secondary deposits, but their architecture is characteristic. Fibrotic tongue worm nodules are more common than most pathologists imagine, and are biopsied for similar reasons, but this would only be included as a difficult case. Some of the variants of hepatocellular carcinoma can be confusing and simulate other entities (e.g. secondary carcinoma). Bile pigment may be present to assist in the diagnosis. Malignant melanoma has very occasionally been included, but is more likely to appear in the surgical histopathology. Searching for ganglion cells in a putative Hirschprung's disease can be tedious if they are not there and ganglion cells can look rather unusual on frozen section so familiarisation with these appearances is advised. Peritoneal endosalpingiosis or endometriosis may be included to trap the inexperienced pathologist who might be tempted to diagnose metastatic adenocarcinoma or even papillary mesothelioma.

Female Reproductive System

- (B)   Ovarian fibrothecoma
- (A)   Serous, mucinous and endometrial carcinoma
- (B)   Borderline tumour
- (A)   Pregnancy luteoma
- (A)   Endometrioma
- (B)   Yolk sac tumour or dysgerminoma of ovary
- (A)   Endometrial adenocarcinoma
- (B)   Mixed Mullerian tumour
- (A)   Choriocarcinoma

The commoner malignant ovarian tumours do not provide many problems although the fibrothecoma can look rather nondescript. It would be unusual for lesions such as granulosa cell tumour to be included and this would certainly fall into the difficult diagnosis category. Although pregnancy luteoma and endometriosis are mentioned, these rarely provide a clinical diagnostic problem. Tumours such as choriocarcinoma are usually diagnosed preoperatively but cryostat section may be requested for confirmation.

Male Reproductive System

- (B/C) Sperm granuloma
- (B)   Adenomatoid tumour
- (C)   Mesothelial proliferation in hernial sac
- (A)   Seminoma
- (A)   Germ cell tumour – choriocarcinoma
- (B)   Germ cell tumour – embryonal carcinoma
- (B/C) Germ cell tumour – yolk sac tumour
- (C)   Interstitial cell tumour
- (B)   Primary testicular lymphoma
- (A)   Prostatic nodular hyperplasia
- (A)   Prostatic carcinoma

The benign entities mentioned are sometimes included because they can be misdiagnosed as malignant and candidates should be aware of this possibility. The other entities mentioned are fairly straightforward diagnostic problems, but seminomas rich in lymphocytes can be misinterpreted as lymphoma and vice versa. Intratubular germ cell neoplasia may be recognisable on the section and help in this respect.

Urinary Tract

- (A)   Renal adenoma/adenocarcinoma
- (B/C) Angiomyolipoma
- (C)   Oncocytoma
- (B/C) Rapidly progressive glomerulonephritis
- (C)   Nephrogenic adenoma of bladder
- (A)   Transitional cell carcinoma of bladder

Most of these lesions are relatively straightforward and of varying degrees of difficulty. Rapidly progressive (crescentic) glomerulonephritis can be recognised on frozen section, which is sometimes requested because of the urgency required in instituting treatment. Nephrogenic adenoma is an example of an 'idiosyncratic' slide which you would be unlikely to encounter.

Skin

- (C)   Juvenile xanthogranuloma
- (C)   Keratoacanthoma
- (C)   Spitz naevus
- (A)   Nodular malignant melanoma – Advanced
- (B/C)   Nodular malignant melanoma – Early
- (B)   Lentigo maligna
- (B)   Paget's disease of nipple

The problems in the diagnosis of melanocytic lesions of the skin have already been discussed and unless the diagnosis is certain there is little to be lost by prevaricating. Paget's disease of the nipple and lentigo maligna are distinctive lesions but there is little clinical value in their recognition on frozen as opposed to paraffin sections.

Nervous System

- (A)   Meningioma
- (B)   Acoustic Schwannoma
- (B)   Glioma
- (B/C)   Retinoblastoma
- (C)   Medulloblastoma
- (C)   Myxopapillary ependymoma

Examiners recognise that not all candidates have had the opportunity to train in a centre specialising in neuropathology but some of the more distinctive or commoner entities are often included. Astrocytomas are the commonest glioma and are usually fairly straightforward with prominent gemistocytes, or as the 'glioblastoma multiforme' type.

The Viva Voce Examination

Introduction

Many candidates have a disproportionate dread of this part of the examination but it helps to remember that in the great majority of cases the fate of the candidate is already sealed by this stage. However, it is a natural tendency for most individuals to believe that they may be just on or below the borderline and that a good performance in the *viva* will tip the balance in their favour. While this is only true in the occasional case, there is still an incentive for candidates who have definitely failed overall, as on rare occasions the examiners might insist that a candidate re-take the written papers; a satisfactory showing in the *viva* could help avert this. For those who are confident they have performed adequately beforehand, it may be an almost enjoyable experience and provides an opportunity to impress examiners. It is not unknown for some pathologists who came to the attention of certain examiners during the Final examination to end up working in their Department!

It is still necessary to have a neat appearance and the bearing of a potential consultant pathologist, as for the situation in general. It is perhaps even more important to have a positive attitude and desire to project an impression of knowledgeability, rather than adopt the attitude of some candidates who try to extract a sympathetic response from the examiners who they hope will understand that their poor showing is merely the result of the stress of the examination and does not reflect their 'true' ability. Unfortunately, most of these candidates tend to overcompensate and end up appearing rather more pathetic than impressive.

One important piece of 'homework' to be done is to try to establish who the internal and external examiners might be. There is no obligation for the centre or the College to give this information but it may be either volunteered by one of the examiners and, if not, it is reasonable to ask discreetly. Obviously, the best time to do this is during the first visit for the necropsy. Alternatively, more senior colleagues who have visited the centre previously may be able to offer advice.

Once having found out who the examiners are to be, either prior to or during the examination, their particular fields of interests should be established. This is essential because some examiners cannot resist the temptation to concentrate on their speciality and it is as well to anticipate this possibility. Moreover, it is advisable to try to direct attention away from these areas and proffer any opinions with some deference to their expertise; it is usually not advisable to argue with examiners on their special subject or claim any particular interest in it unless there is good justification, for the examiner would doubtless ask out of interest. Those who are less than proficient in their reply would create a very bad impression.

The Examination Itself

Most centres allocate about 20–30 minutes to the *viva*, but this may be rather longer for candidates on the borderline or who have performed very badly, and for whom resitting of the written papers may be contemplated. Generally speaking the chief internal and external examiners conduct the interview together.

Many of the recommendations on the approach to this session have already been covered under clinicopathological conferences or mounted specimens and there is no point in repeating them but certain aspects relating to this particular stage merit consideration.

Firstly it is important not to take too much account of other candidates prior to the *viva*, especially of their views on some aspects of the surgical histopathology. Their comments are equally likely to be incorrect as correct and this should not undermine confidence. Similarly, disregard the attitude of those individuals emerging from the *viva*, as their attitude would undoubtedly be affected by the relief at completing the examination. They are unlikely to provide any useful information at this stage, and interrogating them would only serve to increase anxiety.

At the start of the *viva*, the examiners would usually attempt some form of 'undemanding' general questions which might help to put the candidate at greater ease. It is very common to be asked an opinion as to how an individual thinks they have performed and where they thought errors may have occurred. It is advisable to prepare for this eventuality because it is possible to anticipate what answers to give. It is worth reflecting on the surgical histopathology during the subsequent evening, checking on any uncertain cases, and reading up on the differential diagnosis of selected examples. Comments made by other candidates can be taken into account, but must be viewed with particular caution, unless they clearly fit the diagnosis and reveal an obvious mistake. However, it should be noted that the memory can often be deceptive and uncertainties placed in one's own mind by others can overcome the product of a reasoned assessment made at the time. It is worth remembering the idiom 'Empty vessels make the most noise' when listening to fellow candidates! As a general rule, avoid 'post mortems' on the component parts of the examination, particularly the surgical pathology. They sap confidence and rarely do anything but harm. It is good advice to decline, politely, to discuss your answers with fellow candidates. Remember, you are just as likely as they are to be correct and expressed second thoughts about your correct diagnosis will do you no good at all.

Thus, if the examiners ask, take one or two examples where a mistake could definitely be identified and state openly what the assessment should have been and why the error was made. It is possible to redeem a certain amount in this way. It does not help to make generalisations about the whole of the surgical histopathology having been difficult, without subsequently identifying specific examples. The examiners may identify examples they are particularly concerned about, and ask for comments. In this situation it is almost certain that an error has been made and therefore the attitude of the candidate should be humble and introspective, rather than defensive and somewhat arrogantly refusing to consider alternatives.

Of course, there could be many other areas of the examination performance which the examiners would seek to qualify and thus candidates should be prepared to reconsider any aspect they have covered, and explain and discuss their reasoning. If such questions are forthcoming, it should be uppermost in the candidate's mind to try to ascertain what information the examiners are seeking to extract. If in doubt, it is better to admit either that the question is not understood or ask for guidance. It is not a good idea to try to bluff one's way out of answering, or to digress into other subjects; examiners like to pursue candidates who try to evade questions.

In the event that a candidate clearly does not know the answer, but has been honest enough to recognise and admit this, examiners usually move to another topic, as they appreciate that areas of ignorance are almost certain to be uncovered in all but the exceptionally able pathologist. They are more interested in the capacity to be flexible in interpretation and the ability to take a balanced view of certain problems, placing ideas in perspective, rather than in a candidate who is technically bright but is arrogant and somewhat narrow-minded, which is often the recipe leading to potentially dangerous diagnoses.

There are other comments which need to be made on the general attitude to be adopted during the examination, especially in the *viva*. Another common question is what you thought about the examination. Any temptation to criticise the centre, staff or even examiners must be avoided at all costs. Very few candidates turn out to have legitimate grounds for complaint and the mature individual always accepts there are always inequalities in standards, and differences in procedures, with which they might not entirely agree. Therefore it is important not to argue in an aggressive fashion, even when the examiner may appear provocative (which is unusual) or complain that the examination has been unfair, no matter how trivial or serious this may be. Anyone who feels that there are legitimate grounds for a formal complaint should discuss the matter with their Head of Department afterwards. It is very rare for the matter to be taken further, and even when formal complaints are made to the College about examination procedure, it appears to be unusual for any action to be taken. For example, at a certain examination centre, it was customary for the examiner to increase the level of anxiety during the frozen sections by walking among the candidates, continually remarking in a loud voice that surgeons were waiting and time was of the essence. Complaints made on behalf of both successful and unsuccessful candidates were met by acknowledgement of receipt, and the continuation of the same practice by the examination centre. At other centres examiners persist in confronting candidates on a double header in frozen sections, a practice heavily frowned on in the instructions to examiners. So the fact remains: the College make the rules, and the examiners interpret them. Arguing with the referee will not help. It is up to you to win in spite of the referee.

The answers in the *viva* should be positive and clearly spoken, and special care should be taken that an impression of enthusiasm and alertness should be maintained throughout the period of the *viva voce*, as there is a tendency to relax or even despair halfway through. The candidate who becomes gradually more inaudible and reticent will end up being a source of irritation to the examiner.

At the end of the *viva*, it is common courtesy to thank the examiners for their hospitality. In addition, candidates should not expect to be told outright how they have fared. It would embarrass the examiners to be asked by the candidate directly, as they are not permitted to divulge the information. Nevertheless, do listen carefully to the last few remarks made to you: it is certainly not unknown for examiners, particularly if they have partaken of liquid refreshment at lunch time, to forget the College's injunction and drop a distinct hint; usually only if you've passed however.

Notification of Results

The results are published within two weeks of the end of the practical examinations and are available at the College in Carlton House Terrace (and candidates will be informed of the exact time and should receive notification through the post the following day). Results are never given over the telephone.

In the case of unsuccessful candidates, the examiners will send a report to the Regional adviser. These reports are sometimes helpful but for the most part have attracted criticism because of their brevity and vagueness. There are two things you can do which may give more information. Discuss the surgical cases, etc., with successful fellow candidates *after the examination*, especially if they are familiar colleagues. This may be a difficult business but it is valuable because it may give more insight into the material. The second is to ask the Head of Department to contact one of the examiners personally. This will often elicit a helpful reply which will identify particular weaknesses and help in preparing for another attempt.

At present, the regulations allow three sittings of the examination without question but thereafter, entry is conditional upon the support of the Regional adviser. This arrangement is partly to allow deficiencies in training to be identified as some candidates have, perhaps unknown to them, had very lop-sided experience because of a poor rotation or other factors (as discussed earlier in this book). The maximum number of attempts appears to be limited to six, however.

Envoi

So here you are. You've read the books, spotted all the questions you can, polished your autopsy technique, looked at many, many sections and are replete with facts, from asteroid bodies to zoonoses. Tomorrow you sit the papers, and in three weeks' time, if spared, you confront the examiners at the dreaded practical.

Are there any final words of advice? There is a deadly tendency, especially if preparation for an examination has been intense, to feel anti-climactic at its immediate prospect. Try to kick yourself out of this. Remember you've prepared hard and well – 'Train hard, fight easy' has been your maxim. It's all too easy with an examination directly in your sights to think only of those things you do not know, or are unsure of, and forget the many facts of which you are certain. Don't do this. Be confident. Be positive. And pass.

Appendix 1

Reference List of Major Texts

1. Gresham, G.A., Turner, A.F. Post-Mortem Procedures (an illustrated textbook). Wolfe Medical Publications, London (1979).
2. Robbins, S.L., Cotran, R.S., Kumar, V. Pathologic Basis of Disease, 4th edition. W.B. Saunders, Philadelphia (1989).
3. Anderson, J.R. (ed.) Muir's Textbook of Pathology, 12th edition. Edward Arnold, London (1985).
4. Enzinger, F.M., Weiss, S.W. Soft Tissue Tumors. 2nd edition. C.V. Mosby Co, St Louis (1988).
5. Taussig, M.J. Processes in Pathology and Microbiology, 2nd edition. Blackwell Scientific Publications, Oxford (1984).
6. MacSween, R.N.M., Anthony, P.P., Scheuer, P.J. (eds.) Pathology of the Liver, 2nd edition. Churchill Livingstone, Edinburgh (1987).
7. Rosai, J. (ed.) Ackerman's Surgical Pathology, 7th edition. C.V. Mosby Co, St. Louis (1989).
8. Anthony, P.P., Woolf, N. (eds.) Recent Advances in Histopathology 10. Churchill Livingstone, Edinburgh (1978).
9. Anthony, P.P., MacSween, R.N.M. (eds.) Recent Advances in Histopathology 11. Churchill Livingstone, Edinburgh (1981).
10. Anthony, P.P., MacSween, R.N.M. (eds.) Recent Advances in Histopathology 12. Churchill Livingstone, Edinburgh (1984).
11. Anthony, P.P., MacSween, R.N.M. (eds.) Recent Advances in Histopathology 13. Churchill Livingstone, Edinburgh (1987).
12. Fox, H. (ed.) Haines & Taylor. Obstetrical and Gynaecological Pathology, 1, 2. 3rd edition. Churchill Livingstone, Edinburgh (1987).
13. Dunnill, M.S. Pulmonary Pathology. Churchill Livingstone, Edinburgh (1982).
14. Olsen, E.G.J. Pathology of the Heart. Intercontinental Medical Book Corporation, New York (1973).
15. Davies, M.J., Pomerance, A. The Pathology of the Heart. Blackwell Scientific Publications, Oxford (1975).
16. Morson, B.C. (ed.) Alimentary Tract. Systemic Pathology, Volume 3. (general ed. W. St. C. Symmers) Churchill Livingstone, Edinburgh (1987).
17. Department of Health and Social Security. Code of Practice for the Prevention of Infection in Clinical Laboratory and Post-mortem Rooms. 6th Impression. HMSO, London (1987) (NB Currently under review). Also see:
    a) Health Services Advisory Committee. Safety in Health Service Laboratories – Hepatitis B, HMSO London (1985).
    b) Health Services Advisory Committee. The labelling, transport and reception of specimens. HMSO, London (1986).
18. Underwood, J.C.E. Introduction to biopsy interpretation and surgical pathology. 2nd edition. Springer-Verlag, Berlin (1987).
19. Berry, C.L. Paediatric Pathology, 2nd edition. Springer-Verlag, Berlin (1989).

Additional Reading/Reference List

1. Stansfeld, A.G. (ed.) Lymph Node Biopsy Interpretation. Churchill Livingstone, Edinburgh (1985).
2. Lever, W.F., Schaumberg-Lever, G. Histopathology of the Skin, 6th edition. J.B. Lippincott Co, Philadelphia (1983).
3. Wickramasinghe, S.N. (ed.) Blood and Bone Marrow. Systemic Pathology, Volume 2. (general ed. Wt. St. C. Symmers) Churchill Livingstone, Edinburgh (1987).
4. Dahlin, D.C., Unni, K.K. Bone Tumours, 4th edition. Charles C. Thomas, Illinois (1986).
5. Azzopardi, J.G. Problems in Breast Pathology. W.B. Saunders Co Ltd, London (1979).
6. Spencer, H. Pathology of the Lung, 4th edition. Pergamon Press, Oxford (1985).

Appendix 2

Teaching Courses in Histopathology and Morbid Anatomy

1. Royal Postgraduate Medical School

    a) Advanced Histopathology

    Biannual (September and February)

A well-established two week course which many candidates attend just prior to the practical examination, comprising a morning practical examination of comprehensive slide collections on a particular topic (e.g. gastrointestinal tract, dermatopathology, breast, etc.) which are discussed and illustrated by the course teachers in the afternoon session. This course is often oversubscribed.

    b) Diagnostic Liver and Gastrointestinal Pathology

    Annual (November)

A five day set of practical sessions and illustrated discussion, together with guest lectures, intended to provide an intensive coverage of most entities in practical diagnostic pathology in this field. An explanatory course booklet is provided. Maximum benefit would be gained by attending this course at least six months in advance of the examination, but is perhaps of greater benefit for post MRCPath senior registrars and consultants with a specialist interest.

    c) Diagnostic Dermatopathology

    Annual (November)

Another five day intensive course organised in a similar fashion to the above. The standard of the course is high and may be too intensive for candidates just prior to the examination, but candidates would benefit by attending well in advance to allow time for reflection and assimilation of the information.

    d) Diagnostic Haematopathology

    Annual (January)

An advanced five day course for pathologists and clinicians perhaps best suited to those with an interest in the areas or at post MRCPath standard. Practical sessions and lectures are provided on a variety of topics including bone marrow, lymph nodes and spleen.

    e) Diagnostic Pathology of Soft Tissue Tumours

    Annual (February)

A comprehensive five day course which would be of interest to pathologists at all levels of training. Soft tissue tumours comprise a disproportionate number of the more difficult sessions in surgical histopathology at many examination centres.

f) Diagnostic Histopathology and Cytopathology of Breast Disease

Annual (February)

A new course which clearly would be an attraction to most pathologists and is very relevant to the examination. Details: Professor N.A. Wright, Department of Histopathology, Royal Postgraduate Medical School, Du Cane Road, London W12 0HS. Telephone 01-743 2030.

2. The British Postgraduate Medical Federation, University of London

Histopathology Module

This was formerly organised on a day-release basis over a period of six months every two years but is currently under review. It may be re-introduced at a later stage and is more likely to be as a concentrated two or three week course, which aims at a fairly comprehensive coverage. Details: Dr J. Tinker, British Postgraduate Medical Federation, 33 Millman Street, London WC1N 3EJ. Telephone 01-831 6222.

3. London Hospital Histopathology Course

This formerly very popular course was organised on weekly evening sessions with emphasis on diagnostic histopathological problems which were released for participants to review in the week prior to the meeting. The course is presently under review, and may be organised in conjunction with the British Postgraduate Medical Federation. Announcements will be made in the major pathology journals when a decision is taken.

4. The Autopsy

Annual (July)

A three day course providing a fairly comprehensive coverage of most topics associated with autopsy pathology, predominantly on a lecture basis, with some practical demonstrations. The course may well be of greatest value to pathologists in the middle stages of their training to allow them to refine and practise their techniques in accordance with the experience gained. We are not aware of any other nationally available course which specifically deals with these topics. Details: Dr Dennis Cotton, Department of Pathology, University of Sheffield Medical School, Beech Hill Road, Sheffield S10 2RX.

5. Diagnostic Histopathology Course

Annual (July)

A two week residential course consisting of practical sessions followed by discussion of the material, aiming to cover most aspects of general surgical pathology. Each three hour session covers one system, and there is particular emphasis on practical diagnostic problems rather than esoteric entities. Accommodation, meals and a social programme are provided. The course is popular and often oversubscribed. Details: Dr A.J. Howat, Department of Pathology, University of Sheffield Medical School, Beech Hill Road, Sheffield S10 2RX.

6. Cytopathology for Histopathologists
   January/February and mid-September

A very popular five day course which includes both practical sessions and lectures from a variety of specialist cytopathologists. Most candidates would gain maximum benefit by having at least a few months experience in cytopathology and many attend in the session prior to sitting the practical examination. Details: Dr E.A. Hudson, Department of Histopathology, Northwick Park Hospital, Watford Road, Harrow, Middlesex HA1 3UJ.

7. Diagnostic Dermatopathology
   Annual (April)

An established course in this subject which covers many aspects of neoplasia and inflammatory disorders of the skin. Details: Mrs W.E. Scott, Administrative Assistant, West of Scotland Committee for Postgraduate Medicine, University of Glasgow, Glasgow G12 8QQ.

8. Paediatric Pathology
   Annual (April)

Courses which are sponsored by the Association of Clinical Pathologists which are to take place in Sheffield and Birmingham on alternate years. Details: Dr F. Raafat, Consultant Paediatric Pathologist, Department of Histopathology, The Children's Hospital, Ladywood Middleway, Ladywood, Birmingham B16 8ET.

9. Management Course for Junior Pathologists
   April and September

A three day residential course relevant to those intending to work within the National Health Service. Topics covered by a series of lectures include management quality control and funding as related to pathology disciplines, and would be of value in preparation for certain questions in the written paper, but more especially to prospective applicants for consultant posts. Details: Dr D.H. Orrell, Department of Pathology, Lancaster Royal Infirmary, Lancaster LA1 4RP.

10. Regional Courses in Pathology

Most university centres within each Regional Health Authority provide training courses in histopathology and/or morbid anatomy on a regular weekly or monthly basis. Attendance at such courses should be *de rigeur* for candidates within that Region, providing an opportunity to meet colleagues as well as gaining experience. Details: Either from the Regional Adviser in Histopathology (Royal College of Pathologists) or in the A.C.P. Programme of Postgraduate Education, which is automatically sent to associates and members.

11. Secondment Schemes in Pathology

Formal arrangements to attend a wide range of general and specialist pathology units can be made via the Education Secretary of the Association of Clinical Pathologists rather than on an individual basis. These may be of great value to those trainees who have a specific deficiency in their training. Details: Dr J.D. Davies, University Department of Pathology, Bristol Royal Infirmary, Bristol BS2 8HW. Telephone 0272-23000 extension 2582.

12. Symposia organised by the Royal College of Pathologists, Association of
    Clinical Pathologists and the International Academy of Pathologists

Symposia on subjects of topical interest are organised by these bodies and details
are circulated to members and associates, as well as advertised in the society
journals. Attendance at these symposia is highly recommended for trainees, and
many of the topics, especially those organised by the College are not infrequently
used as a basis for a question in the subsequent written examination. Attendance
at all of these symposia would be impossible for most trainees, but a well
organised group of trainees would send one representative to each and pool the
information.

Appendix 3

Professional Societies and Associations

1. The Royal College of Pathologists
    2 Carlton House Terrace, London SW1Y 5AF
    Telephone: 01-930 5861

Society publication – Bulletin of Royal College of Pathologists

2. The Association of Clinical Pathologists
    57 Lower Belgrave Street, London SW1W 0LR
    Telephone: 01-730 0078

Society publication – Journal of Clinical Pathology

3. The Pathological Society of Great Britain and Ireland,
    c/o Department of Pathology, Royal Infirmary, Glasgow G4 0SF
    041-552 3535 ext. 4224

Society publication – Journal of Pathology

4. The British Medical Association
    BMA House, Tavistock Square, London WC1H 9JP
    Telephone: 01-387 4499

Society publication – British Medical Journal

5. The International Academy of Pathologists (British Division),
    Dr M. Wells, Department of Histopathology,
    Leeds University Medical School, Leeds LS2 9JT

Society publication – Histopathology

6. British Association of Clinical Cytology,
    c/o Dr P.A. Trott, Dept of Cytopathology,
    Royal Marsden Hospital, Fulham Road, London SW3 6JJ

Regulations Regarding the Examinations for Membership (Medically-Qualified Candidates)

The Council of the College finalised the regulations for the Membership examinations at its meeting on 24th November 1988. The detailed requirements for the individual specialties will be published together later.

1. A candidate is admitted to the examinations, Part I and Part II, solely at the discretion of Council.
2. The candidate must hold a qualification in medicine that is approved by Council.
3. A candidate holding a medical qualification not registered by the General Medical Council in the United Kingdom must furnish with his/her application form the document or certificate whereby registration or permission to practise is granted in the country or territory of domicile in which the qualification is granted.
4. Entrance to any College examination can be effected only by completion of the printed application form obtainable from the Registrar. The form and entrance fee must be returned to the Registrar not later than the date specified in the public announcement of the examination. Incomplete or later applications cannot be accepted.
5. It can sometimes be arranged for a candidate for the Part I Examination to take the written part of the examination overseas; a candidate who passes the written papers overseas is usually asked to attend for his/her practical and oral components in the United Kingdom at the next session of the examination.
6. A candidate must have held suitable clinical appointments for not less than one year; pre-registration appointments are accepted for this purpose.
7. A candidate shall not be admitted to an examination until he/she has fulfilled the training requirements set out in the appropriate sections of these regulations.
   Training in laboratories outside the United Kingdom will be considered on an individual basis. An applicant who has worked in appropriate laboratories or departments other than pathology laboratories may be admitted to the examination at the discretion of Council.
8. The applicant is responsible for keeping the College office informed of his/her address and telephone number during the time of the examination.
9. The applicant should be sponsored by a Fellow or Member of the College. When sponsorship by a Fellow or Member is impracticable the signature of the head of the department in which the candidate is working may be accepted by Council.
10. **Part I Examination**

(a) *Training requirements:* A candidate entering for the Part I Examination is required to have worked in departments recognised for training in the relevant discipline for a total period of not less than three years, of which two and a half years must have been in the subject in which the candidate elects to be examined. A candidate who has held or hopes to hold part-time posts must obtain the approval of the College for his/her training (*overseas candidates* see Regulation 7).

Up to one year in a relevant clinical or research appointment or in training courses of certain MSc degrees and Diplomas approved by the College may be accepted towards the training period. A full list of approved postgraduate qualifications may be obtained from the Registrar.

(b) *Entrance fee* for the Part I examination is set by Council and details may be obtained from the Registrar; withdrawal from the examination after candidature has been accepted may involve the forfeiture of all or part of the entrance fee.

(c) The candidate must state which one of the following branches of pathology he/she has chosen for the examination: chemical pathology, clinical cytogenetics and molecular genetics, haematology, histopathology, immunology, medical microbiology, neuropathology, oral pathology, toxicology, virology and any other subjects which Council may approve.

(d) *Form of the examination:* the Part I Examination comprises:

(i) two three hour written papers in the chosen branch of pathology which may, at the discretion of the Examiners' Sub-committee, contain an MCQ component;

(ii) a practical and oral examination in the branch of pathology the candidate has chosen (with the exception of haematology). The candidate will be notified of the time and place of the practical and oral examination (see Regulation 8). In Haematology, the Part I examination will comprise written papers only. Candidates selecting histopathology must provide the College with a certificate indicating competence in cutting and staining frozen sections.

(e) A candidate who fails to satisfy the examiners in the written papers will not go forward to the practical and oral stage.

(f) A candidate who obtains an acceptable mark in the written papers and who fails the practical and oral examination by only a small margin may, at the discretion of Council, retain the pass in the written papers.

(g) A candidate will normally be allowed four attempts at the Part I examination in whole or in part, after which he/she may re-enter only for a specified number of attempts to be decided by Council.

11. Part II Examination

(a) *Training requirements:* A candidate may not enter for the Part II Examination until he/she has successfully completed the Part I Examination.

(b) A candidate for the Part II examination is required to have completed the equivalent of five years – full-time approved training of which two years must have been in a post recognised for higher specialist training and four years in the branch of pathology chosen for the examination (*overseas candidates* should see Regulation 7).

The entrance fee for the Part II Examination is set by Council and details may be obtained from the Registrar; withdrawal from the examination after candidature has been accepted may involve the forfeiture of all or part of the entrance fee.

(c) Candidates must state which branch of pathology they have chosen for the examination. A candidate who wishes to sit the Part II examination in a subject other than that passed in Part I must obtain the permission of the Council.

All candidates for the Part II examination in haematology are required to have undertaken training in blood transfusion in an approved blood transfusion centre. This should normally be for a period of at least six months of which three months may be in a hospital centre which is recognised for this purpose.

Application forms are obtainable from the Registrar. Examinations are held twice a year, except in clinical cytogenetics and molecular genetics and toxicology, which are normally held once a year in the Spring.

(d) *Form of the examination:* the Part II examination and completion of the training programme are designed to ensure that the candidate has advanced to a stage of full professional competence in a branch of pathology. The examination comprises:

1. an oral examination and
2. one or more of the following options agreed by Council for the discipline concerned:

    (i) a test of practical competence appropriate to the discipline or subspecialty and agreed by Council;

    (ii) a dissertation;

    (iii) a suitable higher degree;

    (iv) a collection of refereed, published papers with a critical commentary;

    (v) a casebook with a critical commentary.

(e) A candidate who fails to pass the Part II examination in whole or in part after two attempts will only be permitted to re-enter after a review of his/her training programme and on the advice of the Regional Adviser in Postgraduate Education in Pathology. Extenuating circumstances supporting the re-admission of a candidate after four failed attempts to any part of the Part II examination must be referred to Council.

12. These regulations may be varied from time to time by decision of Council.

13. Membership

(a) Every Member of the College shall be held to have agreed to be bound by provisions of the Charter and the Ordinances as amended from time to time and shall be bound to further to the best of his/her ability the objects and interests of the College (Ordinance 2).

(b) Membership of the College may be followed after a twelve year period by an offer, to those Members in good standing, of admission to the Fellowship.

Regulations Regarding the Examinations for Membership (Candidates Without a Medical Qualification)

1. The candidate is admitted to the examinations, Part I and Part II, solely at the discretion of Council.

2. The candidate must hold a qualification that is approved by Council. For the purpose of this regulation Council recognises the qualifications in dental surgery and veterinary medicine that are registrable in the United Kingdom and 1st and 2nd class honours degrees or equivalent qualifications granted in the United Kingdom and Republic of Ireland in appropriate science subjects. Applications may also be considered on an individual basis from those holding other science degrees granted in the United Kingdom and Republic of Ireland and from those holding science degrees from overseas universities.

3. Entrance to any College examination can be effected only by completion of the printed application form obtainable from the Registrar. The form and entrance fee must be returned to the Registrar not later than the date specified in the public announcement of the examination.

Incomplete or late applications cannot be accepted.

4.   It can sometimes be arranged for a candidate for the Part I Examination to take the written part of the examination overseas; a candidate who passes the written papers overseas is usually asked to attend for his/her practical and oral components in the United Kingdom at the next session of the examination.

5.   A candidate shall not be admitted to an examination until he/she has fulfilled the training requirements set out in the appropriate sections of these regulations. Training in laboratories outside the United Kingdom will be considered on an individual basis.

An applicant who has worked in appropriate laboratories or departments other than pathology laboratories may be admitted to the examination at the discretion of Council.

6.   The applicant is responsible for keeping the College office informed of his/her address and telephone number during the time of the examination.

7.   The applicant should be sponsored by a Fellow or Member of the College. When sponsorship by a Fellow or Member is impracticable the signature of the head of the department in which the candidate is working may be accepted by Council.

8. Part I Examination

(a) *Training requirements:* Veterinary and dental candidates cannot enter for the Part I examination until four years after obtaining the qualification laid down in Regulation 2. Non-medical candidates other than veterinary and dental cannot enter for the Part I examination until six years after obtaining the qualifications laid down in Regulation 2. Of these four and six years respectively, three years must have been spent in approved appointments in laboratories recognised for Part I training. A candidate who has held or hopes to hold part-time posts must obtain the approval of the College for his/her training (*overseas candidates* see Regulation 5).

Other laboratory experience up to one year may be accepted towards the training requirements of the College's examinations but only posts held after an acceptable degree (or degree equivalent) has been obtained will be accepted towards the College's training requirements. For each applicant, the nature and suitability of the post must be approved by the Council.

Up to one year in a relevant clinical or research appointment or in training courses of certain MSc degrees and Diplomas approved by the College may be accepted towards the training period. A full list of approved postgraduate qualifications may be obtained from the Registrar.

(b) The *entrance fee* for the Part I examination is set by Council and details may be obtained from the Registrar; withdrawal from the examination after candidature has been accepted may involve the forfeiture of all or part of the entrance fee.

(c) The candidate must state which one of the following branches of pathology he/she has chosen for the examination: chemical pathology, clinical cytogenetics and molecular genetics, immunology, medical microbiology, oral pathology, toxicology, virology.

(d) The examinations are held twice a year, except in clinical cytogenetics and molecular genetics, veterinary pathology and toxicology, which are normally held once a year in the Spring.

(e) *Form of the examination:* The Part I examination comprises:

   (i)   two three hour written papers, which may, at the discretion of the Examiners, contain an MCQ component.
   Special papers for non-medical candidates will be set in certain disciplines.
   (ii) a practical and oral examination in the branch of pathology that the candidate has chosen. The candidate will be notified of the time and place of the practical and oral examination (see *Regulation 6*).

(f) A candidate who fails to satisfy the examiners in the written papers will not go forward to the practical and oral stage.

(g) A candidate who obtains an acceptable mark in the written papers and who fails the practical and oral examination by only a small margin may, at the discretion of the Council, retain the pass in the written papers.

(h) A candidate will normally be allowed four attempts at the Part I examination in whole or part, after which he/she may re-enter only for a specified number of attempts to be decided by Council.

9. Part II Examination

(a) *Training requirements:* A candidate may not enter for the Part II Examination until he/she has successfully completed the Part I Examination.

(b) A dental and veterinary candidate may not enter for the Part II examination until six years after obtaining his/her basic qualification (see Regulation 2) and must have completed the equivalent of five years full-time training in recognised appointments, of which two years must have been in appointments recognised for higher specialist training in pathology.

(c) A science graduate may not enter for the Part II Examination practical and oral examination until eight years after obtaining his/her basic qualification (see Regulation 2) and must have completed the equivalent of five years full-time training in approved appointments of which two years must have been in appointments, approved for higher specialist training and four years in the branch of pathology chosen for the examination.
The entrance fee for the Part II Examination is set by Council and details may be obtained from the Registrar; withdrawal from the examination after candidature has been accepted may involve the forfeiture of all or part of the entrance fee.

(d) Candidates must state which branch of pathology they have chosen for the examination. A candidate who wishes to sit the Part II examination in a subject other than that passed in Part I must obtain the permission of Council.

(e) Examination are held twice a year, except in clinical cytogenetics and molecular genetics, veterinary pathology and toxicology, which are normally held once a year in the Spring.

(f) *Form of the examination:* The Part II examination and completion of the training programme are designed to ensure that the candidate has advanced to a stage of full professional competence in a branch of pathology. The examination comprises:

1.   an oral examination and
2.   one or more of the following options agreed by Council for the discipline concerned:

   (i)   a test of practical competence appropriate to the discipline or subspeciality and agreed by Council;
   (ii) a dissertation;
   (iii) a suitable higher degree;

(iv) a collection of refereed, published papers with a critical commentary;

(v) a casebook with a critical commentary.

(g) A candidate who fails to pass the Part II examination in whole or in part after two attempts will only be permitted to re-enter after a review of his/her training programme and on the advice of the Regional Adviser in Postgraduate Education in Pathology. Extenuating circumstances supporting the re-admission of a candidate after four failed attempts to any part of the Part II examination must be referred to Council.

10. These regulations may be varied from time to time by decision of Council.

11. **Membership**

(a) Every Member of the College shall be held to have agreed to be bound by the provisions of the Charter and the Ordinances as amended from time to time and shall be bound to further to the best of his/her ability the objects and interests of the College (ordinance 2).

(b) Membership of the College may be followed after a twelve year period by an offer, to those Members in good standing, of admission to the Fellowship.